CONTENTS

3

INTRODUCTION

The Mediterranean diet is based on the diets of traditional eating habits from the 1960s of people from countries that surround the Mediterranean Sea, such as Greece, Italy, and Spain, and it encourages the consumption of fresh, seasonal, and local foods. The Mediterranean diet has become popular because individuals show low rate of heart disease, chronic disease, and obesity. The Mediterranean diet profile focuses on whole grains, good fats (fish, olive oil, nuts etc.), vegetables, fruits, fish, and very low consumption of any non-fish meat. Along with food, the Mediterranean diet emphasizes the need to spend time eating with family and physical activity. The Mediterranean diet is not a single prescribed diet, but rather a general food-based eating pattern, which is marked by local and cultural differences throughout the Mediterranean region. The diet is generally characterized by a high intake of plant-based foods (e.g. fresh fruit and vegetables, nuts, and cereals) and olive oil, a moderate intake of fish and poultry, and low intakes of dairy products (mostly yoghurt and cheese), red and processed meats, and sweets. Wine is typically consumed in moderation and, normally, with a meal. A strong focus is placed on social and cultural aspects, such as communal mealtimes, resting after eating, and regular physical activity. Nowadays, however, the diet is no longer followed as widely as it was 30-50 years ago, as the diets of people living in these regions are becoming more 'Westernized' and higher in energy dense foods.

Benefits

The Mediterranean diet is not a weight loss, but increasing fiber intake and cutting out red meat, animal fats, and processed food may lead to weight loss. People who follow the diet may also have a lower risk of various diseases.

Heart health

In the 1950s,an American scientist, found that people living in the poorer areas of southern Italy had a lower risk of heart disease and death than those in wealthier parts of New York. Dr. Keys attributed this to diet. Since then, many studies have indicated that following a Mediterranean diet can help the body maintain healthy cholesterol levels and reduce the risk of high blood pressure and cardiovascular disease. The overall pattern of the Mediterranean diet is similar to their own dietary recommendations. A high proportion of calories on the diet come from fat, which can increase the risk of obesity. However, they also note that this fat is mainly unsaturated, which makes it a more healthful option than that from the typical American diet.

Protection from disease

The Mediterranean diet focuses on plant-based foods, and these are good sources of antioxidants.
The Mediterranean diet might offer protection from various cancers, and especially colorectal cancer. The reduction in risk may stem from the high intake of fruits, vegetables, and whole grains. By sticking to eat Mediterranean meals, people's levels of blood glucose and fats had decreased. During this time, there was also a lower incidence of stroke.

Diabetes

The Mediterranean diet may help prevent type 2 diabetes and improve markers of diabetes in people who already have the condition. Various other studies have concluded that following the Mediterranean diet can reduce the risk of type 2 diabetes and cardiovascular disease, which often occur together.

Food to eat

There is no single definition of the Mediterranean diet, but one group of scientists used the following as their 2015 basis of research.

Vegetables: Include 3 to 9 servings a day.
Fresh fruit: Up to 2 servings a day.
Cereals: Mostly whole grain from 1 to 13 servings a day.
Oil: Up to 8 servings of extra virgin (cold pressed) olive oil a day.

Fat — mostly unsaturated — made up 37% of the total calories. Unsaturated fat comes from plant sources, such as olives and avocado. The Mediterranean diet also provided 33 grams (g) of fiber a day. The baseline diet for this study provided around 2,200 calories a day. Typical ingredients. Here are some examples of ingredients that people often include in the Mediterranean diet.

Vegetables: Tomatoes, peppers, onions, eggplant, zucchini, cucumber, leafy green vegetables, plus others.
Fruits: Melon, apples, apricots, peaches, oranges, and lemons, and so on.
Legumes: Beans, lentils, and chickpeas.
Nuts and seeds: Almonds, walnuts, sunflower seeds, and cashews.
Unsaturated fat: Olive oil, sunflower oil, olives, and avocados.
Dairy products: Cheese and yogurt are the main dairy foods.
Cereals: These are mostly whole grain and include wheat and rice with bread accompanying many meals.
Fish: Sardines and other oily fish, as well as oysters and other shellfish.
Poultry: Chicken or turkey.
Eggs: Chicken, quail, and duck eggs.
Drinks: A person can drink red wine in moderation.
The Mediterranean diet does not include strong liquor or carbonated and sweetened drinks. According to one definition, the diet limits red meat and sweets to less than 2 servings per week.

Food to avoid

Here's a list of foods you should generally limit while eating Mediterranean-style meals. Heavily processed foods. Let's be real: Many, many foods are processed to some degree. A can of beans has been processed, in the sense that the beans have been cooked before being canned. Olive oil has been processed, because olives have been turned into oil. But when we talk about limiting processed foods, this really means avoiding things like frozen meals with tons of sodium. You should also limit soda, desserts and candy. As the adage goes, if the ingredient list includes items that your great-grandparents wouldn't recognize as food, it's probably processed. If you're buying a packaged food that's as close to its whole-food form as possible — such as frozen fruit or veggies with nothing added — you're good to go.

Processed red meat

On the Mediterranean diet, you should minimize your intake of red meat, such as steak. What about processed red meat, such as hot dogs and bacon? You should avoid these foods or limit them as much as possible. A study published in BMJ found that regularly eating red meat, especially processed varieties, was associated with a higher risk of death. Butter. Here's another food that should be limited on the Mediterranean diet. Use olive oil instead, which has many heart-health benefits and contains less saturated fat than butter. According to the USDA National Nutrient Database, butter has 7 grams of saturated fat per tablespoon, while olive oil has about 2 grams.

Refined grains

The Mediterranean diet is centered around whole grains, such as farro, millet, couscous and brown rice. With this eating style, you'll generally want to limit your intake of refined grains such as white pasta and white bread.

Alcohol

When you're following the Mediterranean diet, red wine should be your chosen alcoholic drink. This is because red wine offers health benefits, particularly for the heart. But it's important to limit intake of any type of alcohol to up to one drink per day for women, as well as men older than 65, and up to two drinks daily for men age 65 and younger. The amount that counts as a drink is 5 ounces of wine, 12 ounces of beer or 1.5 ounces of 80-proof liquor.

8 Ways to Follow the Mediterranean Diet for Better Health
1. Cook with Olive Oil

If you've been cooking with vegetable oil or coconut oil, make the switch to extra-virgin olive oil. Olive oil is rich in monounsaturated fatty acids, which may improve HDL cholesterol, the "good" type of cholesterol. HDL cholesterol ferries "bad" LDL particles out of arteries, according to a 2017 study in Circulation. Use olive oil in homemade salad dressings and vinaigrettes. Drizzle it on finished dishes like fish or chicken to boost flavor. Swap butter for olive oil in mashed potatoes, pasta and more.

2. Eat More Fish

The go-to protein in the Mediterranean diet is fish. In particular, this diet emphasizes fatty fish like salmon, sardines and mackerel. These fish are rich in heart- and brain-healthy omega-3 fatty acids. Even those fish that are leaner and have less fat (like cod or tilapia) are still worth it, as they provide a good source of protein. If you currently don't get a lot of fish in your diet, an easy point of entry is to designate one day each week as fish night. Cooking fish in parchment paper or foil packets is one no-fuss, no-mess way to put dinner on the table. Or try incorporating it in some of your favorite foods, like tacos, stir-fries and soups.

3. Eat Veggies All Day Long

If you look at your diet and worry that there's barely a green to be seen, this is the perfect opportunity to fit in more veggies. A good way to do this is to eat one serving at snack time, like crunching on bell pepper strips or throwing a handful of spinach into a smoothie, and one at dinner, like these quick and easy side dishes. Aim for at least two servings per day. More is better. At least three servings can help you bust stress, Australian research notes.

4. Help Yourself to Whole Grains

Experiment with "real" whole grains that are still in their "whole" form and haven't been refined. Quinoa cooks up in just 20 minutes, making it a great side dish for weeknight meals. Barley is full of fiber and it's filling: pair it with mushrooms for a steamy, satisfying soup. A hot bowl of oatmeal is perfect for breakfast on a cold winter morning. Even popcorn is a whole grain-just keep it healthy by eating air-popped corn and forgoing the butter (try a drizzle of olive oil instead). Supplement your intake with other whole-grain products, like whole-wheat bread and pasta. Look for the term "whole" or "whole grain" on the food package and in the ingredient list-it should be listed as the first ingredient. But if you still find it too hard to make the switch from your old refined favorites, phase in a whole grain by using whole-grain blends of pastas and rice or mixing a whole grain half-and-half with a refined one (like half whole-wheat pasta and half white).

5. Snack on Nuts

Nuts are another Mediterranean diet staple. Grabbing a handful, whether that's almonds, cashews or pistachios, can make for a satisfying, on-the-go snack. One study in Nutrition Journal found that if people replaced their standard snack (cookies, chips, crackers, snack mix, cereal bars) with almonds, their diets would be lower in empty calories, added sugar and sodium. Plus, nuts contain more fiber and minerals, such as potassium, than processed snack foods.

6. Enjoy Fruit for Dessert

Generally a good source of fiber, vitamin C and antioxidants, fresh fruit is a healthy way to indulge your sweet tooth. If it helps you to eat more, add a little sugar-drizzle slices of pear with honey or sprinkle a little brown sugar on grapefruit. Keep fresh fruit visible at home and keep a piece or two at work so you have a healthful snack when your stomach starts growling. Lots of grocery stores stock exotic fruit-pick a new one to try each week and expand your fruit horizons.

7. Sip (a Little) Wine

The people who live along the Mediterranean-the Spanish, Italian, French, Greek and others-are not known to shy away from wine, but that doesn't mean you should pour it at your leisure. Dietitians and experts who developed the Mediterranean diet for the New England Journal of Medicine study advised women to stick to a 3-ounce serving, and men to a 5-ounce serving, per day. When you do sip, try to do so with a meal-even better if that meal is shared with loved ones. If you're a teetotaler, you shouldn't start to drink just for this diet.

8. Savor Every Bite

Eating like a Mediterranean is as much lifestyle as it is diet. Instead of gobbling your meal in front of the TV, slow down and sit down at the table with your family and friends to savor what you're eating. Not only will you enjoy your company and your food, eating slowly also allows you to tune in to your body's hunger and fullness signals. You're more apt to eat just until you're satisfied than until you're busting-at-the-seams full.

Building a meal plan

The Mediterranean diet puts a higher focus on plant foods than many other diets. It is not uncommon for vegetables, whole grains, and legumes to make up all or most of a meal. People following the diet typically cook these foods using healthful fats, such as olive oil, and add plenty of flavorful spices. Meals may include small portions of fish, meat, or eggs. Water and sparkling water are common drink choices, as well as moderate amounts of red wine. People on a Mediterranean diet avoid the following foods: refined grains, such as white bread, white pasta, and pizza dough containing white flour. refined oils, which include canola oil and soybean oil. foods with added sugars, such as pastries, sodas, and candies. deli meats, hot dogs, and other processed meats processed or packaged foods.

BREAKFAST RECIPES

1. Zucchini And Quinoa Pan

Servings: 4   Cooking Time: 20 Minutes
Ingredients:

1 tablespoon olive oil
2 garlic cloves, minced
1 zucchini, roughly cubed
2 tablespoons basil, chopped
¼ cup green olives, pitted and chopped
1 cup quinoa
1 tomato, cubed
½ cup feta cheese, crumbled
2 cups water
1 cup canned garbanzo beans, drained and rinsed
A pinch of salt and black pepper

Directions:
Heat up a pan with the oil over medium-high heat, add the garlic and quinoa and brown for 3 minutes. Add the water, zucchinis, salt and pepper, toss, bring to a simmer and cook for 15 minutes.   Add the rest of the ingredients, toss, divide everything between plates and serve for breakfast.
Nutrition Info:calories 310, fat 11, fiber 6, carbs 42, protein 11

2. Peas Omelet

Servings: 6   Cooking Time: 20 Minutes
Ingredients:

4 oz green peas
¼ cup corn kernels
6 eggs, beaten
½ teaspoon of sea salt
¼ cup heavy cream
1 red bell pepper, chopped
1 teaspoon butter
½ teaspoon paprika

Directions:
Toss butter in the skillet and melt it.   Add green peas, bell pepper, and corn kernels. Start to roast the vegetables over the medium heat.   Meanwhile, in the mixing bowl whisk together eggs, heavy cream, sea salt, and paprika.   Pour the mixture over the roasted vegetables and stir well immediately.   Close the lid and cook omelet over the medium-low heat for 15 minutes or until it is solid.   Transfer the cooked omelet in the big plate and cut into the servings.
Nutrition Info: Per Serving:calories 113, fat 7.1, fiber 1.5, carbs 6, protein 7.1

3. Low Carb Green Smoothie

Servings: 2   Cooking Time: 15 Mins
Ingredients:

1/3 cup romaine lettuce
1/3 tablespoon fresh ginger, peeled and chopped
1½ cups filtered water
1/8 cup fresh pineapple, chopped
¾ tablespoon fresh parsley
1/3 cup raw cucumber, peeled and sliced
¼ Hass avocado
¼ cup kiwi fruit, peeled and chopped
1/3 tablespoon Swerve

Directions:
Put all the ingredients in a blender and blend until smooth.   Pour into 2 serving glasses and serve chilled.

Nutrition Info: Calories: 108 Carbs: 7.8g Fats: 8.9g Proteins: 1.6g Sodium: 4mg Sugar: 2.2g

4. Fig With Ricotta Oatmeal

Servings: 1   Cooking Time: 5 Minutes
Ingredients:

2 tablespoons ricotta cheese, part-skim
2 tablespoons dried figs, chopped
1/2 cup old-fashioned rolled oats
2 teaspoons honey
1 tablespoon almonds, toasted, sliced
1 cup water
Pinch of salt

Directions:
Pour the water in a small saucepan and add the salt; bring to a boil.   Stir in the oats and reduce heat to medium. Cook the oats for about 5 minutes, occasionally stirring, until most of the water is absorbed.   Remove the pan from the heat, cover, and let stand for 2-3 minutes.   Serve topped with the figs, almonds, ricotta, and drizzle of honey.
Nutrition Info: Per Serving:315 Cal, 8 g total fat (2 g sat. fat, 4 g mono), 10 mg chol., 194 mg sodium, 359 mg pot., 53 g carb.,7 g fiber, 10 g protein.

5. Raspberry Pudding

Servings: 2   Cooking Time: 30 Minutes
Ingredients:

½ cup raspberries
2 teaspoons maple syrup
1 ½ cup Plain yogurt
¼ teaspoon ground cardamom
1/3 cup Chia seeds, dried

Directions:
Mix up together Plain yogurt with maple syrup and ground cardamom.   Add Chia seeds. Stir it gently. Put the yogurt in the serving glasses and top with the raspberries.   Refrigerate the breakfast for at least 30 minutes or overnight.
Nutrition Info: Per Serving:calories 303, fat 11.2, fiber 11.8, carbs 33.2, protein 15.5

6. Walnuts Yogurt Mix

Servings: 6   Cooking Time: 0 Minutes
Ingredients:

2 and ½ cups Greek yogurt
1 and ½ cups walnuts, chopped
¾ cup honey
1 teaspoon vanilla extract
2 teaspoons cinnamon powder

Directions:
In a bowl, combine the yogurt with the walnuts and the rest of the ingredients, toss, divide into smaller bowls and keep in the fridge for 10 minutes before serving for breakfast.
Nutrition Info:calories 388, fat 24.6, fiber 2.9, carbs 39.1, protein 10.2

7. Mediterranean Egg-feta Scramble

Servings: 4   Cooking Time: 15 Minutes
Ingredients:

3/4 cup crumbled feta cheese
2 tablespoons green onions, minced
2 tablespoons red peppers, roasted,
6 eggs
1/4 cup Greek yogurt
1/2 teaspoon dry oregano
1/2 teaspoon dry basil

diced
1/4 teaspoon kosher salt
1/4 teaspoon garlic powder

1 teaspoon olive oil
A few cracks freshly ground black pepper
Warm whole-wheat tortillas, optional

Directions:
Preheat a skillet over medium heat. In a bowl, whisk the eggs, the sour cream, basil, oregano, garlic powder, salt, and pepper. Gently add the feta. When the skillet is hot, add the olive oil and then the egg mixture; allow the egg mix to set then scrape the bottom of the pan to let the uncooked egg to cook. Stir in the red peppers and the green onions. Continue cooking until the eggs mixture is cooked to your preferred doneness. Serve immediately. If desired, sprinkle with extra feta and then wrap the scrambled eggs in tortillas.
Nutrition Info: Per Serving:260 Cal, 16 g total fat (8 g sat. fat), 350 mg chol., 750 mg sodium, 190 mg pot., 12 g carb.,>1 g fiber, 2 g sugar, 16 g protein.

8. Spiced Chickpeas Bowls

Servings: 4   Cooking Time: 30 Minutes
Ingredients:

15 ounces canned chickpeas, drained and rinsed
1/4 teaspoon cardamom, ground
1/2 teaspoon cinnamon powder
1 and 1/2 teaspoons turmeric powder
1 teaspoon coriander, ground

1 tablespoon olive oil
A pinch of salt and black pepper
3/4 cup Greek yogurt
1/2 cup green olives, pitted and halved
1/2 cup cherry tomatoes, halved
1 cucumber, sliced

Directions:
Spread the chickpeas on a lined baking sheet, add the cardamom, cinnamon, turmeric, coriander, the oil, salt and pepper, toss and bake at 375 degrees F for 30 minutes. In a bowl, combine the roasted chickpeas with the rest of the ingredients, toss and serve for breakfast.
Nutrition Info:calories 519, fat 34.5, fiber 13.3, carbs 49.8, protein 12

9. Orzo And Veggie Bowls

Servings: 4   Cooking Time: 0 Minutes
Ingredients:

2 and 1/2 cups whole-wheat orzo, cooked
14 ounces canned cannellini beans, drained and rinsed
1 yellow bell pepper, cubed
1 green bell pepper, cubed
A pinch of salt and black pepper
3 tomatoes, cubed
1 red onion, chopped

1 cup mint, chopped
2 cups feta cheese, crumbled
2 tablespoons olive oil
1/4 cup lemon juice
1 tablespoon lemon zest, grated
1 cucumber, cubed
1 and 1/4 cup kalamata olives, pitted and sliced
3 garlic cloves, minced

Directions:
In a salad bowl, combine the orzo with the beans, bell peppers and the rest of the ingredients, toss, divide the mix between plates and serve for breakfast.

Nutrition Info:calories 411, fat 17, fiber 13, carbs 51, protein 14

10. Vanilla Oats

Servings: 4   Cooking Time: 10 Minutes
Ingredients:

1/2 cup rolled oats
1 teaspoon vanilla extract
1 teaspoon ground cinnamon

1 cup milk
2 teaspoon honey
2 tablespoons Plain yogurt
1 teaspoon butter

Directions:
Pour milk in the saucepan and bring it to boil. Add rolled oats and stir well. Close the lid and simmer the oats for 5 minutes over the medium heat. The cooked oats will absorb all milk. Then add butter and stir the oats well. In the separated bowl, whisk together Plain yogurt with honey, cinnamon, and vanilla extract. Transfer the cooked oats in the serving bowls. Top the oats with the yogurt mixture in the shape of the wheel.
Nutrition Info: Per Serving:calories 243, fat 20.2, fiber 1, carbs 2.8, protein 13.3

11. Mushroom-egg Casserole

Servings: 3   Cooking Time: 25 Minutes
Ingredients:

1/2 cup mushrooms, chopped
1/2 yellow onion, diced
4 eggs, beaten
1 tablespoon coconut flakes

1/2 teaspoon chili pepper
1 oz Cheddar cheese, shredded
1 teaspoon canola oil

Directions:
Pour canola oil in the skillet and preheat well. Add mushrooms and onion and roast for 5-8 minutes or until the vegetables are light brown. Transfer the cooked vegetables in the casserole mold. Add coconut flakes, chili pepper, and Cheddar cheese. Then add eggs and stir well. Bake the casserole for 15 minutes at 360F.
Nutrition Info: Calories 152, fat 11.1, fiber 0.7, carbs 3, protein 10.4

12. Bacon Veggies Combo

Servings: 2   Cooking Time: 35 Minutes
Ingredients:

1/2 green bell pepper, seeded and chopped
2 bacon slices
1/4 cup Parmesan Cheese

1/2 tablespoon mayonnaise
1 scallion, chopped

Directions:
Preheat the oven to 375 degrees F and grease a baking dish. Place bacon slices on the baking dish and top with mayonnaise, bell peppers, scallions and Parmesan Cheese. Transfer in the oven and bake for about 25 minutes. Dish out to serve immediately or refrigerate for about 2 days wrapped in a plastic sheet for meal prepping.
Nutrition Info: Calories: 197 Fat: 13.8g Carbohydrates: 4.7g Protein: 14.3g Sugar: 1.9g Sodium: 662mg

13. Brown Rice Salad

Servings: 4   Cooking Time: 0 Minutes
Ingredients:

9 ounces brown rice, cooked
7 cups baby arugula
15 ounces canned garbanzo beans, drained and rinsed
4 ounces feta cheese, crumbled

¾ cup basil, chopped
A pinch of salt and black pepper
2 tablespoons lemon juice
¼ teaspoon lemon zest, grated
¼ cup olive oil

Directions:
In a salad bowl, combine the brown rice with the arugula, the beans and the rest of the ingredients, toss and serve cold for breakfast.
Nutrition Info:calories 473, fat 22, fiber 7, carbs 53, protein 13

14. Olive And Milk Bread

Servings: 6   Cooking Time: 50 Minutes
Ingredients:
1 cup black olives, pitted, chopped
1 tablespoon olive oil
½ teaspoon fresh yeast
½ cup milk, preheated
½ teaspoon salt

1 teaspoon baking powder
2 cup wheat flour, whole grain
2 eggs, beaten
1 teaspoon butter, melted
1 teaspoon sugar

Directions:
In the big bowl combine together fresh yeast, sugar, and milk. Stir it until yeast is dissolved.   Then add salt, baking powder, butter, and eggs. Stir the dough mixture until homogenous and add 1 cup of wheat flour. Mix it up until smooth.   Add olives and remaining flour. Knead the non-sticky dough. Transfer the dough into the non-sticky dough mold. Bake the bread for 50 minutes at 350 F.   Check if the bread is cooked with the help of the toothpick. Is it is dry, the bread is cooked.   Remove the bread from the oven and let it chill for 10-15 minutes.   Remove it from the loaf mold and slice.
Nutrition Info: Per Serving:calories 238, fat 7.7, fiber 1.9, carbs 35.5, protein 7.2

15. Breakfast Tostadas

Servings: 6   Cooking Time: 6 Minutes
Ingredients:
½ white onion, diced
1 tomato, chopped
1 cucumber, chopped
1 tablespoon fresh cilantro, chopped
½ jalapeno pepper, chopped
1 tablespoon lime juice
6 corn tortillas

1 tablespoon canola oil
2 oz Cheddar cheese, shredded
½ cup white beans, canned, drained
6 eggs
½ teaspoon butter
½ teaspoon Sea salt

Directions:
Make Pico de Galo: in the salad bowl combine together diced white onion, tomato, cucumber, fresh cilantro, and jalapeno pepper.   Then add lime juice and a ½ tablespoon of canola oil. Mix up the mixture well. Pico de Galo is cooked.   After this, preheat the oven to 390F.   Line the tray with baking paper.   Arrange the corn tortillas on the baking paper and brush with remaining canola oil from both sides.   Bake the tortillas for 10 minutes or until they start to be crunchy.   Chill the cooked crunchy tortillas well.   Meanwhile,

toss the butter in the skillet.   Crack the eggs in the melted butter and sprinkle them with sea salt. Fry the eggs until the egg whites become white (cooked). Approximately for 3-5 minutes over the medium heat.   After this, mash the beans until you get puree texture.   Spread the bean puree on the corn tortillas.   Add fried eggs.   Then top the eggs with Pico de Galo and shredded Cheddar cheese.
Nutrition Info: Calories 246, fat 11.1, fiber 4.7, carbs 24.5, protein 13.7

16. Chicken Souvlaki

Servings: 4   Cooking Time: 2 Minutes
Ingredients:
4 pieces (6-inch) pitas, cut into halves
2 cups roasted chicken breast skinless, boneless, and sliced
1/4 cup red onion, thinly sliced
1/2 teaspoon dried oregano
1/2 cup Greek yogurt, plain
1/2 cup plum tomato, chopped

1/2 cup cucumber, peeled, chopped
1/2 cup (2 ounces) feta cheese, crumbled
1 tablespoon olive oil, extra-virgin, divided
1 tablespoon fresh dill, chopped
1 cup iceberg lettuce, shredded
1 1/4 teaspoons minced garlic, bottled, divided

Directions:
In a small mixing bowl, combine the yogurt, cheese, 1 teaspoon of the olive oil, and 1/4 teaspoon of the garlic until well mixed.   In a large skillet, heat the remaining olive oil over medium-high heat. Add the remaining 1 teaspoon garlic and the oregano; sauté for 20 seconds.   Add the chicken; cook for about 2 minutes or until the chicken are heated through.   Put 1/4 cup chicken into each pita halves. Top with 2 tablespoons yogurt mix, 2 tablespoons lettuce,1 tablespoon tomato, and 1 tablespoon cucumber. Divide the onion between the pita halves.
Nutrition Info: Per Serving:414 Cal, 13.7 g total fat (6.4 g sat. fat, 1.4 g poly. Fat, 4.7 g mono), 81 mg chol., 595 mg sodium, 38 g carb.,2 g fiber, 32.3 g protein.

17. Tahini Pine Nuts Toast

Servings: 2   Cooking Time: 0 Minutes
Ingredients:
2 whole wheat bread slices, toasted
1 tablespoon tahini paste
2 teaspoons feta cheese, crumbled

1 teaspoon water
Juice of ½ lemon
2 teaspoons pine nuts
A pinch of black pepper

Directions:
In a bowl, mix the tahini with the water and the lemon juice, whisk really well and spread over the toasted bread slices.   Top each serving with the remaining ingredients and serve for breakfast.
Nutrition Info:calories 142, fat 7.6, fiber 2.7, carbs 13.7, protein 5.8

18. Eggs And Veggies

Servings: 4   Cooking Time: 15 Minutes
Ingredients:
2 tomatoes, chopped
2 eggs, beaten

¼ cup of water

1 bell pepper, chopped
1 teaspoon tomato paste

1 teaspoon butter
½ white onion, diced
½ teaspoon chili flakes
1/3 teaspoon sea salt

Directions:
Put butter in the pan and melt it. Add bell pepper and cook it for 3 minutes over the medium heat. Stir it from time to time. After this, add diced onion and cook it for 2 minutes more. Stir the vegetables and add tomatoes. Cook them for 5 minutes over the medium-low heat. Then add water and tomato paste. Stir well. Add beaten eggs, chili flakes, and sea salt. Stir well and cook menemen for 4 minutes over the medium-low heat. The cooked meal should be half runny.
Nutrition Info: Per Serving:calories 67, fat 3.4, fiber 1.5, carbs 6.4, protein 3.8

19. Chili Scramble

Servings: 4   Cooking Time: 15 Minutes
Ingredients:
3 tomatoes
¼ teaspoon of sea salt
½ chili pepper, chopped

4 eggs
1 tablespoon butter
1 cup water, for cooking

Directions:
Pour water in the saucepan and bring it to boil. Then remove water from the heat and add tomatoes. Let the tomatoes stay in the hot water for 2-3 minutes. After this, remove the tomatoes from water and peel them. Place butter in the pan and melt it. Add chopped chili pepper and fry it for 3 minutes over the medium heat. Then chop the peeled tomatoes and add into the chili peppers. Cook the vegetables for 5 minutes over the medium heat. Stir them from time to time. After this, add sea salt and crack then eggs. Stir (scramble) the eggs well with the help of the fork and cook them for 3 minutes over the medium heat.
Nutrition Info: Per Serving:calories 105, fat 7.4, fiber 1.1, carbs 4, protein 6.4

20. Pear Oatmeal

Servings: 4   Cooking Time: 25 Minutes
Ingredients:
1 cup oatmeal
1/3 cup milk
1 pear, chopped
1 teaspoon vanilla extract

1 tablespoon Splenda
1 teaspoon butter
½ teaspoon ground cinnamon
1 egg, beaten

Directions:
In the big bowl mix up together oatmeal, milk, egg, vanilla extract, Splenda, and ground cinnamon. Melt butter and add it in the oatmeal mixture. Then add chopped pear and stir it well. Transfer the oatmeal mixture in the casserole mold and flatten gently. Cover it with the foil and secure edges. Bake the oatmeal for 25 minutes at 350F.
Nutrition Info: Per Serving:calories 151, fat 3.9, fiber 3.3, carbs 23.6, protein 4.9

21. Mediterranean Frittata 3

Servings: 6   Cooking Time: 15 Minutes
Ingredients:

9 large eggs, lightly beaten
8 kalamata olives, pitted, chopped
1/4 cup olive oil
1/3 cup parmesan cheese, freshly grated
1/3 cup fresh basil, thinly sliced

1/2 teaspoon salt
1/2 teaspoon pepper
1/2 cup onion, chopped
1 sweet red pepper, diced
1 medium zucchini, cut to 1/2-inch cubes
1 package (4 ounce) feta cheese, crumbled

Directions:
In a 10-inch oven-proof skillet, heat the olive oil until hot. Add the olives, zucchini, red pepper, and the onions, constantly stirring, until the vegetables are tender. Ina bowl, mix the eggs, feta cheese, basil, salt, and pepper; pour in the skillet with vegetables. Adjust heat to medium-low, cover, and cook for about 10-12 minutes, or until the egg mixture is almost set. Remove from the heat and sprinkle with the parmesan cheese. Transfer to the broiler. With oven door partially open, broil 5 1/2 from the source of heat for about 2-3 minutes or until the top is golden. Cut into wedges.
Nutrition Info: Per Serving:288.5 Cal, 22.8 g total fat (7.8 g sat. fat), 301 mg chol., 656 mg sodium, 5.6 g carb.,1.2 g fiber,3.3g sugar, 15.2 g protein.

22. Mediterranean Egg Casserole

Servings: 8   Cooking Time: 50 Minutes
Ingredients:
1 1/2 cups (6 ounces) feta cheese, crumbled
1 jar (6 ounces) marinated artichoke hearts, drained well, coarsely chopped
10 eggs
2 cups milk, low-fat
2 cups fresh baby spinach, packed, coarsely chopped
6 cups whole-wheat baguette, cut into 1-inch cubes
1 tablespoon garlic (about 4 cloves), finely chopped

1 tablespoon olive oil, extra-virgin
1/2 cup red bell pepper, chopped
1/2 cup Parmesan cheese, shredded
1/2 teaspoon pepper
1/2 teaspoon red pepper flakes
1/2 teaspoon salt
1/3 cup kalamata olives, pitted, halved
1/4 cup red onion, chopped
1/4 cup tomatoes (sun-dried) in oil, drained, chopped

Directions:
Preheat oven to 350F. Grease a 9x13-inch baking dish with olive oil cooking spray. In an 8-inch non-stick pan over medium heat, heat the olive oil. Add the onions, garlic, and bell pepper; cook for about 3 minutes, frequently stirring, until slightly softened. Add the spinach; cook for about 1 minute or until starting to wilt. Layer half of the baguette cubes in the prepared baking dish, then 1 cup of the eta, 1/4 cup Parmesan, the bell pepper mix, artichokes, the olives, and the tomatoes. Top with the remaining baguette cubes and then with the remaining 1/2 cup of feta. In a large mixing bowl, whisk the eggs and the low-fat milk together. Beat in the pepper, salt and the pepper. Pour the mix over the bread layer in the baking dish, slightly pressing down. Sprinkle with the remaining 1/4 cup Parmesan. Bake for about 40-45 minutes, or until the center is set and the top is golden brown. Before serving, let stand for 15 minutes.

Nutrition Info: Per Serving:360 Cal, 21 g total fat (9 g sat. fat), 270 mg chol., 880 mg sodium, 24 g carb.,3 g fiber,7 g sugar, 20 g protein.

23. Milk Scones

Servings: 4   Cooking Time: 10 Minutes

Ingredients:

½ cup wheat flour, whole grain

1 teaspoon baking powder

1 tablespoon butter, melted

1 egg, beaten

1 teaspoon vanilla extract

¾ teaspoon salt

3 tablespoons milk

1 teaspoon vanilla sugar

Directions:

In the mixing bowl combine together wheat flour, baking powder, butter, vanilla extract, and egg. Add salt and knead the soft and non-sticky dough. Add more flour if needed.   Then make the log from the dough and cut it into the triangles.   Line the tray with baking paper.   Arrange the dough triangles on the baking paper and transfer in the preheat to the 360F oven.   Cook the scones for 10 minutes or until they are light brown.   After this, chill the scones and brush with milk and sprinkle with vanilla sugar.

Nutrition Info: Per Serving:calories 112, fat 4.4, fiber 0.5, carbs 14.3, protein 3.4

24. Herbed Eggs And Mushroom Mix

Servings: 4   Cooking Time: 20 Minutes

Ingredients:

1 red onion, chopped

1 bell pepper, chopped

1 tablespoon tomato paste

1/3 cup water

½ teaspoon of sea salt

1 tablespoon butter

1 cup cremini mushrooms, chopped

1 tablespoon fresh parsley

1 tablespoon fresh dill

1 teaspoon dried thyme

½ teaspoon dried oregano

½ teaspoon paprika

½ teaspoon chili flakes

½ teaspoon garlic powder

4 eggs

Directions:

Toss butter in the pan and melt it.   Then add chopped mushrooms and bell pepper.   Roast the vegetables for 5 minutes over the medium heat. After this, add red onion and stir well.   Sprinkle the ingredients with garlic powder, chili flakes, dried oregano, and dried thyme. Mix up well After this, add tomato paste and water.   Mix up the mixture until it is homogenous.   Then add fresh parsley and dill.   Cook the mixture for 5 minutes over the medium-high heat with the closed lid.   After this, stir the mixture with the help of the spatula well.   Crack the eggs over the mixture and close the lid.   Cook shakshuka for 10 minutes over the low heat.

Nutrition Info: Per Serving:calories 123, fat 7.5, fiber 1.7, carbs 7.8, protein 7.1

25. Leeks And Eggs Muffins

Servings: 2   Cooking Time: 20 Minutes

Ingredients:

3 eggs, whisked

¼ cup baby spinach

2 tablespoons leeks,

Cooking spray

1 small red bell pepper, chopped

chopped

4 tablespoons parmesan, grated

2 tablespoons almond milk

Salt and black pepper to the taste

1 tomato, cubed

2 tablespoons cheddar cheese, grated

Directions:

In a bowl, combine the eggs with the milk, salt, pepper and the rest of the ingredients except the cooking spray and whisk well.   Grease a muffin tin with the cooking spray and divide the eggs mixture in each muffin mould.   Bake at 380 degrees F for 20 minutes and serve them for breakfast.

Nutrition Info:calories 308, fat 19.4, fiber 1.7, carbs 8.7, protein 24.4

26. Mango And Spinach Bowls

Servings: 4   Cooking Time: 0 Minutes

Ingredients:

1 cup baby spinach, chopped

1 mango, peeled and cubed

1 cup strawberries, halved

1 tablespoon hemp seeds

1 cup baby arugula

1 cucumber, sliced

1 tablespoon lime juice

1 tablespoon tahini paste

1 tablespoon water

Directions:

In a salad bowl, mix the arugula with the rest of the ingredients except the tahini and the water and toss. In a small bowl, combine the tahini with the water, whisk well, add to the salad, toss, divide into small bowls and serve for breakfast.

Nutrition Info:calories 211, fat 4.5, fiber 6.5, carbs 10.2, protein 3.5

27. Veggie Quiche

Servings: 8   Cooking Time: 55 Minutes

Ingredients:

½ cup sun-dried tomatoes, chopped

2 tablespoons avocado oil

1 yellow onion, chopped

2 garlic cloves, minced

2 cups spinach, chopped

1 red bell pepper, chopped

¼ cup kalamata olives, pitted and sliced

1 prepared pie crust

1 teaspoon parsley flakes

1 teaspoon oregano, dried

1/3 cup feta cheese, crumbled

4 eggs, whisked

1 and ½ cups almond milk

1 cup cheddar cheese, shredded

Salt and black pepper to the taste

Directions:

Heat up a pan with the oil over medium-high heat, add the garlic and onion and sauté for 3 minutes. Add the bell pepper and sauté for 3 minutes more. Add the olives, parsley, spinach, oregano, salt and pepper and cook everything for 5 minutes.   Add tomatoes and the cheese, toss and take off the heat. Arrange the pie crust in a pie plate, pour the spinach and tomatoes mix inside and spread.   In a bowl, mix the eggs with salt, pepper, the milk and half of the cheese, whisk and pour over the mixture in the pie crust.   Sprinkle the remaining cheese on top and bake at 375 degrees F for 40 minutes. Cool the quiche down, slice and serve for breakfast.

Nutrition Info: calories 211, fat 14.4, fiber 1.4, carbs 12.5, protein 8.6

28. Tuna And Cheese Bake

Servings: 4   Cooking Time: 15 Minutes

Ingredients:

10 ounces canned tuna, drained and flaked	4 eggs, whisked
	1 tablespoon parsley, chopped
½ cup feta cheese, shredded	Salt and black pepper to the taste
1 tablespoon chives, chopped	3 teaspoons olive oil

Directions:

Grease a baking dish with the oil, add the tuna and the rest of the ingredients except the cheese, toss and bake at 370 degrees F for 15 minutes. Sprinkle the cheese on top, leave the mix aside for 5 minutes, slice and serve for breakfast.

Nutrition Info: calories 283, fat 14.2, fiber 5.6, carbs 12.1, protein 6.4

29. Tomato And Cucumber Salad

Servings: 4   Cooking Time: 5 Minutes

Ingredients:

3 tomatoes, chopped	1 tablespoon capers
2 cucumbers, chopped	1 tablespoon canola oil
1 red onion, sliced	½ teaspoon minced garlic
2 red bell peppers, chopped	
¼ cup fresh cilantro, chopped	1 tablespoon Dijon mustard
1 oz whole-grain bread, chopped	1 teaspoon olive oil
	1 teaspoon lime juice

Directions:

Pour canola oil in the skillet and bring it to boil. Add chopped bread and roast it until crunchy (3-5 minutes).   Meanwhile, in the salad bowl combine together sliced red onion, cucumbers, tomatoes, bell peppers, cilantro, capers, and mix up gently. Make the dressing: mix up together lime juice, olive oil, Dijon mustard, and minced garlic.   Pour the dressing over the salad and stir it directly before serving.

Nutrition Info: Per Serving: calories 136, fat 5.7, fiber 4.1, carbs 20.2, protein 4.1

30. Cream Olive Muffins

Servings: 6   Cooking Time: 20 Minutes

Ingredients:

½ cup quinoa, cooked	1 tomato, chopped
2 oz Feta cheese, crumbled	1 teaspoon butter, softened
2 eggs, beaten	1 tablespoon wheat flour, whole grain
3 kalamata olives, chopped	½ teaspoon salt
¾ cup heavy cream	

Directions:

In the mixing bowl whisk eggs and add Feta cheese. Then add chopped tomato and heavy cream. After this, add wheat flour, salt, and quinoa. Then add kalamata olives and mix up the ingredients with the help of the spoon.   Brush the muffin molds with the butter from inside. Transfer quinoa mixture in the muffin molds and flatten it with the help of the spatula or spoon if needed.   Cook the muffins in the preheated to 355F oven for 20 minutes.

Nutrition Info: Per Serving: calories 165, fat 10.8, fiber 1.2, carbs 11.5, protein 5.8

31. Roasted Asparagus With Prosciu6tto And Poached Egg

Servings: 4   Cooking Time: 25 Minutes

Ingredients:

1 bunch fresh asparagus, trimmed	4 eggs
	1 tablespoon olive oil
1 tablespoon extra-virgin olive oil	1 pinch salt
2 ounces minced prosciutto	1 pinch ground black pepper
1/2 lemon, zested and juiced	1 teaspoon distilled white vinegar
	Ground black pepper

Directions:

Preheat oven to 425F or 220C.   In a baking dish, place the asparagus and drizzle with the extra-virgin olive oil.   In a skillet, heat the olive oil over medium-low heat; add the prosciutto and cook for about 3-4 minutes, stirring, until golden and rendered. Sprinkle over the asparagus in the baking dish and season with black pepper; toss to coat.   Roast for 10 minutes, toss, return to the oven, and continue roasting for 5 minutes or until the asparagus are tender yet firm to the bite.   Fill a large saucepan with about 2-3 inches of water; bring to a boil over high heat. When boiling, reduce the heat to low; pour in the vinegar and a pinch of salt. Crack an egg into a small bowl, then gently slip the egg into the water.   Repeat with the remaining eggs. Poach the eggs for about 4-6 minutes or until the whites are firm and the yolks are thick but not hard. With a slotted spoon, remove the eggs, dab the spoon on a clean kitchen towel to remove excess water from the eggs, and transfer to a warm plate.   Drizzle the asparagus with the lemon juice and transfer divide between 2 plates. Top each asparagus bed with the 2 poached eggs, sprinkle with a pinch of lemon zest, and season with black pepper; serve.

Nutrition Info: Per Serving: 163 Cal, 12.3 g total fat (2.7 g sat. fat), 171 mg chol., 273 mg sodium, 4.3 g carb., 1.9 g fiber, 10.4 g protein.

32. Figs Oatmeal

Servings: 5   Cooking Time: 20 Minutes

Ingredients:

2 cups oatmeal	3 figs, chopped
1 ½ cup milk	1 tablespoon honey
1 tablespoon butter	

Directions:

Pour milk in the saucepan.   Add oatmeal and close the lid.   Cook the oatmeal for 15 minutes over the medium-low heat.   Then add chopped figs and honey.   Add butter and mix up the oatmeal well.   Cook it for 5 minutes more. Close the lid and let the cooked breakfast rest for 10 minutes before serving.

Nutrition Info: Per Serving: calories 222, fat 6, fiber 4.4, carbs 36.5, protein 7.1

33. Mediterranean Freezer Breakfast Wraps

Servings: 4   Cooking Time: 3 Minutes

Ingredients:

1 cup spinach leaves,	4 eggs, beaten

fresh, chopped
1 tablespoon water or low-fat milk
1/2 teaspoon garlic-chipotle seasoning or your preferred seasoning
4 tablespoons tomato chutney (or dried tomatoes, chopped or canned tomatoes)

4 pieces (8-inch) whole-wheat tortillas
4 tablespoons feta cheese, crumbled (or goat cheese)
Optional: prosciutto, chopped or bacon, cooked, crumbled
Salt and pepper, to taste

Directions:
In a mixing bowl, whisk the eggs, water or milk, and seasoning together. Heat a skillet with a little olive oil; pour the eggs and scramble for about 3-4 minutes, or until just cooked. Lay the tortillas in a clean surface; divide the eggs between them, arranging the scrambled eggs in a line and leaving the tortilla edges free to fold later. Top the egg layer with about 1 tablespoon of cheese, 1 tablespoon tomatoes, and 1/4 cup spinach. If using, layer with prosciutto or bacon. In a burrito-style, roll up the tortillas, folding both of the ends in the process. In a panini maker or a clean skillet, cook for about 1 minute, turning once, until the tortilla wraps are crisp and brown; serve.
Nutrition Info: Per Serving:450 Cal, 15 g total fat (5 g sat. fat), 220 mg chol., 1, 280 mg sodium, 960 mg pot., 64 g carb.,6 g fiber,20 g sugar, 17 g protein.

34. Cheesy Olives Bread

Servings: 10   Cooking Time: 30 Minutes
Ingredients:
4 cups whole-wheat flour
3 tablespoons oregano, chopped
2 teaspoons dry yeast
¼ cup olive oil

1 and ½ cups black olives, pitted and sliced
1 cup water
½ cup feta cheese, crumbled

Directions:
In a bowl, mix the flour with the water, the yeast and the oil, stir and knead your dough very well. Put the dough in a bowl, cover with plastic wrap and keep in a warm place for 1 hour. Divide the dough into 2 bowls and stretch each ball really well. Add the rest of the ingredients on each ball and tuck them inside well kneading the dough again. Flatten the balls a bit and leave them aside for 40 minutes more. Transfer the balls to a baking sheet lined with parchment paper, make a small slit in each and bake at 425 degrees F for 30 minutes. Serve the bread as a Mediterranean breakfast.
Nutrition Info:calories 251, fat 7.3, fiber 2.1, carbs 39.7, protein 6.7

35. Scrambled Eggs

Servings: 2   Cooking Time: 10 Minutes
Ingredients:
1 yellow bell pepper, chopped
8 cherry tomatoes, cubed
2 spring onions, chopped
1 tablespoon olive oil
1 tablespoon capers, drained

2 tablespoons black olives, pitted and sliced
4 eggs
A pinch of salt and black pepper
¼ teaspoon oregano, dried

1 tablespoon parsley, chopped

Directions:
Heat up a pan with the oil over medium-high heat, add the bell pepper and spring onions and sauté for 3 minutes. Add the tomatoes, capers and the olives and sauté for 2 minutes more. Crack the eggs into the pan, add salt, pepper and the oregano and scramble for 5 minutes more. Divide the scramble between plates, sprinkle the parsley on top and serve.
Nutrition Info:calories 249, fat 17, fiber 3.2, carbs 13.3, protein 13.5

36. Paprika Salmon Toast

Servings: 2   Cooking Time: 3 Minutes
Ingredients:
4 whole grain bread slices
2 oz smoked salmon, sliced
2 teaspoons cream cheese
½ teaspoon paprika

1 teaspoon fresh dill, chopped
½ teaspoon lemon juice
4 lettuce leaves
1 cucumber, sliced

Directions:
Toast the bread in the toaster (1-2 minutes totally). In the bowl, mix up together fresh dill, cream cheese, lemon juice, and paprika. Then spread the toasts with the cream cheese mixture. Slice the smoked salmon and place it on 2 bread slices. Add sliced cucumber and lettuce leaves. Top the lettuce with remaining bread toasts and pin with the toothpick.
Nutrition Info: Per Serving:calories 202, fat 4.7, fiber 5.1, carbs 31.5, protein 12.7

37. Creamy Fritatta

Servings: 4   Cooking Time: 15 Minutes
Ingredients:
5 eggs, beaten
1 poblano chile, chopped, raw
1 oz scallions, chopped
1/3 cup heavy cream

½ teaspoon butter
½ teaspoon salt
½ teaspoon chili flakes
1 tablespoon fresh cilantro, chopped

Directions:
Mix up together eggs with heavy cream and whisk until homogenous. Add chopped poblano chile, scallions, salt, chili flakes, and fresh cilantro. Toss butter in the skillet and melt it. Add egg mixture and flatten it in the skillet if needed. Close the lid and cook the frittata for 15 minutes over the medium-low heat. When the frittata is cooked, it will be solid.
Nutrition Info: Per Serving:calories 131, fat 10.4, fiber 0.2, carbs 1.3, protein 8.2

38. Egg And Pepper Bake

Servings: 4   Cooking Time: 28 Minutes
Ingredients:
2 eggs, beaten
1 red bell pepper, chopped
1 chili pepper, chopped
½ red onion, diced
1 teaspoon canola oil

1 teaspoon paprika
1 tablespoon fresh cilantro, chopped
1 garlic clove, diced
1 teaspoon butter, softened
¼ teaspoon chili

½ teaspoon salt   flakes

Directions:
Brush the casserole mold with canola oil and pour beaten eggs inside. After this, toss the butter in the skillet and melt it over the medium heat. Add chili pepper and red bell pepper. After this, add red onion and cook the vegetables for 7-8 minutes over the medium heat. Stir them from time to time. Transfer the vegetables in the casserole mold. Add salt, paprika, cilantro, diced garlic, and chili flakes. Stir gently with the help of a spatula to get a homogenous mixture. Bake the casserole for 20 minutes at 355F in the oven. Then chill the meal well and cut into servings. Transfer the casserole in the serving plates with the help of the spatula.
Nutrition Info: Per Serving:calories 68, fat 4.5, fiber 1, carbs 4.4, protein 3.4

39. Mediterranean Chicken Salad Pitas

Servings: 6   Cooking Time: 15 Minutes
Ingredients:
6 slices (1/8-inch-thick) tomato, cut into halves
1 can (15-ounce) chickpeas (garbanzo beans), no-salt-added, rinsed, drained
3 cups chicken cooked, chopped
2 tablespoons lemon juice
12 Bibb lettuce leaves
1/4 teaspoon red pepper, crushed

6 pieces (6-inch) whole-wheat pitas, cut into halves
1/4 cup fresh cilantro, chopped
1/2 teaspoon ground cumin
1/2 cup red onion, diced
1/2 cup (about 20 small) green olives, chopped, pitted
1 cup Greek yogurt, plain, whole-milk
1 cup (about 1 large) red bell pepper, chopped

Directions:
In a small bowl, combine the yogurt, lemon juice, cumin, and red pepper; set aside. In a large mixing bowl, combine the chicken, red bell pepper, olives, red onion, cilantro, and chickpeas. Add the yogurt mixture into the chicken mixture; gently toss to coat. Line each pita half with 1 lettuce leaf and then with 1 tomato slice. Fill each pita half with 1/2 cup of the chicken mixture.
Nutrition Info: Per Serving:404 Cal, 10.2 g total fat (3.8 g sat. fat, 1.5 g poly. Fat, 4 g mono), 66 mg chol., 575 mg sodium, 46.4 g carb.,6 g fiber,33.6 g protein.

40. Raspberries And Yogurt Smoothie

Servings: 2   Cooking Time: 0 Minutes
Ingredients:
2 cups raspberries
½ cup Greek yogurt
½ cup almond milk
½ teaspoon vanilla extract

Directions:
In your blender, combine the raspberries with the milk, vanilla, and the yogurt, pulse well, divide into 2 glasses and serve for breakfast.
Nutrition Info:calories 245, fat 9.5, fiber 2.3, carbs 5.6, protein 1.6

41. Farro Salad

Servings: 2   Cooking Time: 4 Minutes
Ingredients:
1 tablespoon olive oil
A pinch of salt and black pepper
1 bunch baby spinach, chopped
1 avocado, pitted, peeled and chopped

1 garlic clove, minced
2 cups farro, already cooked
½ cup cherry tomatoes, cubed

Directions:
Heat up a pan with the oil over medium heat, add the spinach, and the rest of the ingredients, toss, cook for 4 minutes, divide into bowls and serve.
Nutrition Info:calories 157, fat 13.7, fiber 5.5, carbs 8.6, protein 3.6

42. Chili Avocado Scramble

Servings: 4   Cooking Time: 15 Minutes
Ingredients:
4 eggs, beaten
1 tablespoon avocado oil
1 avocado, finely chopped
½ teaspoon chili flakes

1 white onion, diced
1 oz Cheddar cheese, shredded
½ teaspoon salt
1 tablespoon fresh parsley

Directions:
Pour avocado oil in the skillet and bring it to boil. Then add diced onion and roast it until it is light brown. Meanwhile, mix up together chili flakes, beaten eggs, and salt. Pour the egg mixture over the cooked onion and cook the mixture for 1 minute over the medium heat. After this, scramble the eggs well with the help of the fork or spatula. Cook the eggs until they are solid but soft. After this, add chopped avocado and shredded cheese. Stir the scramble well and transfer in the serving plates. Sprinkle the meal with fresh parsley.
Nutrition Info: Per Serving:calories 236, fat 20.1, fiber 4, carbs 7.4, protein 8.6

43. Tapioca Pudding

Servings: 3   Cooking Time: 15 Minutes
Ingredients:
¼ cup pearl tapioca
¼ cup maple syrup
½ cup coconut flesh, shredded

2 cups almond milk
1 and ½ teaspoon lemon juice

Directions:
In a pan, combine the milk with the tapioca and the rest of the ingredients, bring to a simmer over medium heat, and cook for 15 minutes. Divide the mix into bowls, cool it down and serve for breakfast.
Nutrition Info:calories 361, fat 28.5, fiber 2.7, carbs 28.3, protein 2.8

44. Feta And Eggs Mix

Servings: 4   Cooking Time: 5 Minutes
Ingredients:
4 eggs, beaten
½ teaspoon ground black pepper
2 oz Feta, scrambled

½ teaspoon salt
1 teaspoon butter
1 teaspoon fresh parsley, chopped

Directions:
Melt butter in the skillet and add beaten eggs. Then add parsley, salt, and scrambled eggs. Cook

the eggs for 1 minute over the high heat. Add ground black pepper and scramble eggs with the help of the fork. Cook the eggs for 3 minutes over the medium-high heat.
Nutrition Info: Per Serving:calories 110, fat 8.4, fiber 0.1, carbs 1.1, protein 7.6

45. Mediterranean Breakfast Quiche

Servings: ⅛ Quiche   Cooking Time: 1 Hour
Ingredients:

1 1/2 cups all-purpose flour	2 cups spinach, chopped
1 tsp. dried oregano	4 large eggs
1/2 tsp. garlic powder	1/2 cup heavy cream
2 tsp. salt	1 cup ricotta cheese
5 TB. cold butter	1/3 cup grated Parmesan cheese
3 TB. vegetable shortening	1 tsp. paprika
1/4 cup ice water	1/2 tsp. cayenne
3 TB. extra-virgin olive oil	1/2 tsp. ground black pepper
1 medium yellow onion, chopped	1/4 cup fresh basil, chopped
1 TB. minced garlic	1/4 cup fresh parsley, chopped
4 stalks asparagus, chopped	1/3 cup sun-dried tomatoes, chopped

Directions:
In a food processor fitted with a chopping blade, pulse together 1 1/2 cups all-purpose flour, oregano, garlic powder, and 1/2 teaspoon salt five times. Add cold butter and vegetable shortening, and pulse for 1 minute or until mixture resembles coarse meal. Continue to pulse while adding ice water, about 1 minute. Test dough—if it holds together when you pinch it, it doesn't need any more water. If it doesn't come together, add 3 more tablespoons cold water. Remove dough from the food processor, put into a plastic bag, and form into a flat disc. Refrigerate for 30 minutes. Preheat the oven to 400°F. Flour a rolling pin and your counter. Roll out dough to 1/4 inch thickness. Fit dough into an 8- or 9-inch tart pan. Using a fork, slightly puncture bottom of piecrust. Bake for 15 minutes. Remove from the oven, and set aside. In a large skillet over medium heat, add extra-virgin olive oil, yellow onion, garlic, and asparagus, and sauté for 5 minutes. Add spinach, and cook for 3 or 4 more minutes. Remove from heat, and set aside. In a large bowl, whisk together eggs, heavy cream, and ricotta cheese. Add remaining 1 1/2 teaspoons salt, Parmesan cheese, paprika, cayenne, black pepper, basil, parsley, and sun-dried tomatoes, and stir to combine. Pour filling into piecrust, and bake for 40 minutes. Remove from the oven, and let rest for 20 minutes before serving warm.

46. Ricotta Tartine And Honey-roasted Cherry

Servings: 4   Cooking Time: 15 Minutes
Ingredients:

4 slices (1/2 inch thick) artisan bread, whole-grain	1 teaspoon fresh thyme
2 cups fresh cherries, pitted	1 tablespoon lemon juice
2 teaspoons extra-virgin olive oil	1 tablespoon honey, plus more for serving
	1 cup ricotta cheese,
1/4 cup slivered almonds, toasted	part-skim
1 teaspoon lemon zest	Pinch of flaky sea salt, such as Maldon
	Pinch of salt

Directions:
Preheat oven to 400F. Line a rimmed baking sheet with parchment paper; set aside. In a mixing bowl, toss the cherries with the honey, oil, lemon juice, and salt. Transfer into pan. Roast for about 15 minutes, shaking the pan once or twice during roasting, until the cherries are very soft and warm. Toast the bread. Top with the cheese, the cherries, thyme, lemon zest, almonds, and season with sea salt. If desired, drizzle more honey.
Nutrition Info: Per Serving:320 Cal, 13 g total fat (6 g sat. fat, 6 g mono), 19 mg chol., 272 mg sodium, 401 g pot., 39 g carb.,6 g fiber,2 g sugar, 15 g protein.

47. Breakfast Spanakopita

Servings: 6   Cooking Time: 1 Hour
Ingredients:

2 cups spinach	1 teaspoon ground paprika
1 white onion, diced	
1/2 cup fresh parsley	2 eggs, beaten
1 teaspoon minced garlic	1/3 cup butter, melted
3 oz Feta cheese, crumbled	2 oz Phyllo dough

Directions:
Separate Phyllo dough into 2 parts. Brush the casserole mold with butter well and place 1 part of Phyllo dough inside. Brush its surface with butter too. Put the spinach and fresh parsley in the blender. Blend it until smooth and transfer in the mixing bowl. Add minced garlic, Feta cheese, ground paprika, eggs, and diced onion. Mix up well. Place the spinach mixture in the casserole mold and flatten it well. Cover the spinach mixture with remaining Phyllo dough and pour remaining butter over it. Bake spanakopita for 1 hour at 350F. Cut it into the servings.
Nutrition Info: Calories 190, fat 15.4, fiber 1.1, carbs 8.4, protein 5.4

48. Creamy Parsley Soufflé

Servings: 2   Cooking Time: 25 Minutes
Ingredients:

2 fresh red chili peppers, chopped	4 tablespoons light cream
Salt, to taste	2 tablespoons fresh parsley, chopped
4 eggs	

Directions:
Preheat the oven to 375 degrees F and grease 2 soufflé dishes. Combine all the ingredients in a bowl and mix well. Put the mixture into prepared soufflé dishes and transfer in the oven. Cook for about 6 minutes and dish out to serve immediately. For meal prepping, you can refrigerate this creamy parsley soufflé in the ramekins covered in a foil for about 2-3 days.
Nutrition Info: Calories: 108 Fat: 9g Carbohydrates: 1.1g Protein: 6g Sugar: 0.5g Sodium: 146mg

49. Berry Oats

Servings: 2   Cooking Time: 0 Minutes
Ingredients:

½ cup rolled oats
1 cup almond milk
A pinch of cinnamon powder
¼ cup chia seeds
2 teaspoons honey
1 cup berries, pureed
1 tablespoon yogurt

Directions:
In a bowl, combine the oats with the milk and the rest of the ingredients except the yogurt, toss, divide into bowls, top with the yogurt and serve cold for breakfast.

Nutrition Info: calories 420, fat 30.3, fiber 7.2, carbs 35.3, protein 6.4

50. Mediterranean Eggs 2

Servings: 2   Cooking Time: 15 Minutes

Ingredients:
4 medium (1/4 cup) green onions, chopped
1 tablespoon fresh basil leaves, chopped (or 1 teaspoon dried basil leaves)
4 eggs
1 teaspoon olive oil
1 medium (3/4 cup) tomato, chopped
Freshly ground pepper

Directions:
In an 8-inch non-stick skillet, heat the olive oil over medium heat. Add onions; cook for about 2 minutes, occasionally stirring. Stir in the tomato and the basil; cook for 1 minute, occasionally stirring, until the tomato is heated through.   In a bowl, whisk the eggs; pour over the mixture in the skillet.   As the egg mix starts to set, lift with a spatula to allow the uncooked egg to flow underneath; cook for about 3-4 minutes, or until the eggs are thick but still moist. Sprinkle with pepper.

Nutrition Info: Per Serving:190 Cal, 13 g total fat (3.5 g sat. fat), 425 mg chol., 130 mg sodium, 5 g carb.,1 g fiber,3 g sugar, 13 g protein.

51. Avocado Chickpea Pizza

Servings: 2   Cooking Time: 20 Minutes

Ingredients:
1 and ¼ cups chickpea flour
A pinch of salt and black pepper
2 tablespoons olive oil
1 teaspoon onion powder
1 teaspoon garlic, minced
1 and ¼ cups water
1 tomato, sliced
1 avocado, peeled, pitted and sliced
2 ounces gouda, sliced
¼ cup tomato sauce
2 tablespoons green onions, chopped

Directions:
In a bowl, mix the chickpea flour with salt, pepper, water, the oil, onion powder and the garlic, stir well until you obtain a dough, knead a bit, put in a bowl, cover and leave aside for 20 minutes.   Transfer the dough to a working surface, shape a bit circle, transfer it to a baking sheet lined with parchment paper and bake at 425 degrees F for 10 minutes. Spread the tomato sauce over the pizza, also spread the rest of the ingredients and bake at 400 degrees F for 10 minutes more.   Cut and serve for breakfast.

Nutrition Info: calories 416, fat 24.5, fiber 9.6, carbs 36.6, protein 15.4

52. Feta And Quinoa Egg Muffins

Servings: 12   Cooking Time: 30 Minutes

Ingredients:
8 eggs
2 teaspoons olive oil
2 cups baby spinach, finely chopped
1/2 cup onion, finely chopped
1/2 cup kalamata olives, chopped, pitted
1/4 teaspoon salt
1 tablespoon fresh oregano, chopped
1 cup quinoa*, cooked
1 cup grape or cherry tomatoes, sliced or chopped
1 cup feta cheese, crumbled

Directions:
Preheat oven to 350F.   Grease a 12 muffin with oil or place 12 silicone muffin holders on a baking sheet.   Heat a skillet over medium heat. Add the olive oil. Add onions; sauté for about 2 minutes. Add the tomatoes, sauté for 1 minute more. Add the spinach; sauté for about 1 minute or until wilted. Turn the heat off. Stir in the olives and the oregano; set aside.   Put the eggs in a bowl and whisk. Add the feta, quinoa, vegetable mixture, and salt; stir until well mixed. Pour the mixture into the prepared muffin tins or silicone cups, dividing equally; bake for about 30 minutes or until the eggs are set and light golden brown.   Cool for 5 minutes then serve. You can eat these warm, chilled, or cold. To reheat left overs, just microwave.

Nutrition Info: Per Serving:120 Cal, 3 g total fat (150 g sat. fat), 150 mg chol., 290 mg sodium, 170 mg pot.,6 g carb.,1 g fiber,2 g sugar, 7 g protein.

53. Cauliflower Skillet

Servings: 5   Cooking Time: 25 Minutes

Ingredients:
1 cup cauliflower, chopped
1 tablespoon olive oil
½ red onion, diced
1 tablespoon Plain yogurt
½ teaspoon ground black pepper
1 teaspoon dried cilantro
1 teaspoon dried oregano
1 bell pepper, chopped
1/3 cup milk
½ teaspoon Za'atar
1 tablespoon lemon juice
1 russet potato, chopped

Directions:
Pour olive oil in the skillet and preheat it.   Add chopped russet potato and roast it for 5 minutes. After this, add cauliflower, ground black pepper, cilantro, oregano, and bell pepper. Roast the mixture for 10 minutes over the medium heat. Then add milk, Za'atar, and Plain Yogurt. Stir it well.   Saute the mixture 10 minutes.   Top the cooked meal with diced red onion and sprinkle with lemon juice.   It is recommended to serve the breakfast hot.

Nutrition Info: Per Serving:calories 112, fat 3.4, fiber 2.6, carbs 18.1, protein 3.1

54. Cheese Pies

Servings: 6   Cooking Time: 20 Minutes

Ingredients:
7 oz yufka dough/phyllo dough
1 cup Cheddar cheese, shredded
1 cup fresh cilantro, chopped
2 eggs, beaten
1 teaspoon paprika
¼ teaspoon chili flakes
½ teaspoon salt
2 tablespoons sour cream
1 teaspoon olive oil

Directions:

In the mixing bowl, combine together sour cream, salt, chili flakes, paprika, and beaten eggs. Brush the springform pan with olive oil. Place ¼ part of all yufka dough in the pan and sprinkle it with ¼ part of the egg mixture. Add a ¼ cup of cheese and ¼ cup of cilantro. Cover the mixture with 1/3 part of remaining yufka dough and repeat the all the steps again. You should get 4 layers. Cut the yufka mixture into 6 pies and bake at 360F for 20 minutes. The cooked pies should have a golden brown color.

Nutrition Info: Per Serving:calories 213, fat 11.4, fiber 0.8, carbs 18.2, protein 9.1

55. Spinach Pie

Servings: 6   Cooking Time: 1 Hour

Ingredients:

2 cups spinach	1 teaspoon ground
1 white onion, diced	paprika
½ cup fresh parsley	2 eggs, beaten
1 teaspoon minced garlic	1/3 cup butter, melted
3 oz Feta cheese, crumbled	2 oz Phyllo dough

Directions:

Separate Phyllo dough into 2 parts. Brush the casserole mold with butter well and place 1 part of Phyllo dough inside. Brush its surface with butter too. Put the spinach and fresh parsley in the blender. Blend it until smooth and transfer in the mixing bowl. Add minced garlic, Feta cheese, ground paprika, eggs, and diced onion. Mix up well. Place the spinach mixture in the casserole mold and flatten it well. Cover the spinach mixture with remaining Phyllo dough and pour remaining butter over it. Bake spanakopita for 1 hour at 350F. Cut it into the servings.

Nutrition Info: Per Serving:calories 190, fat 15.4, fiber 1.1, carbs 8.4, protein 5.4

56. Bacon, Spinach And Tomato Sandwich

Servings: 1   Cooking Time: 0 Minutes

Ingredients:

2 whole-wheat bread slices, toasted	Salt and black pepper to the taste
1 tablespoon Dijon mustard	2 tomato slices
3 bacon slices	¼ cup baby spinach

Directions:

Spread the mustard on each bread slice, divide the bacon and the rest of the ingredients on one slice, top with the other one, cut in half and serve for breakfast.

Nutrition Info:calories 246, fat 11.2, fiber 4.5, carbs 17.5, protein 8.3

57. Watermelon Pizza

Servings: 2   Cooking Time: 10 Minutes

Ingredients:

1 tablespoon Pomegranate sauce	9 oz watermelon slice
2 oz Feta cheese, crumbled	1 tablespoon fresh cilantro, chopped

Directions:

Place the watermelon slice in the plate and sprinkle with crumbled Feta cheese. Add fresh cilantro.

After this, sprinkle the pizza with Pomegranate juice generously. Cut the pizza into the servings.

Nutrition Info: Calories 143, fat 6.2, fiber 0.6, carbs 18.4, protein 5.1

58. Artichokes And Cheese Omelet

Servings: 1   Cooking Time: 8 Minutes

Ingredients:

1 teaspoon avocado oil	2 tablespoons kalamata olives, pitted and sliced
1 tablespoon almond milk	1 artichoke heart, chopped
2 eggs, whisked	1 tablespoon tomato sauce
A pinch of salt and black pepper	1 tablespoon feta cheese, crumbled
2 tablespoons tomato, cubed	

Directions:

In a bowl, combine the eggs with the milk, salt, pepper and the rest of the ingredients except the avocado oil and whisk well. Heat up a pan with the avocado oil over medium-high heat, add the omelet mix, spread into the pan, cook for 4 minutes, flip, cook for 4 minutes more, transfer to a plate and serve.

Nutrition Info:calories 303, fat 17.7, fiber 9.9, carbs 21.9, protein 18.2

59. Creamy Oatmeal With Figs

Servings: 5   Cooking Time: 20 Minutes

Ingredients:

2 cups oatmeal	3 figs, chopped
1 ½ cup milk	1 tablespoon honey
1 tablespoon butter	

Directions:

Pour milk in the saucepan. Add oatmeal and close the lid. Cook the oatmeal for 15 minutes over the medium-low heat. Then add chopped figs and honey. Add butter and mix up the oatmeal well. Cook it for 5 minutes more. Close the lid and let the cooked breakfast rest for 10 minutes before serving.

Nutrition Info: Calories 222, fat 6, fiber 4.4, carbs 36.5, protein 7.1

60. Cheesy Breakfast Pizza (cheese Manakish)

Servings: 1 Pizza   Cooking Time: 10 Minutes

Ingredients:

1 batch Multipurpose Dough (recipe in Chapter 12)	2 cups kashkaval cheese, grated
1/4 cup all-purpose flour	2 cups mozzarella cheese, grated

Directions:

Preheat the oven to 400°F. Flour a rolling pin and your counter. Divide Multipurpose Dough into 6 equal portions, and roll out dough into 6- to 8-inch-diameter circles. In a medium bowl, combine kashkaval cheese and mozzarella cheese. Divide cheese mixture into 6 portions, and sprinkle on each dough circle. Place pizzas onto a baking sheet, and bake for 8 to 10 minutes or until cheese begins to bubble. Remove pizzas from the oven, fold each pizza in half, and enjoy as is or with Yogurt Spread (Labne; recipe in Chapter 3).

61. Blueberries Quinoa

Servings: 4   Cooking Time: 0 Minutes

Ingredients:

2 cups almond milk
2 cups quinoa, already cooked
½ teaspoon cinnamon powder
1 tablespoon honey
1 cup blueberries
¼ cup walnuts, chopped

Directions:
In a bowl, mix the quinoa with the milk and the rest of the ingredients, toss, divide into smaller bowls and serve for breakfast.

Nutrition Info:calories 284, fat 14.3, fiber 3.2, carbs 15.4, protein 4.4

62. Creamy Chorizo Bowls

Servings: 4   Cooking Time: 15 Minutes

Ingredients:

9 oz chorizo
1 tablespoon almond butter
½ cup corn kernels
1 tomato, chopped
¾ cup heavy cream
1 teaspoon butter
¼ teaspoon chili pepper
1 tablespoon dill, chopped

Directions:
Chop the chorizo and place in the skillet.   Add almond butter and chili pepper.   Roast the chorizo for 3 minutes.   After this, add tomato and corn kernels.   Add butter and chopped the dill. Mix up the mixture well. Cook for 2 minutes. Close the lid and simmer the meal for 10 minutes over the low heat.   Transfer the cooked meal into the serving bowls.

Nutrition Info: Per Serving:calories 422, fat 36.2, fiber 1.2, carbs 7.3, protein 17.6

63. Mediterranean Omelet

Servings: 1 Omelet   Cooking Time: 10 Minutes

Ingredients:

2 TB. extra-virgin olive oil
2 TB. yellow onion, finely chopped
1 small clove garlic, minced
1/2 tsp. salt
1 cup fresh spinach, chopped
1/2 medium tomato, diced
2 large eggs
2 TB. whole or 2 percent milk
4 kalamata olives, pitted and chopped
1/2 tsp. ground black pepper
3 TB. crumbled feta cheese
1 TB. fresh parsley, finely chopped

Directions:
In a nonstick pan over medium heat, cook extra-virgin olive oil, yellow onion, and garlic for 3 minutes.   Add salt, spinach, and tomato, and cook for 4 minutes.   In a small bowl, whisk together eggs and whole milk.   Add kalamata olives and black pepper to the pan, and pour in eggs over sautéed vegetables.   Using a rubber spatula, slowly push down edges of eggs, letting raw egg form a new layer, and continue for about 2 minutes or until eggs are cooked.   Fold omelet in half, and slide onto a plate. Top with feta cheese and fresh parsley, and serve warm.

64. Hummus And Tomato Sandwich

Servings: 3   Cooking Time: 2 Minutes

Ingredients:

6 whole grain bread slices
1 tomato
3 Cheddar cheese
slices
½ teaspoon dried oregano
1 teaspoon green chili paste
½ red onion, sliced
1 teaspoon lemon juice
1 tablespoon hummus
3 lettuce leaves

Directions:
Slice tomato into 6 slices.   In the shallow bowl mix up together dried oregano, green chili paste, lemon juice, and hummus.   Spread 3 bread slices with the chili paste mixture.   After this, place the sliced tomatoes on them.   Add sliced onion, Cheddar cheese, and lettuce leaves.   Cover the lettuce leaves with the remaining bread slices to get the sandwiches.   Preheat the grill to 365F. Grill the sandwiches for 2 minutes.

Nutrition Info: Per Serving:calories 269, fat 12.1, fiber 5.1, carbs 29.6, protein 13.9

65. Sage Omelet

Servings: 8   Cooking Time: 25 Minutes

Ingredients:

8 eggs, beaten
6 oz Goat cheese, crumbled
½ teaspoon salt
3 tablespoons sour cream
1 teaspoon butter
½ teaspoon canola oil
¼ teaspoon sage
¼ teaspoon dried oregano
1 teaspoon chives, chopped

Directions:
Put butter in the skillet. Add canola oil and preheat the mixture until it is homogenous.   Meanwhile, in the mixing bowl combine together salt, sour cream, sage, dried oregano, and chives. Add eggs and stir the mixture carefully with the help of the spoon/fork.   Pour the egg mixture in the skillet with butter-oil liquid.   Sprinkle the omelet with goat cheese and close the lid.   Cook the breakfast for 20 minutes over the low heat. The cooked omelet should be solid.   Slice it into the servings and transfer in the plates.

Nutrition Info: Per Serving:calories 176, fat 13.7, fiber 0, carbs 0, protein 12.2

66. Red Pepper And Artichoke Frittata

Servings: 2   Cooking Time: 15 Minutes

Ingredients:

4 large eggs
1 can (14-ounce) artichoke hearts, rinsed, coarsely chopped
1 medium red bell pepper, diced
1 teaspoon dried oregano
1/4 cup Parmesan cheese, freshly grated
1/4 teaspoon red pepper, crushed
1/4 teaspoon salt, or to taste
2 garlic cloves, minced
2 teaspoons extra-virgin olive oil, divided
Freshly ground pepper, to taste

Directions:
In a 10-inch non-stick skillet, heat 1 teaspoon of the olive oil over medium heat. Add the bell pepper; cook for about 2 minutes or until tender. Add the garlic and the red pepper; cook for about 30 seconds, stirring. Transfer the mixture to a plate and wipe the skillet clean.   In a medium mixing bowl, whisk the eggs. Stir in the artichokes, cheese, the bell pepper mixture, and season with salt and pepper.   Place an oven rack 4 inches from the

source of heat; preheat broiler. Brush the skillet with the remaining 1 teaspoon olive oil and heat over medium heat. Pour the egg mixture into the skillet and tilt to evenly distribute. Reduce the heat to medium low; cook for about 3-4 minutes, lifting the edges to allow the uncooked egg to flow underneath, until the bottom of the frittata is light golden. Transfer the pan into the broiler, cook for about 1 1/2-2 1/2 minutes, or until the top is set. Slide into a platter; cut into wedges and serve.

Nutrition Info: Per Serving:305 Cal, 18 g total fat (6 g sat. fat, 8 g mono), 432 mg chol., 734 mg sodium, 1639 mg pot., 18 g carb.,8 g fiber, 21 g protein.

67. Stuffed Figs

Servings: 2   Cooking Time: 15 Minutes

Ingredients:

7 oz fresh figs	4 bacon slices
1 tablespoon cream cheese	¼ teaspoon paprika
½ teaspoon walnuts, chopped	¼ teaspoon salt
	½ teaspoon canola oil
	½ teaspoon honey

Directions:

Make the crosswise cuts in every fig. In the shallow bowl mix up together cream cheese, walnuts, paprika, and salt. Fill the figs with cream cheese mixture and wrap in the bacon. Secure the fruits with toothpicks and sprinkle with honey. Line the baking tray with baking paper. Place the prepared figs in the tray and sprinkle them with olive oil gently. Bake the figs for 15 minutes at 350F.

Nutrition Info: Calories 299, fat 19.4, fiber 2.3, carbs 16.7, protein 15.2

68. Keto Egg Fast Snickerdoodle Crepes

Servings: 2   Cooking Time: 15 Minutes

Ingredients:

5 oz cream cheese, softened	2 tablespoons granulated Swerve
6 eggs	8 tablespoons butter, softened
1 teaspoon cinnamon	1 tablespoon cinnamon
Butter, for frying	
1 tablespoon Swerve	

Directions:

For the crepes: Put all the ingredients together in a blender except the butter and process until smooth. Heat butter on medium heat in a non-stick pan and pour some batter in the pan. Cook for about 2 minutes, then flip and cook for 2 more minutes. Repeat with the remaining mixture. Mix Swerve, butter and cinnamon in a small bowl until combined. Spread this mixture onto the centre of the crepe and serve rolled up.

Nutrition Info: Calories: 543 Carbs: 8g Fats: 51.6g Proteins: 15.7g Sodium: 455mg Sugar: 0.9g

69. Cauliflower Hash Brown Breakfast Bowl

Servings: 2   Cooking Time: 30 Minutes

Ingredients:

1 tablespoon lemon juice	½ green onion, chopped

1 egg	¼ cup salsa
1 avocado	¾ cup cauliflower rice
1 teaspoon garlic powder	½ small handful baby spinach
2 tablespoons extra virgin olive oil	Salt and black pepper, to taste
2 oz mushrooms, sliced	

Directions:

Mash together avocado, lemon juice, garlic powder, salt and black pepper in a small bowl. Whisk eggs, salt and black pepper in a bowl and keep aside. Heat half of olive oil over medium heat in a skillet and add mushrooms. Sauté for about 3 minutes and season with garlic powder, salt, and pepper. Sauté for about 2 minutes and dish out in a bowl. Add rest of the olive oil and add cauliflower, garlic powder, salt and pepper. Sauté for about 5 minutes and dish out. Return the mushrooms to the skillet and add green onions and baby spinach. Sauté for about 30 seconds and add whisked eggs. Sauté for about 1 minute and scoop on the sautéed cauliflower hash browns. Top with salsa and mashed avocado and serve.

Nutrition Info: Calories: 400 Carbs: 15.8g Fats: 36.7g Proteins: 8g Sodium: 288mg Sugar: 4.2g

70. Pumpkin Coconut Oatmeal

Servings: 6   Cooking Time: 13 Minutes

Ingredients:

2 cups oatmeal	2 tablespoons pumpkin puree
1 cup of coconut milk	1 tablespoon Honey
1 cup milk	½ teaspoon butter
1 teaspoon Pumpkin pie spices	

Directions:

Pour coconut milk and milk in the saucepan. Add butter and bring the liquid to boil. Add oatmeal, stir well with the help of a spoon and close the lid. Simmer the oatmeal for 7 minutes over the medium heat. Meanwhile, mix up together honey, pumpkin pie spices, and pumpkin puree. When the oatmeal is cooked, add pumpkin puree mixture and stir well. Transfer the cooked breakfast in the serving plates.

Nutrition Info: Per Serving:calories 232, fat 12.5, fiber 3.8, carbs 26.2, protein 5.9

71. Bacon, Vegetable And Parmesan Combo

Servings: 2   Cooking Time: 25 Minutes

Ingredients:

2 slices of bacon, thick-cut	½ tbsp mayonnaise
½ of medium green bell pepper, deseeded, chopped	1 scallion, chopped
	¼ cup grated Parmesan cheese
	1 tbsp olive oil

Directions:

Switch on the oven, then set its temperature to 375°F and let it preheat. Meanwhile, take a baking dish, grease it with oil, and add slices of bacon in it. Spread mayonnaise on top of the bacon, then top with bell peppers and scallions, sprinkle with Parmesan cheese and bake for about 25 minutes until cooked thoroughly. When done, take out the baking dish and serve immediately. For meal prepping, wrap bacon in a plastic sheet

and refrigerate for up to 2 days. When ready to eat, reheat bacon in the microwave and then serve.
Nutrition Info: Calories 197, Total Fat 13.8g, Total Carbs 4.7g, Protein 14.3g, Sugar 1.9g, Sodium 662mg

72. Mediterranean Crostini

Servings: 4   Cooking Time: 15 Minutes
Ingredients:

12 slices (1/3-inch thick) whole-wheat baguette, toasted
Coarse salt and freshly ground pepper
1 can chickpeas (15 1/2 ounces), drained, rinsed
1/4 cup olive oil, extra-virgin
1 tablespoon lemon juice, freshly squeezed

For the spread:
1 small clove garlic, minced
2 tablespoons olive oil, extra-virgin, divided
2 tablespoons celery, finely diced, plus celery leaves for garnish
8 large green olives, pitted, cut into 1/8-inch slivers

Directions:
In a food processor, combine the spread ingredients and season with salt and pepper; set aside. In a small mixing bowl, combine 1 tablespoon of olive oil and the remaining ingredients. Season with salt and pepper. Set aside. Divide the spread between the toasted baguette slices, top with the relish. Drizzle the remaining1 tablespoon of olive oil over each and season with pepper. If desired, garnish with the celery leaves. Serve immediately.
Nutrition Info: Per Serving:603 Cal, 3.7 g total fat (3.7 g sat. fat), 0 mg chol., 781 mg sodium, 483 mg pot, 79.2 g carb.,9.6 g fiber,6.8 g sugar, 19.1 g protein.

73. Heavenly Egg Bake With Blackberry

Servings: 4   Cooking Time: 15 Minutes
Ingredients:

Chopped rosemary
1 tsp lime zest
½ tsp salt
¼ tsp vanilla extract, unsweetened
1 tsp grated ginger
3 tbsp coconut flour

1 tbsp unsalted butter
5 organic eggs
1 tbsp olive oil
½ cup fresh blackberries
Black pepper to taste

Directions:
Switch on the oven, then set its temperature to 350°F and let it preheat. Meanwhile, place all the ingredients in a blender, reserving the berries and pulse for 2 to 3 minutes until well blended and smooth. Take four silicon muffin cups, grease them with oil, evenly distribute the blended batter in the cups, top with black pepper and bake for 15 minutes until cooked through and the top has golden brown. When done, let blueberry egg bake cool in the muffin cups for 5 minutes, then take them out, cool them on a wire rack and then serve. For meal prepping, wrap each egg bake with aluminum foil and freeze for up to 3 days. When ready to eat, reheat blueberry egg bake in the microwave and then serve.
Nutrition Info: Calories 144, Total Fat 10g, Total Carbs 2g, Protein 8.5g

74. Quick Cream Of Wheat

Servings: 1 Cup   Cooking Time: 12 Minutes
Ingredients:

4 cups whole milk
1/2 cup farina
1/2 tsp. salt

3 TB. sugar
3 TB. butter
3 TB. pine nuts

Directions:
In a large saucepan over medium heat, bring whole milk to a simmer, and cook for about 4 minutes. Do not allow milk to scorch. Whisk in farina, salt, and sugar, and bring to a slight boil. Cook for 2 minutes, reduce heat to low, and cook for 3 more minutes. Stay close to the pan to ensure it doesn't boil over. Pour mixture into 4 bowls, and let cool for 5 minutes. Meanwhile, in a small pan over low heat, cook butter and pine nuts for about 3 minutes or until pine nuts are lightly toasted. Evenly spoon butter and pine nuts over each bowl, and serve warm.

75. Herbed Spinach Frittata

Servings: 4   Cooking Time: 20 Minutes
Ingredients:

5 eggs, beaten
1 cup fresh spinach
2 oz Parmesan, grated
1/3 cup cherry tomatoes

½ teaspoon dried oregano
1 teaspoon dried thyme
1 teaspoon olive oil

Directions:
Chop the spinach into the tiny pieces and or use a blender. Then combine together chopped spinach with eggs, dried oregano and thyme. Add Parmesan and stir frittata mixture with the help of the fork. Brush the springform pan with olive oil and pour the egg mixture inside. Cut the cherry tomatoes into the halves and place them over the egg mixture. Preheat the oven to 360F. Bake the frittata for 20 minutes or until it is solid. Chill the cooked breakfast till the room temperature and slice into the servings.
Nutrition Info: Per Serving:calories 140, fat 9.8, fiber 0.5, carbs 2.1, protein 11.9

76. Ham Spinach Ballet

Servings: 2   Cooking Time: 40 Minutes
Ingredients:

4 teaspoons cream
¾ pound fresh baby spinach
7-ounce ham, sliced

Salt and black pepper, to taste
1 tablespoon unsalted butter, melted

Directions:
Preheat the oven to 360 degrees F. and grease 2 ramekins with butter. Put butter and spinach in a skillet and cook for about 3 minutes. Add cooked spinach in the ramekins and top with ham slices, cream, salt and black pepper. Bake for about 25 minutes and dish out to serve hot. For meal prepping, you can refrigerate this ham spinach ballet for about 3 days wrapped in a foil.
Nutrition Info: Calories: 188 Fat: 12.5g Carbohydrates: 4.9g Protein: 14.6g Sugar: 0.3g Sodium: 1098mg

77. Banana Quinoa

Servings: 4   Cooking Time: 12 Minutes
Ingredients:

1 cup quinoa
1 teaspoon honey

2 cup milk
1 teaspoon vanilla extract

2 bananas, sliced
¼ teaspoon ground cinnamon

Directions:
Pour milk in the saucepan and add quinoa. Close the lid and cook it over the medium heat for 12 minutes or until quinoa will absorb all liquid. Then chill the quinoa for 10-15 minutes and place in the serving mason jars. Add honey, vanilla extract, and ground cinnamon. Stir well. Top quinoa with banana and stir it before serving.
Nutrition Info: Calories 279, fat 5.3, fiber 4.6, carbs 48.4, protein 10.7

78. Quinoa And Potato Bowl

Servings: 4   Cooking Time: 20 Minutes
Ingredients:

1 sweet potato, peeled, chopped
1 tablespoon olive oil
½ teaspoon chili flakes

½ teaspoon salt
1 cup quinoa
2 cups of water
1 teaspoon butter
1 tablespoon fresh cilantro, chopped

Directions:
Line the baking tray with parchment. Arrange the chopped sweet potato in the tray and sprinkle it with chili flakes, salt, and olive oil. Bake the sweet potato for 20 minutes at 355F. Meanwhile, pour water in the saucepan. Add quinoa and cook it over the medium heat for 7 minutes or until quinoa will absorb all liquid. Add butter in the cooked quinoa and stir well. Transfer it in the bowls, add baked sweet potato and chopped cilantro.
Nutrition Info: Per Serving:calories 221, fat 7.1, fiber 3.9, carbs 33.2, protein 6.6

79. Almond Cream Cheese Bake

Servings: 4   Cooking Time: 2 Hours
Ingredients:

1 cup cream cheese
4 tablespoons honey
½ teaspoon vanilla extract

1 oz almonds, chopped
3 eggs, beaten
1 tablespoon semolina

Directions:
Put beaten eggs in the mixing bowl. Add cream cheese, semolina, and vanilla extract. Blend the mixture with the help of the hand mixer until it is fluffy. After this, add chopped almonds and mix up the mass well. Transfer the cream cheese mash in the non-sticky baking mold. Flatten the surface of the cream cheese mash well. Preheat the oven to 325F. Cook the breakfast for 2 hours. The meal is cooked when the surface of the mash is light brown. Chill the cream cheese mash little and sprinkle with honey.
Nutrition Info: Per Serving:calories 352, fat 27.1, fiber 1, carbs 22.6, protein 10.4

80. Slow-cooked Peppers Frittata

Servings: 6   Cooking Time: 3 Hours
Ingredients:

½ cup almond milk
Salt and black pepper to the taste
1 teaspoon oregano, dried

8 eggs, whisked
½ cup red onion, chopped
4 cups baby arugula

1 and ½ cups roasted peppers, chopped

1 cup goat cheese, crumbled
Cooking spray

Directions:
In a bowl, combine the eggs with salt, pepper and the oregano and whisk. Grease your slow cooker with the cooking spray, arrange the peppers and the remaining ingredients inside and pour the eggs mixture over them. Put the lid on and cook on Low for 3 hours. Divide the frittata between plates and serve.
Nutrition Info:calories 259, fat 20.2, fiber 1, carbs 4.4, protein 16.3

81. Apricots With Yogurt, Honey, And Pistachios

Servings: 1   Cooking Time: 5 Minutes
Ingredients:

1 ripe apricot, halved, pitted
1 tablespoon roasted pistachios, unsalted, roughly chopped

4 tablespoons Greek yogurt, plain
Honey (try wildflower or lavender)

Directions:
Top each apricot with 2 tablespoons of Greek yogurt, drizzle with honey, and sprinkle with the chopped pistachios. Serve.
Nutrition Info: Per Serving:143 Cal, 6 g total fat (2 g sat. fat), 7 mg chol., 27 mg sodium, 19 g carb., 1 g fiber, 6 g protein.

82. Mediterranean Garbanzo Chili

Servings: 6   Cooking Time: 15 Minutes
Ingredients:

1 can (14 1/2 ounces) chicken broth, reduced-sodium
3 cans (15 ounces each) garbanzo beans or chickpeas, rinsed, drained
1 large (about 1 1/4 cups) sweet green pepper, cut into bite-size strips
1 pint grape tomatoes, halved
1/2 cup feta cheese, crumble, plus more for sprinkling

1/3 cup Kalamata olives, pitted, halved
1/4 teaspoon red pepper, crushed
2 large (about 2 cups) onions, sliced
2 tablespoons olive oil, extra-virgin
2 teaspoons dried basil, crushed
2 teaspoons lemon peel, finely shredded
5 garlic cloves, minced

Directions:
Over medium-high heat, heat the olive oil in a Dutch oven. Add the garlic, onions, basil, and red pepper; cook for about 4-5 minutes, frequently stirring, until softened. Add the sweet peppers; cook, stirring, for about 2 minutes. Add the garbanzo beans; cook for about 2 minutes, occasionally stirring. Add the broth and the olives; bring to a boil, reduce the heat to medium, and simmer uncovered for about 5 minutes, occasionally stirring. Add the grape tomatoes in; cook, stirring, for about 2 minutes, or just until heated through and wilted. Remove the Dutch oven from the heat. Add in the feta cheese and the lemon peel. Stir until the cheese is melted. Divide the chili between 6 bowls. If desired, trop with additional crumbled feta cheese.
Nutrition Info: Per Serving:385 Cal, 11 g total fat (3 g sat. fat, 2 g poly. Fat, 4 g mono), 11 mg chol.,

812 mg sodium, 59 g carb.,12 g fiber,15 g sugar, 15 g protein.

83. Veggie Salad

Servings: 4   Cooking Time: 0 Minutes
Ingredients:

2 tomatoes, cut into wedges	1 red onion, sliced
2 red bell peppers, chopped	¼ cup lime juice
1 cucumber, chopped	½ cup olive oil
½ cup kalamata olives, pitted and sliced	2 garlic cloves, minced
2 ounces feta cheese, crumbled	1 tablespoon oregano, chopped
	Salt and black pepper to the taste

Directions:
In a large salad bowl, combine the tomatoes with the peppers and the rest of the ingredients except the cheese and toss.   Divide the salad into smaller bowls, sprinkle the cheese on top and serve for breakfast.
Nutrition Info:calories 327, fat 11.2, fiber 4.4, carbs 16.7, protein 6.4

84. Fennel Bruschetta

Servings: 20   Cooking Time: 10 Minutes
Ingredients:

6 large-sized tomatoes, diced	1 loaf (20 ounces) French bread, sliced into 1/2-inch thick pieces
2 garlic cloves, minced	1 1/2 tablespoons fennel seed
1/4 cup olive oil, extra-virgin, for brushing	1/3 cup olive oil, extra-virgin
1/3 cup fresh basil, minced	Salt and black pepper, to taste
1/2 large Bermuda onion, diced	

Directions:
In a mixing bowl, combine the tomatoes, fennel seeds, garlic, onion, basil, the 1/3 cup of olive oil, and season of salt and then pepper. Refrigerate for a minimum of 1 hour to allow the flavors to blend. Preheat the oven to 350F or 175C.   Brush the sides of the slices of bread with a little of the1/4 cup olive oil. Place them into baking sheet, and toast for 3 minutes each side until golden brown.   To serve, scoop the chilled tomato toppings into each toasted bread slice, arrange them on a serving plate.
Nutrition Info: Per Serving:146 Cal, 6.6 g total fat (1 g sat. fat), 0 mg chol., 188 mg sodium, 18.8 g carb., 1.6 g fiber, 4 g protein.

85. Cheesy Eggs Ramekins

Servings: 2   Cooking Time: 10 Minutes
Ingredients:

1 tablespoon chives, chopped	2 tablespoons cheddar cheese, grated
1 tablespoon dill, chopped	1 tomato, chopped
A pinch of salt and black pepper	2 eggs, whisked
	Cooking spray

Directions:
In a bowl, mix the eggs with the tomato and the rest of the ingredients except the cooking spray and whisk well.   Grease 2 ramekins with the cooking spray, divide the mix into each ramekin, bake at 400 degrees F for 10 minutes and serve.

Nutrition Info:calories 104, fat 7.1, fiber 0.6, carbs 2.6, protein 7.9

86. Mediterranean Frittata

Servings: 6   Cooking Time: 15 Minutes
Ingredients:

8 eggs	1/4 cup fresh basil, slivered
3 tablespoons olive oil, divided	1/2 cup onion-and-garlic croutons, purchased, coarsely crushed
2 tablespoons Parmesan cheese, finely shredded	
1/8 teaspoon ground black pepper	1/2 cup kalamata or ripe olives, sliced, pitted
1/4 cup low-fat milk	
1/2 of a 7-ounce jar (about 1/2 cup) roasted red sweet peppers, drained, chopped	1/2 cup (2 ounces) feta cheese, crumbled
	1 teaspoon garlic, bottled minced
	1 cup onion, chopped

Directions:
Preheat broiler.   In a cast-iron skillet over medium heat, heat 2 tablespoons of the olive oil. Add the garlic and the onion; cook until the onions are just tender.   In a large bowl, combine the eggs and the milk; beat. Stir in the feta, sweet peppers, basil, olives, and black pepper. Pour the egg mixture into the skillet and cook. As the mixture sets, using a spatula, lift the egg mixture to allow the uncooked liquid to flow underneath. Continue cooking and lifting until the egg is almost set but the surface is still moist. Reduce the heat, if necessary, to prevent overcooking.   In a small-sized bowl, combine the parmesan, croutons, and the remaining 1 tablespoon of olive oil; sprinkle the mixture over the frittata.   Transfer the skillet under the broiler about 4-5 inches from the source of heat; broil for about 1-2 minutes, or until the top is set.
Nutrition Info: Per Serving:242 Cal, 19 g total fat (6 g sat. fat), 297 mg chol., 339 mg sodium, 7g carb.,1 g fiber,12 g protein.

87. Cinnamon Apple And Lentils Porridge

Servings: 4   Cooking Time: 10 Minutes
Ingredients:

½ cup walnuts, chopped	½ cup red lentils
2 green apples, cored, peeled and cubed	½ teaspoon cinnamon powder
3 tablespoons maple syrup	½ cup cranberries, dried
3 cups almond milk	1 teaspoon vanilla extract

Directions:
Put the milk in a pot, heat it up over medium heat, add the walnuts, apples, maple syrup and the rest of the ingredients, toss, simmer for 10 minutes, divide into bowls and serve.
Nutrition Info:calories 150, fat 2, fiber 1, carbs 3, protein 5

88. Creamy Oatmeal

Servings: 2   Cooking Time: 15 Minutes
Ingredients:

1 ½ cup oatmeal	1 teaspoon vanilla extract
1 tablespoon cocoa	

powder
1 tablespoon butter
½ cup heavy cream
2 tablespoons
¼ cup of water
Splenda

Directions:
Mix up together oatmeal with cocoa powder and Splenda. Transfer the mixture in the saucepan. Add vanilla extract, water, and heavy cream. Stir it gently with the help of the spatula. Close the lid and cook it for 10-15 minutes over the medium-low heat. Remove the cooked cocoa oatmeal from the heat and add butter. Stir it well.
Nutrition Info: Per Serving:calories 230, fat 10.6, fiber 3.5, carbs 28.1, protein 4.6

89. Stuffed Sweet Potato

Servings: 8   Cooking Time: 40 Minutes
Ingredients:
8 sweet potatoes, pierced with a fork
1 teaspoon garlic, minced
14 ounces canned chickpeas, drained and rinsed
1 tablespoon oregano, chopped
1 small red bell pepper, chopped
2 tablespoons parsley, chopped
1 tablespoon lemon zest, grated
A pinch of salt and black pepper
2 tablespoons lemon juice
1 avocado, peeled, pitted and mashed
3 tablespoons olive oil
¼ cup water
¼ cup tahini paste

Directions:
Arrange the potatoes on a baking sheet lined with parchment paper, bake them at 400 degrees F for 40 minutes, cool them down and cut a slit down the middle in each. In a bowl, combine the chickpeas with the bell pepper, lemon zest, half of the lemon juice, half of the oil, half of the garlic, oregano, half of the parsley, salt and pepper, toss and stuff the potatoes with this mix. In another bowl, mix the avocado with the water, tahini, the rest of the lemon juice, oil, garlic and parsley, whisk well and spread over the potatoes. Serve cold for breakfast.
Nutrition Info:calories 308, fat 2, fiber 8, carbs 38, protein 7

90. Couscous And Chickpeas Bowls

Servings: 4   Cooking Time: 6 Minutes
Ingredients:
¾ cup whole wheat couscous
1 cup water
1 yellow onion, chopped
15 ounces canned tomatoes, chopped
1 tablespoon olive oil
14 ounces canned artichokes, drained and chopped
2 garlic cloves, minced
½ cup Greek olives, pitted and chopped
15 ounces canned chickpeas, drained and rinsed
½ teaspoon oregano, dried
A pinch of salt and black pepper
1 tablespoon lemon juice

Directions:
Put the water in a pot, bring to a boil over medium heat, add the couscous, stir, take off the heat, cover the pan, leave aside for 10 minutes and fluff with a fork. Heat up a pan with the oil over medium-high heat, add the onion and sauté for 2 minutes. Add the rest of the ingredients, toss and cook for 4 minutes more. Add the couscous, toss, divide into bowls and serve for breakfast.
Nutrition Info:calories 340, fat 10, fiber 9, carbs 51, protein 11

91. Vegetarian Three Cheese Quiche Stuffed Peppers

Servings: 2   Cooking Time: 50 Minutes
Ingredients:
2 large eggs
¼ cup ricotta cheese
¼ cup mozzarella, shredded
½ teaspoon garlic powder
1 medium bell peppers, sliced in half and seeds removed
1/8 cup baby spinach leaves
¼ cup grated Parmesan cheese
¼ teaspoon dried parsley
1 tablespoon Parmesan cheese, to garnish

Directions:
Preheat oven to 375 degrees F. Blend all the cheeses, eggs, garlic powder and parsley in a food processor and process until smooth. Pour the cheese mixture into each sliced bell pepper and top with spinach leaves. Stir with a fork, pushing them under the cheese mixture and cover with foil. Bake for about 40 minutes and sprinkle with Parmesan cheese. Broil for about 5 minutes and dish out to serve.
Nutrition Info: Calories: 157 Carbs: 7.3g Fats: 9g Proteins: 12.7g Sodium: 166mg Sugar: 3.7g

92. Sweet Bread With Dates

Servings: 1 Roll   Cooking Time: 30 Minutes
Ingredients:
23/4 cups all-purpose flour
3 large eggs
1/4 cup dry milk
10 TB. butter
1/4 cup sugar
12 medjool dates, pitted
11/4 tsp. salt
1 TB. orange blossom water
1 TB. instant yeast
1/3 cup plus 1 TB. water
1/2 tsp. cinnamon
1 large egg white

Directions:
In a food processor fitted with a dough attachment or in a blender, knead all-purpose flour, dry milk, sugar, salt, instant yeast, eggs, 1/3 cup water, and 8 tablespoons butter for 15 minutes. Transfer dough to a bowl lightly sprayed with olive oil spray, cover the bowl with plastic wrap, and let rise in the refrigerator for 24 hours. In a food processor fitted with a chopping blade, blend medjool dates, orange blossom water, and cinnamon for 2 minutes or until smooth. Grease a 12-cup muffin tin with remaining 2 tablespoons butter. Form dough into 12 equal pieces. Spoon 1 tablespoon date mixture into center of each dough piece, tightly seal dough around date mixture, and place seal side down into the prepared muffin tin. Set aside dough to rise for 1 hour. Preheat the oven to 375°F. In a small bowl, whisk together egg white and remaining 1 tablespoon water. Brush each roll with egg wash. Bake for 30 minutes. Remove rolls from the oven, and let rest for 20 minutes before serving.

93. Shrimp Toast

Servings: 4   Cooking Time: 10 Minutes

Ingredients:

13 oz shrimps, peeled
1 tablespoon tomato sauce
½ teaspoon Splenda
¼ teaspoon garlic powder
1 teaspoon fresh parsley, chopped
½ teaspoon olive oil
1 teaspoon lemon juice
4 whole-grain bread slices
1 cup water, for cooking

Directions:

Pour water in the saucepan and bring it to boil. Add shrimps and boil them over the high heat for 5 minutes.   After this, drain shrimps and chill them to the room temperature.   Mix up together shrimps with Splenda, garlic powder, tomato sauce, and fresh parsley.   Add lemon juice and stir gently.   Preheat the oven to 360F.   Brush the bread slices with olive oil and bake for 3 minutes. Then place the shrimp mixture on the bread. Bruschetta is cooked.

Nutrition Info: Per Serving:calories 199, fat 3.7, fiber 2.1, carbs 15.3, protein 24.1

94. Breakfast Beans (ful Mudammas)

Servings: 1 Cup   Cooking Time: 10 Minutes

Ingredients:

1 (15-oz.) can chickpeas, rinsed and drained
1 (15-oz.) can fava beans, rinsed and drained
1 cup water
1 TB. minced garlic
1/2 cup fresh lemon juice
1 tsp. salt
1/2 tsp. cayenne
1/2 cup fresh parsley, chopped
1 large tomato, diced
3 medium radishes, sliced
1/4 cup extra-virgin olive oil

Directions:

In a 2-quart pot over medium-low heat, combine chickpeas, fava beans, and water. Simmer for 10 minutes.   Pour bean mixture into a large bowl, and add garlic, salt, and lemon juice. Stir and smash half of beans with the back of a wooden spoon.   Sprinkle cayenne over beans, and evenly distribute parsley, tomatoes, and radishes over top. Drizzle with extra-virgin olive oil, and serve warm or at room temperature.

95. Seeds And Lentils Oats

Servings: 4   Cooking Time: 50 Minutes

Ingredients:

½ cup red lentils
¼ cup pumpkin seeds, toasted
2 teaspoons olive oil
¼ cup coconut flesh, shredded
¼ cup rolled oats
1 tablespoon honey
1 tablespoon orange zest, grated
1 cup Greek yogurt
1 cup blackberries

Directions:

Spread the lentils on a baking sheet lined with parchment paper, introduce in the oven and roast at 370 degrees F for 30 minutes.   Add the rest of the ingredients except the yogurt and the berries, toss and bake at 370 degrees F for 20 minutes more. Transfer this to a bowl, add the rest of the ingredients, toss, divide into smaller bowls and serve for breakfast.

Nutrition Info:calories 204, fat 7.1, fiber 10.4, carbs 27.6, protein 9.5

96. Couscous With Artichokes, Sun-dried Tomatoes And Feta

Servings: 6   Cooking Time: 15 Minutes

Ingredients:

3 cups chicken breast, cooked, chopped
2 1/3 cups water, divided
2 jars (6-ounces each) marinated artichoke hearts, undrained
1/4 teaspoon black pepper, freshly ground
1/2 cup tomatoes, sun-dried
1/2 cup (2 ounces) feta cheese, crumbled
1 cup flat-leaf parsley, fresh, chopped
1 3/4 cups whole-wheat Israeli couscous, uncooked
1 can (14 1/2 ounces) vegetable broth

Directions:

In a microwavable bowl, combine 2 cups of the water and the tomatoes. Microwave on HIGH for about 3 minutes or until the water boils. When water is boiling, remove from the microwave, cover, and let stand for about 3 minutes or until the tomatoes are soft; drain, chop, and set aside.   In a large saucepan, place the vegetable broth and the remaining 1/3 cup of water; bring to boil. Stir in the couscous, cover, reduce heat, and simmer for about 8 minutes or until tender. Remove the pan from the heat; add the tomatoes and the remaining ingredients. Stir to combine.

Nutrition Info: Per Serving:419 Cal, 14.1 g total fat (3.9 g sat. fat, 0.8 g poly. Fat, 1.4 g mono), 64 mg chol.,677 mg sodium, 42.5 g carb.,2.6 g fiber, 30.2 g protein.

97. Cinnamon Roll Oats

Servings: 4   Cooking Time: 10 Minutes

Ingredients:

½ cup rolled oats
1 teaspoon vanilla extract
1 teaspoon ground cinnamon
1 cup milk
2 teaspoon honey
2 tablespoons Plain yogurt
1 teaspoon butter

Directions:

Pour milk in the saucepan and bring it to boil. Add rolled oats and stir well.   Close the lid and simmer the oats for 5 minutes over the medium heat. The cooked oats will absorb all milk.   Then add butter and stir the oats well.   In the separated bowl, whisk together Plain yogurt with honey, cinnamon, and vanilla extract.   Transfer the cooked oats in the serving bowls.   Top the oats with the yogurt mixture in the shape of the wheel.

Nutrition Info: Calories 243, fat 20.2, fiber 1, carbs 2.8, protein 13.3

98. Mediterranean Wrap

Servings: 4   Cooking Time: 10 Minutes

Ingredients:

4 pieces (10-inch) spinach wraps (or whole wheat tortilla or sun-dried tomato wraps)
1 pound chicken tenders
1 cup cucumber,
1/3 cup couscous, whole-wheat
2 teaspoons garlic, minced
1/4 teaspoon salt, divided
1/4 teaspoon freshly ground pepper

chopped
3 tablespoons extra-virgin olive oil
1 medium tomato, chopped

1/4 cup lemon juice
1/2 cup water
1/2 cup fresh mint, chopped
1 cup fresh parsley, chopped

Directions:
In a small saucepan, pour the water and bring to a boil. Stir in the couscous, remove pan from heat, cover, and allow to stand for 5 minutes, then fluff using a fork; set aside.   Meanwhile, in a small mixing bowl, combine the mint, parsley, oil, lemon juice, garlic, 1/8 teaspoon of the salt, and the pepper.   In a medium mixing bowl, toss the chicken with the 1 tablespoon of the mint mixture and the remaining 1/8 teaspoon of salt.   Place the chicken mixture into a large non-stick skillet; cook for about 3-5 minutes each side, or until heated through. Remove from the skillet, allow to cool enough to handle, and cut into bite-sized pieces. Stir the remaining mint mixture, the cucumber, and the tomato into the couscous.   Spread about 3/4 cup of the couscous mix onto each wrap and divide the chicken between the wraps, roll like a burrito, tucking the sides in to hold to secure the ingredients in. Cut in halves and serve.
Nutrition Info: Per Serving:479 Cal, 17 g total fat (3 g sat. fat, 11 g mono), 67 mg chol., 653 mg sodium, 382 pot., 49 g carb.,5 g fiber, 15 g protein.

99. Chicken Liver

Servings: ¾ Cup   Cooking Time: 7 Minutes
Ingredients:
2 lb. chicken liver

1 tsp. salt

3 TB. extra-virgin olive oil
3 TB. minced garlic
1/2 tsp. ground black pepper

1 cup fresh cilantro, finely chopped
1/4 cup fresh lemon juice

Directions:
Cut chicken livers in half, rinse well, and pat dry with paper towels.   Preheat a large skillet over medium heat. Add extra-virgin olive oil and garlic, and cook for 2 minutes.   Add chicken liver and salt, and cook, tossing gently, for 5 minutes. Remove the skillet from heat, and spoon liver onto a plate.   Add black pepper, cilantro, and lemon juice. Lightly toss, and serve warm.

100.	Avocado Spread

Servings: 8   Cooking Time: 0 Minutes
Ingredients:
2 avocados, peeled, pitted and roughly chopped
1 tablespoon sun-dried tomatoes, chopped
2 tablespoons lemon juice
3 tablespoons cherry tomatoes, chopped

¼ cup red onion, chopped
1 teaspoon oregano, dried
2 tablespoons parsley, chopped
4 kalamata olives, pitted and chopped
A pinch of salt and black pepper

Directions:
Put the avocados in a bowl and mash with a fork. Add the rest of the ingredients, stir to combine and serve as a morning spread.
Nutrition Info:calories 110, fat 10, fiber 3.8, carbs 5.7, protein 1.2

Lunch & Dinner Recipes

101. Chili Oregano Baked Cheese

Servings: 4   Cooking Time: 35 Minutes

Ingredients:

8 oz. feta cheese	1 teaspoon dried
4 oz. mozzarella, crumbled	oregano
1 chili pepper, sliced	2 tablespoons olive oil

Directions:

Place the feta cheese in a small deep dish baking pan.   Top with the mozzarella then season with pepper slices and oregano.   Cover the pan with aluminum foil and cook in the preheated oven at 350F for 20 minutes.   Serve the cheese right away.

Nutrition Info: Per Serving:Calories:292 Fat:24.2g Protein:16.2g Carbohydrates:3.7g

102. Mediterranean-style Vegetable Casserole

Servings: 4   Cooking Time: 1 Hour

Ingredients:

1 aubergine or eggplant, sliced lengthwise	100 ml vegetable stock
1 clove garlic, finely chopped	3 sprigs rosemary
1 spring onion, very finely chopped	4-5 tomatoes, sliced
2 courgettes or zucchini, sliced lengthwise	5 tablespoons olive oil, divided
	8 anchovy fillets, chopped
	8 black olives

Directions:

Heat the oven to 325F.   In a greased oven-safe dish, layer the vegetables, adding the anchovies between each vegetable layers. Sprinkle the olives over the veggie layer, drizzle with 4 tablespoons of the olive oil, and then season with salt and pepper. Pour the stock; bake for 1 hour.   About 15 minutes before the end of baking, sprinkle the rosemary. When cooked, mix the green onion, garlic, and the remaining 1 tablespoon olive oil together; drizzle al over the baked veggies. Serve hot.

Nutrition Info: Per Serving:250 cal., 18 g total fat (2.5 g sat fat), <5 mg chol., 190 mg sodium, 980 mg potassium, 19 g carb., 7 g fiber, 11 g sugar, and 6 g protein.

103. Creamy Smoked Salmon Pasta

Servings: 4   Cooking Time: 30 Minutes

Ingredients:

2 tablespoons olive oil	1 cup green peas
2 garlic cloves, chopped	1 cup heavy cream
1 shallot, chopped	Salt and pepper to taste
4 oz. smoked salmon, chopped	1 pinch chili flakes
	8 oz. penne

Directions:

Heat the oil in a skillet and add the garlic and shallot. Cook for 5 minutes until softened.   Add the salmon and peas, as well as salt and chili flakes. Cook for 5 more minutes then add the cream. Lower the heat and cook for 5 more minutes.   In the meantime, cook the penne in a large pot of water just until al dente.   Drain well then mix the pasta with the salmon sauce.   Serve the pasta fresh.

Nutrition Info: Per Serving:Calories:393 Fat:20.8g Protein:14.3g Carbohydrates:38.0g

104. Spiced Eggplant Stew

Servings: 4   Cooking Time: 45 Minutes

Ingredients:

Salt and black pepper to the taste	4 eggplants, cubed
2 yellow onions, chopped	½ teaspoon cinnamon powder
2 red bell peppers, chopped	1 teaspoon oregano, dried
30 ounces canned tomatoes, chopped	A drizzle of olive oil
1 cup black olives, pitted and chopped	A pinch of red chili flakes
¼ teaspoon allspice, ground	3 tablespoons Greek yogurt

Directions:

Heat up a pot with the oil over medium high heat, add the onions, bell pepper, oregano, cinnamon and the allspice and sauté fro 5 minutes.   Add the rest of the ingredients except the flakes and the yogurt, bring to a simmer and cook the stew over medium heat for 40 minutes.   Divide the stew into bowls, top each serving with the flakes and the yogurt and serve.

Nutrition Info: calories 256, fat 3.5, fiber 25.4, carbs 53.3, protein 8.8

105. Shrimp Soup

Servings: 6   Cooking Time: 5 Minutes

Ingredients:

1 cucumber, chopped	3 cups tomato juice
3 roasted red peppers, chopped	Salt and black pepper to the taste
3 tablespoons olive oil	½ teaspoon cumin, ground
2 tablespoons balsamic vinegar	1 pounds shrimp, peeled and deveined
1 garlic clove, minced	1 teaspoon thyme, chopped

Directions:

In your blender, mix cucumber with tomato juice, red peppers, 2 tablespoons oil, the vinegar, cumin, salt, pepper and the garlic, pulse well, transfer to a bowl and keep in the fridge for 10 minutes.   Heat up a pot with the rest of the oil over medium heat, add the shrimp, salt, pepper and the thyme and cook for 2 minutes on each side.   Divide cold soup into bowls, top with the shrimp and serve.

Nutrition Info: calories 263, fat 11.1, fiber 2.4, carbs 12.5, protein 6.32

106. Halloumi, Grape Tomato And Zucchini Skewers With Spinach-basil Oil

Servings: 16   Cooking Time: 10 Minutes

Ingredients:

1 large zucchini halved lengthways,	2 cups baby spinach leaves

cut into 8 pieces
16 grape tomatoes
180 g halloumi cheese, cut into 16 pieces
Olive oil spray
For the spinach-basil oil:

2 cups fresh basil leaves
185 ml (3/4 cup) extra-virgin olive oil
125 ml (1/2 cup) light olive oil

Directions:
In a saucepan of boiling water, cook the spinach and the basil for about 30 seconds or until just wilted. Drain and cool under running cold water. Place the cooked spinach and basil into a food processor. Add the light olive oil and the extra-virgin olive oil; process until the mixture is smooth. Transfer into an airtight container, refrigerate for 8 hours to develop the flavors. Preheat the barbecue grill to medium-high. Thread a piece of zucchini, halloumi cheese, and tomato into each skewer. Lightly spray with the olive oil spray. Grill for about4 minutes per side or until cooked through and golden brown. Arrange the grilled skewers on to serving platter; serve immediately with the prepared spinach-basil oil.
Nutrition Info: Per Serving:192.2Cal, 20 g total fat (4 g sat. fat), 1 g carb., 1 g fiber, 1 g sugar, 3 g protein, and 328.8 mg sodium.

107. Beef Bourguignon

Servings: 8   Cooking Time: 2 Hours
Ingredients:

3 tablespoons olive oil
2 pounds beef roast, cubed
1 tablespoon all-purpose flour
3 sweet onions, chopped
2 carrots, sliced
4 garlic cloves, minced

1 chili pepper, sliced
1 pound button mushrooms
1 ½ cups beef stock
½ cup dark beer
2 bay leaves
1 thyme sprig
1 rosemary sprig
Salt and pepper to taste

Directions:
Sprinkle the beef with flour. Heat the oil in a deep heavy pot and add the beef roast. Cook on all sides for 5 minutes or until browned. Add the onions, carrots and chili and cook for 5 more minutes. Add the mushrooms, stock, beer, bay leaves, thyme, rosemary, salt and pepper. Cover the pot and cook on low heat for 1 ½ hours. Serve the stew warm and fresh.
Nutrition Info: Per Serving:Calories:306 Fat:12.6g Protein:37.6g Carbohydrates:9.0g

108. Mediterranean Flank Steak

Servings: 4   Cooking Time: 40 Minutes
Ingredients:

4 flank steaks
1 lemon, juiced
1 orange, juiced
4 garlic cloves, chopped
1 teaspoon Dijon mustard

1 teaspoon chopped thyme
1 teaspoon dried sage
2 tablespoons olive oil
Salt and pepper to taste

Directions:
Combine the flank steaks and the rest of the ingredients in a zip lock bag. Refrigerate for 30 minutes. Heat a grill pan over medium flame and place the steaks on the grill. Cook on each side for 6-7 minutes. Serve the steaks warm and fresh.
Nutrition Info: Per Serving:Calories:234 Fat:13.4g Protein:21.6g Carbohydrates:6.7g

109. Spiced Grilled Flank Steak

Servings: 4   Cooking Time: 40 Minutes
Ingredients:

1 teaspoon chili powder
1 teaspoon ground coriander
1 teaspoon ground cumin

4 flank steaks
1 teaspoon mustard powder
Salt and pepper to taste

Directions:
Season the steaks with salt and pepper then sprinkle with chili, coriander, cumin and mustard powder. Allow to rest for 20 minutes then heat a grill pan over medium flame and place the steaks on the grill. Cook on each side for 5-7 minutes and serve the steaks warm and fresh.
Nutrition Info: Per Serving:Calories:202 Fat:8.8g Protein:28.2g Carbohydrates:0.9g

110.Pan Roasted Chicken With Olives And Lemon

Servings: 4   Cooking Time: 50 Minutes
Ingredients:

4 chicken legs
Salt and pepper to taste
3 tablespoons olive oil
1 lemon, juiced
1 orange, juiced
1 jalapeno, sliced

2 garlic cloves, chopped
½ cup green olives, sliced
¼ cup black olives, pitted and sliced
1 thyme sprig
1 rosemary sprig

Directions:
Season the chicken with salt and pepper. Heat the oil in a skillet and add the chicken. Cook on each side for 5 minutes until golden brown then add the rest of the ingredients and continue cooking on medium heat for15 minutes. Serve the chicken and the sauce warm.
Nutrition Info: Per Serving:Calories:319 Fat:18.9g Protein:29.7g Carbohydrates:8.0g

111. Creamy Salmon Soup

Servings: 6   Cooking Time: 15 Minutes
Ingredients:

2 tablespoon olive oil
1 red onion, chopped
Salt and white pepper to the taste
3 gold potatoes, peeled and cubed
2 carrots, chopped

4 cups fish stock
4 ounces salmon fillets, boneless and cubed
½ cup heavy cream
1 tablespoon dill, chopped

Directions:
Heat up a pan with the oil over medium heat, add the onion, and sauté for 5 minutes. Add the rest of the ingredients expect the cream, salmon and the dill, bring to a simmer and cook for 5-6 minutes more. Add the salmon, cream and the dill, simmer for 5 minutes more, divide into bowls and serve.
Nutrition Info:calories 214, fat 16.3, fiber 1.5, carbs 6.4, protein 11.8

112. Grilled Salmon With Cucumber Dill Sauce

Servings: 4   Cooking Time: 40 Minutes
Ingredients:

4 salmon fillets
1 teaspoon smoked paprika
1 teaspoon dried sage
Salt and pepper to taste
4 cucumbers, sliced
2 tablespoons chopped dill
½ cup Greek yogurt
1 tablespoon lemon juice
1 tablespoon olive oil

Directions:
Season the salmon with salt, pepper, paprika and sage.   Heat a grill pan over medium flame and place the salmon on the grill.   Cook on each side for 4 minutes.   For the sauce, mix the cucumbers, dill, yogurt, lemon juice and oil in a bowl. Add salt and pepper and mix well.   Serve the salmon with the cucumber sauce.
Nutrition Info: Per Serving:Calories:224 Fat:10.3g Protein:26.3g Carbohydrates:8.9g

113. Grilled Basil-lemon Tofu Burgers

Servings: 6   Cooking Time: 6 Minutes
Ingredients:

6 slices (1/4-inch thick each) tomato
6 pieces (1 1/2-ounce) whole-wheat hamburger buns
1 pound tofu, firm or extra-firm, drained
1 cup watercress, trimmed
Cooking spray
1/3 cup fresh basil, finely chopped
2 tablespoons Dijon mustard
1/4 cup freshly squeezed lemon juice
2 teaspoons grated lemon rind
2 tablespoons honey
1 tablespoon olive oil, extra-virgin,
1/2 teaspoon salt
1/4 teaspoon black pepper (freshly ground)
3 garlic cloves, minced
1 garlic cloves, minced
1/3 cup Kalamata olives, finely, chopped pitted
3 tablespoons sour cream, reduced-fat
3 tablespoons light mayonnaise

Directions:
Combine the marinade ingredients in a small-sized bowl. In a crosswise direction, cut the tofu into 6 slices. Pat each piece dry using paper towels. Place them in a jelly roll pan and brush both sides of the slices with the marinade mixture; reserve any leftover marinade. Marinate for 1 hour.   Preheat the grill and coated the grill rack with cooking spray. Place the tofu slices; grill for about 3 minutes per side, brushing the tofu with the reserved marinade mixture.   In a small-sized bowl, combine the garlic-olive mayonnaise ingredients. Spread about 1 1/2 tablespoons of the mixture over the bottom half of the hamburger buns. Top each with 1 slice tofu, 1 slice tomato, about 2 tablespoons of watercress, and top with the top buns.
Nutrition Info: Per Serving:276 Cal, 11.3 g total fat (1.9 g sat. fat, 5.7 g mono fat, 2.2 g poly fat), 10.5 g protein, 34.5 g carb., 1.5 g fiber, 5 mg chol., 2.4 mg iron, 743 mg sodium, and 101 mg calcium.

114. Creamy Green Pea Pasta

Servings: 4   Cooking Time: 25 Minutes
Ingredients:

8 oz. whole wheat spaghetti
1 cup green peas
1 avocado, peeled and cubed
2 tablespoons olive oil
2 garlic cloves, chopped
2 mint leaves
1 tablespoon lemon juice
¼ cup heavy cream
2 tablespoons vegetable stock
Salt and pepper to taste

Directions:
Pour a few cups of water in a deep pot and bring to a boil with a pinch of salt.   Add the spaghetti and cook for 8 minutes then drain well.   For the sauce, combine the remaining ingredients in a blender and pulse until smooth.   Mix the cooked the spaghetti with the sauce and serve the pasta fresh.
Nutrition Info: Per Serving:Calories:294 Fat:20.1g Protein:6.4g Carbohydrates:25.9g

115. Meat Cakes

Servings: 4   Cooking Time: 10 Minutes
Ingredients:

1 cup broccoli, shredded
½ cup ground pork
2 eggs, beaten
1 tablespoon Italian seasonings
1 teaspoon salt
1 teaspoon olive oil
3 tablespoons wheat flour, whole grain
1 tablespoon dried dill

Directions:
In the mixing bowl combine together shredded broccoli and ground pork,   Add salt, Italian seasoning, flour, and dried dill.   Mix up the mixture until homogenous.   Then add eggs and stir until smooth.   Heat up olive oil in the skillet. With the help of the spoon make latkes and place them in the hot oil.   Roast the latkes for 4 minutes from each side over the medium heat. The cooked latkes should have a light brown crust. Dry the latkes with the paper towels if needed.
Nutrition Info: Per Serving:calories 143, fat 6, fiber 0.9, carbs 7, protein 15.1

116. Herbed Roasted Cod

Servings: 4   Cooking Time: 45 Minutes
Ingredients:

4 cod fillets
4 parsley sprigs
2 cilantro sprigs
2 basil sprigs
1 lemon, sliced
Salt and pepper to taste
2 tablespoons olive oil

Directions:
Season the cod with salt and pepper.   Place the parsley, cilantro, basil and lemon slices at the bottom of a deep dish baking pan.   Place the cod over the herbs and cook in the preheated oven at 350F for 15 minutes.   Serve the cod warm and fresh with your favorite side dish.
Nutrition Info: Per Serving:Calories:192 Fat:8.1g Protein:28.6g Carbohydrates:0.1g

117. Mushroom Soup

Servings: 2   Cooking Time: 20 Minutes
Ingredients:

1 cup cremini mushrooms, chopped
1 cup Cheddar cheese, shredded
2 cups of water
½ teaspoon salt
1 teaspoon dried
½ teaspoon dried oregano
1 tablespoon fresh parsley, chopped
1 tablespoon olive oil
1 bell pepper,

thyme   chopped

Directions:
Pour olive oil in the pan.   Add mushrooms and bell pepper. Roast the vegetables for 5 minutes over the medium heat.   Then sprinkle them with salt, thyme, and dried oregano.   Add parsley and water. Stir the soup well.   Cook the soup for 10 minutes.   After this, blend the soup until it is smooth and simmer it for 5 minutes more.   Add cheese and stir until cheese is melted.   Ladle the cooked soup into the bowls. It is recommended to serve soup hot.

Nutrition Info: Per Serving:calories 320, fat 26, fiber 1.4, carbs 7.4, protein 15.7

118. Salmon Parmesan Gratin

Servings: 4   Cooking Time: 45 Minutes

Ingredients:

4 salmon fillets, cubed	1 fennel bulb, sliced
2 garlic cloves, chopped	½ cup vegetable stock
½ teaspoon ground coriander	1 cup heavy cream
½ teaspoon Dijon mustard	2 eggs
	Salt and pepper to taste
	1 cup grated Parmesan cheese

Directions:
Combine the salmon, garlic, fennel, coriander and mustard in a small deep dish baking pan.   Mix the eggs with cream and stock and pour the mixture over the fish.   Top with Parmesan cheese and bake in the preheated oven at 350F for 25 minutes.   Serve the gratin right away.

Nutrition Info: Per Serving:Calories:414 Fat:25.9g Protein:41.0g Carbohydrates:6.1g

119. Chicken Souvlaki 2

Servings: 4-6   Cooking Time: 12-15 Minutes

Ingredients:

4-6 chicken breasts, boneless, skinless	For the marinade:
1 tablespoon dried oregano (use Greek or Turkish oregano)	1 tablespoon red wine vinegar
	1 teaspoon dried thyme
1 tablespoon garlic, finely minced (or garlic puree from a jar)	1/2 cup lemon juice, freshly squeezed
	1/2 cup olive oil

Directions:
If there are any visible fat on the chicken, trim them off. Cut each breasts into 5-6 pieces 1-inch thick crosswise strips. Put them in a Ziploc bag or a container with tight lid.   Whisk the marinade ingredients together until combined. Pour into the bag or container with the chicken, seal, and shake the bag or the container to coat the chicken. Marinade for 6 to 8 hours or more in the refrigerator.   When marinated, remove the chicken from the fridge, let thaw to room temperature, and drain; discard the marinade. Thread the chicken strips into skewers, about 6 pieces on each skewer, the meat folded over to it would not spin around on the skewers.   Mist the grill with olive oil. Preheat the charcoal or gas grill to medium high.   Grill the skewers for about 12-15 minutes, turning once as soon as you see grill marks. Souvlaki is done when the chicken is slightly browned and firm, but not hard to the touch.

Nutrition Info: Per Serving:Per Serving:360 cal., 26 g total fat (4.5 g sat fat), 90 mg chol., 170 mg sodium, 570 mg potassium, 3 g carb., 0 g fiber, <1 g sugar, and 30 g protein.

120.   Rosemary Roasted New Potatoes

Servings: 6   Cooking Time: 1 Hour

Ingredients:

2 pounds new potatoes, washed	4 garlic cloves, crushed
3 tablespoons olive oil	Salt and pepper to taste
2 rosemary sprigs	

Directions:
Place the new potatoes in a large pot and cover them with water. Cook for 15 minutes then drain well.   Heat the oil in a skillet and add the rosemary and garlic.   Stir in the potatoes and continue cooking on medium flame for 20 minutes or until evenly golden brown.   Serve the potatoes warm.

Nutrition Info: Per Serving:Calories:168 Fat:7.2g Protein:2.7g Carbohydrates:24.6g

121. Artichoke Feta Penne

Servings: 4   Cooking Time: 40 Minutes

Ingredients:

8 oz. penne pasta	1 shallot, chopped
2 tablespoons olive oil	1 cup diced tomatoes
4 garlic cloves, chopped	¼ cup white wine
1 jar artichoke hearts, drained and chopped	½ cup vegetable stock
	Salt and pepper to taste
	4 oz. feta cheese, crumbled

Directions:
Heat the oil in a skillet and stir in the shallot and garlic. Cook for 2 minutes until softened.   Add the artichoke hearts, tomatoes, wine and stock, as well as salt and pepper to taste.   Cook on low heat for 15 minutes.   In the meantime, cook the penne in a large pot of water until al dente, not more than 8 minutes.   Drain the pasta well and mix it with the artichoke sauce.   Serve the penne with crumbled feta cheese.

Nutrition Info: Per Serving:Calories:325 Fat:14.4g Protein:11.1g Carbohydrates:35.8g

122.   Grilled Chicken And Rustic Mustard Cream

Servings: 4   Cooking Time: 12 Minutes

Ingredients:

1 tablespoon plus 1 teaspoon whole-grain Dijon mustard, divided	1/4 teaspoon of salt
	3 tablespoons light mayonnaise
1 tablespoon water	4 pieces (6-ounces each) chicken breast halves, skinless, boneless
1 teaspoon fresh rosemary, chopped	
1/4 teaspoon black pepper	Rosemary sprigs (optional)
1 tablespoon olive oil	Cooking spray

Directions:
Preheat the grill.   In a small-sized bowl, combine the olive oil, 1-teaspoon of mustard; brush evenly

over each chicken breast. Coat the grill rack with the cooking spray, place and chicken, and grill for 6 minutes per side or until cooked. While the chicken is grilling, combine the mayonnaise, the 1 tablespoon of mustard, and the water in a bowl. Serve the grilled chicken with the mustard cream. If desired garnish with some rosemary sprigs.

Nutrition Info: Per Serving:262 Cal, 10 g total fat (1 g sat. fat, 4 g mono fat, 3 g poly fat), 39.6 g protein, 1.7 g carb., 0.2 g fiber, 102 mg chol., 1.4 mg iron, 448 mg sodium, and 25 mg calcium.

123. Balsamic Steak With Feta, Tomato, And Basil

Servings: 4   Cooking Time: 23 Minutes
Ingredients:

1 tablespoon balsamic vinegar	4 sirloin steaks, trimmed
1/4 cup basil leaves	4 whole garlic cloves, skin on
175 g Greek fetta, crumbled	6 roma tomatoes, halved
2 tablespoons olive oil	Olive oil spray
2 teaspoons baby capers	Salt and cracked black pepper

Directions:
Preheat the oven to 200C. Line a baking tray with baking paper. Place the tomatoes and then scatter with the capers, crumbled feta, and the garlic cloves. Drizzle with 1 tablespoon of the olive oil and season with salt and pepper; cook for about 15 minutes or until the tomatoes are soft. Remove from the oven, set aside. In a large non-metallic bowl, toss the steak with the remaining 1 tablespoon of olive oil, vinegar, salt and pepper; cover and refrigerate for 5 minutes. Preheat the grill pan to high heat; grill the steaks for about 4 minutes per side or until cooked to your preference. Serve with the prepared tomato mixture and sprinkle with basil.

Nutrition Info: Per Serving:520.3 Cal, 30 g total fat (12 g sat. fat), 3 g carb., 2 g fiber, 2 g sugar, 59 g protein, and 622.82 mg sodium.

124. Fried Chicken With Tzatziki Sauce

Servings: 4   Cooking Time: 45 Minutes
Ingredients:

4 chicken breasts, cubed	Salt and pepper to taste
4 tablespoons olive oil	1 cucumber, grated
1 teaspoon dried basil	4 garlic cloves, minced
1 teaspoon dried oregano	1 teaspoon lemon juice
1/2 teaspoon chili flakes	1 teaspoon chopped mint
1 cup Greek yogurt	2 tablespoons chopped parsley

Directions:
Season the chicken with salt, pepper, basil, oregano and chili. Heat the oil in a skillet and add the chicken. Cook on each side for 5 minutes on high heat just until golden brown. Cover the chicken with a lid and continue cooking for 15-20 more minutes. For the sauce, mix the yogurt, cucumber, garlic, lemon juice, mint and parsley, as well as salt and pepper. Serve the chicken and the sauce fresh.

Nutrition Info: Per Serving:Calories:366 Fat:22.6g Protein:34.8g Carbohydrates:6.2g

125. Spiced Lamb Patties

Servings: 8   Cooking Time: 1 Hour
Ingredients:

4 garlic cloves, minced	2 pounds ground lamb
1 shallot, finely chopped	1 teaspoon dried mint
1 teaspoon ground coriander	2 tablespoons pine nuts, crushed
1 teaspoon ground cumin	Salt and pepper to taste
1/2 teaspoon chili powder	2 tablespoons chopped parsley
	1 tablespoon chopped cilantro

Directions:
Mix the lamb meat and the remaining ingredients in a bowl. Add salt and pepper and mix well. Form small patties and place them on a chopping board. Heat a grill pan over medium flame and cook on each side for 4-5 minutes or until browned and the juices run out clean. Serve the patties warm.

Nutrition Info: Per Serving:Calories:231 Fat:9.9g Protein:32.4g Carbohydrates:1.3g

126. Chicken And Orzo Soup

Servings: 4   Cooking Time: 11 Minutes
Ingredients:

1/2 cup carrot, chopped	2 cups kale, chopped
1 yellow onion, chopped	1 cup orzo
12 cups chicken stock	1/4 cup lemon juice
3 cups chicken meat, cooked and shredded	1 tablespoon olive oil

Directions:
Heat up a pot with the oil over medium heat, add the onion and sauté for 3 minutes. Add the carrots and the rest of the ingredients, stir, bring to a simmer and cook for 8 minutes more. Ladle into bowls and serve hot.

Nutrition Info:calories 300, fat 12.2, fiber 5.4, carbs 16.5, protein 12.2

127. Sweet And Sour Chicken Fillets

Servings: 4   Cooking Time: 40 Minutes
Ingredients:

4 chicken fillets	1 tablespoon honey
3 tablespoons olive oil	Salt and pepper to taste
1 red pepper, sliced	Chopped parsley for serving
1 lemon, juiced	

Directions:
Season the chicken with salt and pepper. Heat the oil in a skillet and add the chicken. Cook on each side for 10 minutes. Add the red pepper, lemon juice and honey and cook just for 1 additional minute. Serve the chicken and the sauce warm and fresh.

Nutrition Info: Per Serving:Calories:309 Fat:18.0g Protein:29.4g Carbohydrates:7.5g

128. Salt Crusted Salmon

Servings: 6   Cooking Time: 40 Minutes
Ingredients:

1 whole salmon (3 pounds)
3 cups salt

½ cup chopped parsley
3 tablespoons olive oil

Directions:
Spread a very thin layer of salt in a baking tray. Place the salmon over the salt and top with parsley. Drizzle with oil then top with the rest of the salt. Cook in the preheated oven at 350F for 30 minutes. Serve the salmon warm.
Nutrition Info: Per Serving:Calories:362 Fat:21.0g Protein:44.1g Carbohydrates:0.3g

129.   Sun-dried Tomato Pesto Penne

Servings: 4   Cooking Time: 20 Minutes
Ingredients:

8 oz. penne
½ cup sun-dried tomatoes, drained well
2 tablespoons olive oil
4 garlic cloves, minced

2 tablespoons lemon juice
2 tablespoons pine nuts
2 tablespoons grated Parmesan cheese
1 pinch chili flakes

Directions:
Cook the penne in a large pot of salty water for 8 minutes or as long as it says on the package, just until al dente.   Drain the penne well.   For the pesto, combine the remaining ingredients in a blender and pulse until well mixed and smooth. Mix the pesto with the penne and serve right away.
Nutrition Info: Per Serving:Calories:308 Fat:14.4g Protein:11.9g Carbohydrates:34.1g

130.   Herbed Marinated Sardines

Servings: 4   Cooking Time: 50 Minutes
Ingredients:

8 sardines
2 tablespoons chopped cilantro
2 tablespoons pesto sauce
2 tablespoons olive oil

½ cup chopped parsley
2 garlic cloves
Salt and pepper to taste
2 tablespoons lemon juice

Directions:
Combine the herbs, pesto, oil, garlic, salt and pepper in a blender and pulse until smooth. Spread the herb mixture over the sardines and season with salt and pepper.   Place the sardines in the fridge for 30 minutes.   Heat a grill pan over medium flame and place the sardines on the grill.   Cook on each side for 5-7 minutes.   Serve the sardines warm and fresh with your favorite side dish.
Nutrition Info: Per Serving:Calories:201 Fat:15.9g Protein:13.0g Carbohydrates:1.7g

131. Spicy Tomato Poached Eggs

Servings: 4   Cooking Time: 30 Minutes
Ingredients:

2 tablespoons olive oil
2 garlic cloves, chopped
2 red bell peppers, cored and sliced
2 yellow bell peppers,

2 shallots, chopped
2 tomatoes, peeled and diced
1 cup vegetable stock
1 jalapeno, chopped
Salt and pepper to taste

cored and sliced   4 eggs
Directions:
Heat the oil in a saucepan and stir in the shallots, garlic, bell peppers and jalapeno. Cook for 5 minutes.   Add the tomatoes, stock, thyme and bay leaf, as well as salt and pepper to taste.   Cook for 10 minutes on low heat.   Crack open the eggs and drop them in the hot sauce.   Cook on low heat for 5 additional minutes.   Serve the eggs and the sauce fresh and warm.
Nutrition Info: Per Serving:Calories:179 Fat:11.9g Protein:7.6g Carbohydrates:11.7g

132.   Mediterranean Scones

Servings: 8   Cooking Time: 15-20 Minutes
Ingredients:

1 egg, beaten, to glaze
1 tablespoon baking powder
1 tablespoon olive oil
10 black olives, pitted, halved
100 g feta cheese, cubed

1/4 tsp salt
300 ml full-fat milk
350 g self-rising whole-wheat flour
50 g butter, cut in pieces
8 halves Italian sundried tomatoes, coarsely chopped

Directions:
Preheat the oven to 220C, gas to 7, or fan to 200C. Grease a large-sized baking sheet with butter.   In a large mixing bowl, mix the flour, the baking powder, and the salt. Rub in the oil and the butter, until the flour mix resembles fine crumbs. Add the cheese, tomatoes, and the olives.   Create a well in the center of the flour mix, pour the milk, and with a knife, mix using cutting movements, until the flour mixture is a stickyish, soft dough. Make sure that you do not over mix the dough.   Flour the work surface and your hands well; shape the dough into 3 to 4-cm think round. Cut into 8 wedges; place the wedges well apart in the prepared baking sheet.   Brush the wedges with the beaten egg; bake for about 15-20 minutes, until the dough has risen, golden, and springy.   Transfer into a wire rack; cover with a clean tea towel to keep them soft. Serve warm and buttered.   Store in airtight container for up to 2 to 3 days.
Nutrition Info: Per Serving:293 Cal, 14 g total fat (7 g sat. fat), 36 g carb.,0 g sugar, 2 g fiber, 8 g protein, and 2 g sodium.

133.   Mixed Olives Braised Chicken

Servings: 4   Cooking Time: 1 Hour
Ingredients:

4 chicken breasts
2 shallots, sliced
4 garlic cloves, chopped
2 red bell peppers, cored and sliced
½ cup black olives
½ cup green olives
½ cup kalamata olives

2 tablespoons olive oil
¼ cup white wine
½ cup vegetable stock
Salt and pepper to taste
1 bay leaf
1 thyme sprig

Directions:
Combine the shallots, garlic, bell peppers, olives, oil, wine and stock in a deep dish baking pan. Season with salt and pepper and place the chicken in the pan over the olives.   Cook in the preheated oven at 350F for 45 minutes.   Serve the chicken warm and fresh.

Nutrition Info: Per Serving:Calories:280 Fat:16.3g Protein:22.9g Carbohydrates:7.9g

134. Coconut Chicken Meatballs

Servings: 4   Cooking Time: 10 Minutes

Ingredients:

2 cups ground chicken	1 egg, beaten
1 teaspoon minced garlic	1 tablespoon olive oil
1 teaspoon dried dill	¼ cup coconut flakes
1/3 carrot, grated	½ teaspoon salt

Directions:

In the mixing bowl mix up together ground chicken, minced garlic, dried dill, carrot, egg, and salt. Stir the chicken mixture with the help of the fingertips until homogenous.   Then make medium balls from the mixture.   Coat every chicken ball in coconut flakes.   Heat up olive oil in the skillet.   Add chicken balls and cook them for 3 minutes from each side. The cooked chicken balls will have a golden brown color.

Nutrition Info: Per Serving:calories 200, fat 11.5, fiber 0.6, carbs 1.7, protein 21.9

135. Grilled Turkey With White Bean Mash

Servings: 4   Cooking Time: 45 Minutes

Ingredients:

4 turkey breast fillets	4 garlic cloves, minced
1 teaspoon chili powder	2 tablespoons lemon juice
1 teaspoon dried parsley	3 tablespoons olive oil
Salt and pepper to taste	2 sweet onions, sliced
2 cans white beans, drained	2 tablespoons tomato paste

Directions:

Season the turkey with salt, pepper and dried parsley.   Heat a grill pan over medium flame and place the turkey on the grill. Cook on each side for 7 minutes.   For the mash, combine the beans, garlic, lemon juice, salt and pepper in a blender and pulse until well mixed and smooth.   Heat the oil in a skillet and add the onions. Cook for 10 minutes until caramelized. Add the tomato paste and cook for 2 more minutes.   Serve the grilled turkey with bean mash and caramelized onions.

Nutrition Info: Per Serving:Calories:337 Fat:8.2g Protein:21.1g Carbohydrates:47.2g

136. Vegetable Turkey Casserole

Servings: 8   Cooking Time: 1 ¼ Hours

Ingredients:

3 tablespoons olive oil	3 carrots, sliced
2 pounds turkey breasts, cubed	½ teaspoon cumin powder
1 sweet onion, chopped	½ teaspoon dried thyme
2 celery stalks, sliced	2 cans diced tomatoes
2 garlic cloves, chopped	1 cup chicken stock
	1 bay leaf
	Salt and pepper to taste

Directions:

Heat the oil in a deep heavy pot and stir in the turkey.   Cook for 5 minutes until golden on all sides then add the onion, carrot, celery and garlic. Cook for 5 more minutes then add the rest of the ingredients.   Season with salt and pepper and cook in the preheated oven at 350F for 40 minutes. Serve the casserole warm and fresh.

Nutrition Info: Per Serving:Calories:186 Fat:7.3g Protein:20.1g Carbohydrates:9.9g

137. Mediterranean Grilled Pork With Tomato Salsa

Servings: 4   Cooking Time: 1 Hour

Ingredients:

4 pork chops	1 jalapeno, chopped
1 teaspoon dried oregano	1 shallot, chopped
1 teaspoon dried basil	2 garlic cloves, minced
1 teaspoon dried marjoram	1 green onion, chopped
Salt and pepper to taste	2 tablespoons chopped parsley
4 tomatoes, peeled and diced	1 tablespoon lemon juice

Directions:

Season with salt and pepper, oregano, basil and marjoram.   Heat a grill pan over medium flame and place the pork chops on the grill.   Cook on each side for 5-6 minutes.   For the salsa, mix the tomatoes, jalapeno, shallot, garlic, onion and parsley. Add salt and pepper to taste. Add the lemon juice as well.   Serve the pork chops with salsa.

Nutrition Info: Per Serving:Calories:286 Fat:20.3g Protein:19.4g Carbohydrates:6.3g

138. Beef And Macaroni Soup

Servings: 6   Cooking Time: 30 Minutes

Ingredients:

½ cup elbow macaroni	1 teaspoon salt
1 teaspoon coconut oil	1 teaspoon chili flakes
1/3 teaspoon minced garlic	3 oz Mozzarella, shredded
2 oz yellow onion, diced	1 teaspoon dried basil
1 ½ cup ground beef	5 cups beef broth
½ teaspoon dried oregano	1 tablespoon cream cheese
½ teaspoon dried thyme	1 cup water, for cooking macaroni

Directions:

Pour water in the pan and bring it to boil.   Add elbow macaroni and cook them according to the manufacturer directions.   Then drain water from the cooked elbow macaroni.   Put coconut oil in the big pot and melt it.   Add minced garlic, yellow onion, ground beef, dried oregano, dried thyme, salt, chili flakes, and dried basil.   Cook the ingredients for 10 minutes over the medium-low heat. Stir the mixture from time to time.   Add beef broth and cream cheese. Stir the soup until it is homogenous.   Cook the soup for 10 minutes.   Then add cooked elbow macaroni and stir well.   Bring the soup to boil and remove from the heat.   Ladle the cooked soup in the serving bowls and garnish with Mozzarella.

Nutrition Info: Per Serving:calories 180, fat 9.2, fiber 0.5, carbs 7.6, protein 15.7

139. Provencal Beef Stew

Servings: 8   Cooking Time: 1 ½ Hours

Ingredients:

3 tablespoons olive oil	2 carrots, diced
2 pounds beef roast, cubed	1 can diced tomatoes
2 sweet onions, chopped	2 tomatoes, peeled and diced
4 garlic cloves, chopped	1 cup vegetable stock
2 celery stalks, diced	1 jalapeno, chopped
	1 bay leaf
	1 thyme sprig
	Salt and pepper to taste

Directions:

Heat the oil in a skillet and stir in the beef. Cook for 10 minutes on all sides.   Add the onions and garlic and cook for 5 more minutes.   Stir in the remaining ingredients and season with salt and pepper.   Place a lid on and cook on low heat for 1 hour.   Serve the stew warm and fresh.

Nutrition Info: Per Serving:Calories:284 Fat:12.5g Protein:35.4g Carbohydrates:6.5g

140. Greek Beef Meatballs

Servings: 8   Cooking Time: 1 Hour

Ingredients:

2 pounds ground beef	1 carrot, grated
6 garlic cloves, minced	1 egg
1 teaspoon dried mint	1 tablespoon tomato paste
1 teaspoon dried oregano	3 tablespoons chopped parsley
1 shallot, finely chopped	Salt and pepper to taste

Directions:

Combine all the ingredients in a bowl and mix well. Season with salt and pepper then form small meatballs and place them in a baking tray lined with baking paper.   Bake in the preheated oven at 350F for 25 minutes.   Serve the meatballs warm and fresh.

Nutrition Info: Per Serving:Calories:229 Fat:7.7g Protein:35.5g Carbohydrates:2.4g

141. Sausage And Beans Soup

Servings: 4   Cooking Time: 20 Minutes

Ingredients:

1 pound Italian pork sausage, sliced	4 cups chicken stock
¼ cup olive oil	28 ounces canned cannellini beans, drained and rinsed
1 carrot, chopped	1 bay leaf
1 yellow onion, chopped	1 teaspoon rosemary, dried
1 celery stalk, chopped	Salt and black pepper to the taste
2 garlic cloves, minced	½ cup parmesan, grated
½ pound kale, chopped	

Directions:

Heat up a pot with the oil over medium heat, add the sausage and brown for 5 minutes.   Add the onion, carrots, garlic and celery and sauté for 3 minutes more.   Add the rest of the ingredients except the parmesan, bring to a simmer and cook over medium heat for 30 minutes.   Discard the bay leaf, ladle the soup into bowls, sprinkle the parmesan on top and serve.

Nutrition Info:calories 564, fat 26.5, fiber 15.4, carbs 37.4, protein 26.6

142. Jalapeno Grilled Salmon With Tomato Confit

Servings: 4   Cooking Time: 30 Minutes

Ingredients:

4 salmon fillets	Salt and pepper to taste
1 jalapeno	2 cups cherry tomatoes, halved
4 garlic cloves	1 shallot, chopped
2 tablespoons tomato paste	1 tablespoon olive oil
2 tablespoons olive oil	

Directions:

Combine the jalapeno, garlic, tomato paste and oil in a mortar. Mix well until a smooth paste is formed.   Spread the spicy paste over the salmon and season it with salt and pepper.   Heat a grill pan over medium flame then place the fish on the grill.   Cook on each side for 5-6 minutes.   For the confit, heat 1 tablespoon of oil in a skillet. Add the shallot and cook for 1 minute then stir in the cherry tomatoes, salt and pepper. Cook for 2 minutes on high heat.   Serve the grilled salmon with the tomatoes.

Nutrition Info: Per Serving:Calories:237 Fat:14.5g Protein:24.0g Carbohydrates:4.4g

143. Chicken And Rice Soup

Servings: 4   Cooking Time: 35 Minutes

Ingredients:

6 cups chicken stock	1 egg, whisked
1 and ½ cups chicken meat, cooked and shredded	Juice of ½ lemon
1 bay leaf	1 cup asparagus, trimmed and halved
1 yellow onion, chopped	1 cup carrots, chopped
2 tablespoons olive oil	½ cup dill, chopped
1/3 cup white rice	Salt and black pepper to the taste

Directions:

Heat up a pot with the oil over medium heat, add the onions and sauté for 5 minutes.   Add the stock, dill, the rice and the bay leaf, stir, bring to a boil over medium heat and cook for 10 minutes.   Add the rest of the ingredients except the egg and the lemon juice, stir and cook for 15 minutes more. Add the egg whisked with the lemon juice gradually, whisk the soup, cook for 2 minutes more, divide into bowls an serve.

Nutrition Info:calories 263, fat 18.5, fiber 4.5, carbs 19.8, protein 14.5

144. Spicy Salsa Braised Beef Ribs

Servings: 12   Cooking Time: 4 Hours

Ingredients:

6 pounds beef ribs	1 cup chopped parsley
4 tomatoes, diced	2 tablespoons balsamic vinegar
2 jalapenos, chopped	1 teaspoon Worcestershire sauce
2 shallots, chopped	Salt and pepper to taste
½ cup chopped cilantro	
3 tablespoons olive oil	

Directions:

Combine the tomatoes, jalapenos, shallots, parsley, cilantro, oil, vinegar, sauce, salt and pepper in a

deep dish baking pan.   Place the ribs in the pan and cover with aluminum foil.   Cook in the preheated oven at 300F for 3 1/3 hours.   Serve the ribs warm.
Nutrition Info: Per Serving:Calories:464 Fat:17.8g Protein:69.4g Carbohydrates:2.5g

---

145.   Pork And Prunes Stew

Servings: 8   Cooking Time: 1 ¼ Hours
Ingredients:

2 pounds pork tenderloin, cubed	1 cup vegetable stock
2 tablespoons olive oil	½ cup white wine
1 sweet onions, chopped	1 pound prunes, pitted
4 garlic cloves, chopped	1 bay leaf
2 carrots, diced	1 thyme sprig
2 celery stalks, chopped	1 teaspoon mustard seeds
2 tomatoes, peeled and diced	1 teaspoon coriander seeds
	Salt and pepper to taste

Directions:
Combine all the ingredients in a deep dish baking pan.   Add salt and pepper to taste and cook in the preheated oven at 350F for 1 hour, adding more liquid as it cooks if needed.   Serve the stew warm and fresh.
Nutrition Info: Per Serving:Calories:363 Fat:7.9g Protein:31.7g Carbohydrates:41.4g

---

146.   Low-carb And Paleo Mediterranean Zucchini Noodles

Servings: 4   Cooking Time: 10 Minutes
Ingredients:

4 medium (about 8 inches long) zucchini	1/2 teaspoon Italian herb blend
3-4 garlic cloves, peeled	Red pepper flakes, to taste (1/2 teaspoon, less or more)
1 tablespoon olive oil (or slightly more if you have a lot of noodles)	1/4 cup parsley, chopped
2 tablespoons olive oil	2 cups cherry tomatoes, cut into halves
1/4 cup red onion, finely chopped	1/2 cup Kalamata olives, drained, cut in half (or regular black olives)
1 tablespoon garlic, finely minced, plus	1/4 cup capers, drained, chopped
1/2 teaspoon dried oregano	

Directions:
Except for the zucchini, prepare and ready the rest of the ingredients.   Wash the zucchini well and pat dry with paper towel. Spiralize the noodles using a spiralizer. With a kitchen shear, cut through the pile of zoodles (zucchini noodles) a few times to shorten them.   For the sauce: In a medium-frying pan, heat the 2 tablespoons olive oil over medium-high heat. Add the red onions; cook for 2 minutes. Add the minced garlic and the dried herbs, cook for 1 minute. Add the tomatoes; cook for 2 minutes. Add the capers, olives, and red pepper flakes; cook for about 1-2 minutes. Turn the heat off; stir the parsley in to mix.   For the zoodles: In a large-sized-sized nonstick wok or pan, heat the remaining 1 tablespoon olive oil. When hot, add the whole garlic cloves, cook for

about 30 seconds, or just until fragrant, discard the garlic. Add the zoodles; cook for 2 to 3 minutes on high heat, stirring a couple of times, just until the zoodles are beginning to soften and hot.   Divide the zoodles between 4 bowls. Top each serve with a generous scoop of the sauce. Best when freshly made and served. However, if there are any leftovers, you can keep them in the fridge and reheat gently in a pan.
Nutrition Info: Per Serving:190 cal., 13 g total fat (1.5 g sat fat), 0 mg chol., 420 mg sodium, 8400 mg potassium, 16 g carb., 5 g fiber, 9 g sugar, and 4 g protein.

147.Pork And Rice Soup

Servings: 4   Cooking Time: 7 Hours
Ingredients:

2 pounds pork stew meat, cubed	3 tablespoons olive oil
A pinch of salt and black pepper	1 cup white rice
6 cups water	2 cups yellow onion, chopped
1 leek, sliced	½ cup lemon juice
2 bay leaves	1 tablespoon cilantro, chopped
1 carrot, sliced	

Directions:
In your slow cooker, combine the pork with the water and the rest of the ingredients except the cilantro, put the lid on and cook on Low for 7 hours. Stir the soup, ladle into bowls, sprinkle the cilantro on top and serve.
Nutrition Info:calories 300, fat 15, fiber 7.6, carbs 17.4, protein 22.4

---

148.   Tomato Roasted Feta

Servings: 4   Cooking Time: 45 Minutes
Ingredients:

2 tomatoes, peeled and diced	8 oz. feta cheese
2 garlic cloves, chopped	1 cup tomato juice
	1 thyme sprig
	1 oregano sprig

Directions:
Mix the tomatoes, garlic, tomato juice, thyme and oregano in a small deep dish baking pan.   Place the feta in the pan as well and cover with aluminum foil.   Cook in the preheated oven at 350F for 10 minutes.   Serve the feta and the sauce fresh.
Nutrition Info: Per Serving:Calories:173 Fat:12.2g Protein:9.2g Carbohydrates:7.8g

---

149.   Fettuccine With Spinach And Shrimp

Servings: 4-6   Cooking Time: 10 Minutes
Ingredients:

8 ounces whole-wheat fettuccine pasta, uncooked	1/4 teaspoon crushed red pepper flakes
3 garlic cloves, peeled, chopped	1/2 cup crumbled feta cheese
2 teaspoons dried basil, crushed	1 teaspoon salt
12 ounces medium raw shrimp, peeled, deveined	1 package (10 ounce) frozen spinach, thawed
	1 cup sour cream

Directions:
In a large-sized mixing bowl, combine sour cream, the feta, basil, garlic, salt, and red pepper.

44

According to the package instructions, cook the fettucine. After the first 8 minutes of cooking, add the spinach and the shrimp to the boiling water with pasta; boil for 2 minutes more and then drain thoroughly. Add the hot pasta, spinach, and shrimp mixture into the bowl with the sour cream mix; lightly toss and serve immediately.
Nutrition Info: Per Serving:417.9 Cal, 18 g total fat (9.8 g sat. fat), 197.6 mg chol., 1395.6 mg sodium, 39.7 g carb., 2.5 g fiber, 3.3 g sugar, and 25.2 g protein.

150. Sage Pork And Beans Stew

Servings: 4   Cooking Time: 4 Hours And 10 Minutes

Ingredients:

2 pounds pork stew meat, cubed	2 teaspoons sage, dried
2 tablespoons olive oil	4 ounces canned white beans, drained
1 sweet onion, chopped	1 cup beef stock
1 red bell pepper, chopped	2 zucchinis, chopped
3 garlic cloves, minced	2 tablespoons tomato paste
	1 tablespoon cilantro, chopped

Directions:

Heat up a pan with the oil over medium-high heat, add the meat, brown for 10 minutes and transfer to your slow cooker. Add the rest of the ingredients except the cilantro, put the lid on and cook on High for 4 hours. Divide the stew into bowls, sprinkle the cilantro on top and serve.
Nutrition Info:calories 423, fat 15.4, fiber 9.6, carbs 27.4, protein 43

151. Broccoli Pesto Spaghetti

Servings: 4   Cooking Time: 35 Minutes

Ingredients:

8 oz. spaghetti	4 basil leaves
1 pound broccoli, cut into florets	2 tablespoons blanched almonds
2 tablespoons olive oil	1 lemon, juiced
4 garlic cloves, chopped	Salt and pepper to taste

Directions:

For the pesto, combine the broccoli, oil, garlic, basil, lemon juice and almonds in a blender and pulse until well mixed and smooth. Cook the spaghetti in a large pot of salty water for 8 minutes or until al dente. Drain well. Mix the warm spaghetti with the broccoli pesto and serve right away.
Nutrition Info: Per Serving:Calories:284 Fat:10.2g Protein:10.4g Carbohydrates:40.2g

152. Chorizo Stuffed Chicken Breasts

Servings: 4   Cooking Time: 1 ¼ Hours

Ingredients:

4 chicken breasts	2 garlic cloves, minced
2 chorizo links, diced	
4 oz. mozzarella, shredded	1 can diced tomatoes
3 tablespoons olive oil	½ cup dry white wine
1 shallot, chopped	½ cup vegetable stock
	Salt and pepper to

taste

Directions:

Mix the chorizo and mozzarella in a bowl. Cut a small pocket into each chicken breast and stuff it with the chorizo. Season the chicken with salt and pepper. Heat the oil in a skillet and add the chicken. Cook on each side for 5 minutes or until golden brown. Add the shallot, garlic and tomatoes, as well as wine, stock, salt and pepper. Cook on low heat for 40 minutes. Serve the chicken and the sauce warm.
Nutrition Info: Per Serving:Calories:435 Fat:30.8g Protein:30.2g Carbohydrates:4.2g

153. Grilled Mediterranean-style Chicken Kebabs

Servings: 10   Cooking Time: 10-15 Minutes

Ingredients:

3 chicken filets, diced in 1-inch cubes	1 red onion
2 green bell peppers	2/3 cup extra virgin olive oil, divided
2 red bell peppers	4 teaspoon oregano, divided
2 teaspoon black pepper (freshly ground), divided	4 teaspoon of salt, divided
2 teaspoon paprika, divided	6 cloves of garlic (minced), divided
2 teaspoon thyme, divided	Juice of 1 lemon, divided

Directions:

Mix 1/2 amount of all the marinade ingredients in a small bowl, place the chicken in a Ziploc bag and add the marinade. Refrigerate for at least 30 minutes to marinate   Mix the remaining 1/2 amount of the marinade ingredients in the same bowl. Pour in the Ziploc bag and add the vegetables. Refrigerate for at least 30 minutes to marinate. When marinated, thread the chicken, the peppers, and the onions into skewers, about 5 to 6 pieces chicken with a combination of onion and peppers between each chicken cubes. Heat an indoor or outdoor grill pan over medium high heat. Lightly oil the grates. Grill the chicken for about 5 minutes per side, or until the center of the cubes are no longer pink. Serve with favorite Mediterranean side dish, salad, or baked potato slices or fries.
Nutrition Info: Per Serving:150 cal., 15 g total fat (2 g sat fat), 0 mg chol., 950 mg sodium, 150 mg potassium, 6 g carb., 2 g fiber, 2 g sugar, and <1 g protein.

154. Sumac Salmon And Grapefruit

Servings: 4   Cooking Time: 5 Minutes

Ingredients:

1 cup parsley leaves, flat-leaf	2 pink grapefruits, peeled, segmented
1 teaspoon ground cumin	2 tablespoons sumac
1/4 cup (60ml) olive oil, plus more to brush	4 pieces (180 g each) salmon fillets, skinless, pin-boned
2 oranges, peeled, segmented	Juice of 1/2 lemon, and wedges to serve

Directions:

In a mixing bowl, combine the sumac and the cumin. Brush the fillets with the olive oil; season with the sumac mixture. In a large frying pan, heat 1 tablespoon olive oil over medium heat. Add the fish fillets; cook for about 2 minutes per side, or until charred on the outside and almost cooked through, but still pink in the middle. Transfer to a plate and loosely cover with foil.   Meanwhile, whisk the remaining 2 tablespoons of olive oil and lemon juice; season. Add the fruits and the parsley, toss to coat. Serve the fish fillets with the salad and wedges of lemon.

Nutrition Info: Per Serving:567.9 Cal, 34 g total fat (7 g sat. fat), 16 g carb., 7 g fiber, 47 g protein, and 95.39 mg sodium.

155.Bean Patties With And Salsa Avocado

Servings: 4   Cooking Time: 10 Minutes

Ingredients:

60 g mixed salad leaves, washed, dried	1 small red onion, finely chopped
5 pieces 13-cm round pocket bread (whole wheat pita bread)	1 can (750 g) red kidney beans, rinsed, drained
1/4 cup chopped fresh coriander	1 avocado, halved, seed removed,
1 egg white	peeled, sliced lengthways
1 container (170 g) chunky tomato salsa dip	1 1/2 tablespoons olive oil

Directions:

Tear 1 round of pita into pieces; place in the bowl of the food processor and process until breadcrumb-like in texture. Transfer into a medium-sized bowl; set aside.   Reserve 185 g (or 1 cup) of the beans; place the remaining beans into the bowl of a food processor. In short bursts, process until roughly mashed.   Transfer into a bowl. Add the coriander, onion, reserved beans, egg white, and the pita crumbs; stir well until combined. With damp hands, divide the mixture into 4 portions, and shape into 8-cm thick and 8-cm wide diameter.   In a large nonstick frying pan, heat the oil over medium heat. Add the patties; cook for 4 minutes per side or until golden brown and the patties are heated through.   Meanwhile, preheat grill to medium-high. Grill the remaining pita under the preheated grill for about 1 to 2 minutes per side or until toasted.   Place the toasted pita into serving plates, top with the mixed salad, the slices of avocado, the bean patties, and the salsa; serve immediately.

Nutrition Info: Per Serving:549 cal., 22 g fat (4 g sat fat), 62 g carb., 8 g sugar, 18 g protein, and 964.9 mg sodium.

156.   Raisin Stuffed Lamb

Servings: 10   Cooking Time: 2 ½ Hours

Ingredients:

4 pounds lamb shoulder	1 cup golden raisins
1 teaspoon garlic powder	2 red apples, cored and diced
1 teaspoon onion powder	1 teaspoon mustard powder
1 teaspoon chili powder	1 teaspoon cumin powder
Salt and pepper to taste	2 tablespoons pine nuts
	1 cup dry white wine

Directions:

Season the lamb with garlic powder, onion powder, chili, salt and pepper.   Cut a pocket into the lamb.

Mix the raisins, red apples, mustard, cumin and pine nuts and stuff the mixture into the lamb. Place the lamb in a deep dish baking pan and cover with aluminum foil.   Cook in the preheated oven at 330F for 2 hours.   Serve the lamb warm and fresh.

Nutrition Info: Per Serving:Calories:436 Fat:14.8g Protein:52.0g Carbohydrates:18.1g

157.Spinach Orzo Stew

Servings: 8   Cooking Time: 1 Hour

Ingredients:

3 tablespoons olive oil	1 cup orzo, rinsed
1 sweet onion, chopped	2 cups vegetable stock
2 garlic cloves, minced	Salt and pepper to taste
1 celery stalk, diced	4 cups baby spinach
2 carrots, diced	1 tablespoon lemon juice

Directions:

Heat the oil in a skillet and stir in the onion, garlic, celery and carrots. Cook for 2 minutes until softened then add the orzo.   Cook for another 5 minutes then pour in the stock.   Add the salt and pepper and cook on low heat for 20 minutes. Add the spinach and lemon juice and cook for another 5 minutes.   Serve the stew warm and fresh.

Nutrition Info: Per Serving:Calories:143 Fat:5.8g Protein:3.5g Carbohydrates:19.8g

158.   Grapes, Cucumbers And Almonds Soup

Servings: 4   Cooking Time: 0 Minutes

Ingredients:

¼ cup almonds, chopped and toasted	6 scallions, sliced
3 cucumbers, peeled and chopped	3 tablespoons olive oil
3 garlic cloves, minced	Salt and white pepper to the taste
½ cup warm water	1 teaspoon lemon juice
¼ cup white wine vinegar	½ cup green grapes, halved

Directions:

In your blender, combine the almonds with the cucumbers and the rest of the ingredients except the grapes and lemon juice, pulse well and divide into bowls.   Top each serving with the lemon juice and grapes and serve cold.

Nutrition Info:calories 200, fat 5.4, fiber 2.4, carbs 7.6, protein 3.3

159.   Nutmeg Beef Soup

Servings: 8   Cooking Time: 30 Minutes

Ingredients:

1 yellow onion, chopped	1 pound eggplant, chopped
1 tablespoon olive oil	¾ cup carrots, chopped
1 garlic clove, minced	
1 pound beef meat, ground	Salt and black pepper to the taste
30 ounces canned tomatoes, drained and chopped	1 quart beef stock
	½ teaspoon nutmeg, ground
	2 teaspoons parsley,

chopped

Directions:
Heat up a pot with the oil over medium heat, add the meat, onion and the garlic and brown for 5 minutes. Add the rest of the ingredients except the parsley, bring to a boil and cook over medium heat for 25 minutes. Add the parsley, divide the soup into bowls and serve.
Nutrition Info:calories 232, fat 5.4, fiber 7.6, carbs 20.1, protein 6.5

160.	**Parsnip Chickpea Veal Stew**

Servings: 10   Cooking Time: 2 Hours
Ingredients:

2 pounds veal meat, cubed	4 parsnips, peeled and sliced
3 tablespoons olive oil	2 carrots, sliced
2 shallots, chopped	1 can diced tomatoes
4 garlic cloves, chopped	1 ½ cups beef stock
2 red bell peppers, cored and sliced	1 bay leaf
	1 rosemary sprig
2 yellow bell peppers, cored and sliced	1 oregano sprig
	1 can chickpeas, drained
	Salt and pepper to taste

Directions:
Heat the oil in a heavy saucepan and stir in the veal. Cook for 5 minutes until slightly browned. Add the shallots, garlic, bell peppers, parsnips and carrots. Cook for another 5 minutes then stir in the rest of the ingredients. Season with salt and pepper and cook for 1 ½ hours on low heat. Serve the stew warm and fresh.
Nutrition Info: Per Serving:Calories:332 Fat:12.7g Protein:27.8g Carbohydrates:26.9g

161.	**Tuna And Couscous**

Servings: 4   Cooking Time: 0 Minutes
Ingredients:

1 cup chicken stock	½ cup pepperoncini, sliced
1 and ¼ cups couscous	1/3 cup parsley, chopped
A pinch of salt and black pepper	1 tablespoon olive oil
10 ounces canned tuna, drained and flaked	¼ cup capers, drained
1 pint cherry tomatoes, halved	Juice of ½ lemon

Directions:
Put the stock in a pan, bring to a boil over medium-high heat, add the couscous, stir, take off the heat, cover, leave aside for 10 minutes, fluff with a fork and transfer to a bowl. Add the tuna and the rest of the ingredients, toss and serve for lunch right away.
Nutrition Info:calories 253, fat 11.5, fiber 3.4, carbs 16.5, protein 23.2

162.	**Olive Oil Lemon Broiled Cod**

Servings: 4   Cooking Time: 35 Minutes
Ingredients:

4 cod fillets	1 lemon, juiced
1 teaspoon dried marjoram	1 thyme sprig
4 tablespoons olive oil	Salt and pepper to taste

Directions:
Season the cod with salt, pepper and marjoram. Heat the oil in a large skillet and place the cod in the hot oil. Fry on medium heat on both sides until golden brown then add the lemon juice. Place the thyme sprig on top and cover with a lid. Cook for 5 more minutes then remove from heat. Serve the cod and sauce fresh.
Nutrition Info: Per Serving:Calories:304 Fat:15.5g Protein:40.0g Carbohydrates:0.1g

163.	**Chicken And Spaghetti Soup**

Servings: 5   Cooking Time: 35 Minutes
Ingredients:

4 chicken drumsticks, skinless	1 tablespoon chives, chopped
3 oz whole grain spaghetti	1 onion, chopped
3 cups chicken stock	1 tablespoon canola oil
1 teaspoon salt	½ teaspoon cilantro, chopped
½ teaspoon dried oregano	2 potatoes, chopped

Directions:
Pour chicken stock in the pan. Add chicken drumsticks and simmer them for 20 minutes. Meanwhile, roast together onion with canola oil. When the onion is light brown, add the potato and roast the vegetables for 3-4 minutes more. Stir them from time to time. Then add the roasted vegetables in the pan with drumsticks. Sprinkle soup with chives, salt, and cilantro. When the potato is half-cooked, add spaghetti, stir well, and cook soup for 10 minutes. Ladle the cooked soup in the bowls.
Nutrition Info: Per Serving:calories 287, fat 6.6, fiber 6.8, carbs 39.4, protein 17.6

164.	**Mediterranean Flounder**

Servings: 4   Cooking Time: 30 Minutes
Ingredients:

6 leaves fresh basil, chopped	2 garlic cloves, chopped
5 roma tomatoes, chopped or 1 (15 ounce) can chopped tomatoes	¼ cup white wine
	½ onion, chopped
	1 teaspoon lemon juice, freshly squeezed
4 tablespoons capers	
3 tablespoons parmesan cheese	1 pound flounder (or sole, halibut, mahi-mahi or tilapia fillet
24 Kalamata olives, pitted, chopped	
2 tablespoons olive oil	1 pinch Italian seasoning

Directions:
Preheat the oven to 425F. Bring water to a boil and place a bowl of ice water near the oven. Plunge the tomatoes into the boiling water, immediately remove them and plunge into the ice water; peel the skins. Alternatively, you can chop them with the skins on or you can use canned if you prefer. In a medium-sized skillet, heat the olive oil over medium flame or heat. Add the onion; sauté until tender. Add the garlic and the Italian seasoning, stirring to combine. Add the tomatoes; cook until tender. Mix in the wine, capers, olives, 1/2 of the basil, and lemon juice. Alternatively, you can use a couple teaspoons of dried basil. However, fresh is preferred. Reduce the heat, add the parmesan

cheese; cook until the mixture is bubbly and hot. If you want a thicker sauce, cook for about 15 minutes or up to thick. Place the fish in a shallow baking dish, pour the sauce over the fish, and bake for about 15 to 20 minutes until it easily flakes with a fork. Take note, the mah-mahi will not easily flake even when it is done.

Nutrition Info: Per Serving:221.9 Cal, 13.1 g total fat (2.5 g sat. fat), 54.4 mg chol., 848.1 mg sodium, 7.5 g carb., 2.3 g fiber, 2.9 g sugar, and 16.9 g protein.

165. Crunchy Baked Mussels

Servings: 4   Cooking Time: 45 Minutes

Ingredients:

2 pounds mussels	1 teaspoon lemon zest
½ cup breadcrumbs	½ teaspoon chili flakes
4 garlic cloves, minced	2 tablespoons butter, melted
2 tablespoons chopped parsley	

Directions:

Mix the breadcrumbs, lemon zest, garlic, parsley, chili and butter in a bowl. Wash the mussels well and place them in a steamer. Cook for a few minutes until they all open up. Carefully remove them from the steamer and place the opened up ones in a baking tray. Top each mussel with the breadcrumb mixture and cook in the preheated oven at 400F for 5 minutes. Serve right away.

Nutrition Info: Per Serving:Calories:305 Fat:11.6g Protein:29.1g Carbohydrates:19.3g

166. Mediterranean-style Tuna Wrap

Servings: 4   Cooking Time: 13 Minutes

Ingredients:

1/2 teaspoon lemon zest	2 large tomatoes, sliced
1/4 cup fresh parsley, chopped	3 tablespoons olive oil
1/4 cup Kalamata olives, chopped	4 whole-grain (about 2 ounces each) wrap breads
1/4 cup red onion, finely diced	6 cups (about 3 ounces) mixed greens, pre-washed
2 cans (6-ounce each) chunk light tuna in water, drained well	Freshly ground black pepper
2 tablespoons lemon juice, freshly squeezed	Salt

Directions:

In a medium mixing bowl, combine the tuna, parsley, onion, and olives. In a small mixing bowl, whisk the olive oil, lemon juice, lemon zest, salt, and pepper. Pour about 2/3 of the dressing over the tuna mixture; toss to incorporate. In another bowl, combine the greens and the remaining 1/3 dressing; toss to coat. Into each piece of wrap bread, top tuna salad, then with 1 1/2 cup greens, and a few slices of tomatoes. Roll the wrap; serve.

Nutrition Info: Per Serving:379 Cal, 16.5 g total fat (2 g sat. fat), 29 g carb., 4 g sugar, 5 g fiber, 26 g protein, and 701 mg sodium.

167.Pear Braised Pork

Servings: 10   Cooking Time: 2 ¼ Hours

Ingredients:

3 pounds pork shoulder	2 shallots, sliced
4 pears, peeled and sliced	1 bay leaf
	1 thyme sprig
4 garlic cloves, minced	½ cup apple cider
	Salt and pepper to taste

Directions:

Season the pork with salt and pepper. Combine the pears, shallots, garlic, bay leaf, thyme and apple cider in a deep dish baking pan. Place the pork over the pears then cover the pan with aluminum foil. Cook in the preheated oven at 330F for 2 hours. Serve the pork and the sauce fresh.

Nutrition Info: Per Serving:Calories:455 Fat:29.3g Protein:32.1g Carbohydrates:14.9g

168. Yogurt Baked Eggplants

Servings: 4   Cooking Time: 45 Minutes

Ingredients:

4 garlic cloves, minced	2 eggplants
1 teaspoon dried basil	Salt and pepper to taste
2 tablespoons lemon juice	1 cup Greek yogurt
	2 tablespoons chopped parsley

Directions:

Cut the eggplants in half and score the halves with a sharp knives. Season the eggplants with salt and pepper, as well as the basil then drizzle with lemon juice and place the eggplant halves on a baking tray. Spread the garlic over the eggplants and bake in the preheated oven at 350F for 20 minutes. When done, place the eggplants on serving plates and top with yogurt and parsley. Serve the eggplants right away.

Nutrition Info: Per Serving:Calories:113 Fat:1.6g Protein:8.1g Carbohydrates:19.4g

169. Pancetta-wrapped Cod With Rosemary New Potatoes

Servings: 6   Cooking Time: 1 ¼ Hours

Ingredients:

6 cod fillets	6 pancetta slices
1 pound new potatoes, rinsed	2 tablespoons lemon juice
½ green beans, trimmed and halved	2 rosemary sprigs
3 tablespoons olive oil	Salt and pepper to taste

Directions:

Season the fish with salt and pepper and wrap it in pancetta. Combine the new potatoes, beans, oil, lemon juice and rosemary in a deep dish baking pan. Season with salt and pepper. Place the cod over the vegetables and cover the pan with aluminum foil. Cook in the preheated oven at 350F for 40 minutes. Serve the fish and the veggies warm and fresh.

Nutrition Info: Per Serving:Calories: 291 Fat: 8.6g Protein: 39.5g Carbohydrates: 12.5g

170. Stuffed Peppers With Basil And Tomato Cream Sauce

Servings: 4   Cooking Time: 50 Minutes

Ingredients:

1 1/2 cups cooked brown rice	1/3 cup heavy cream
	1 tablespoon olive oil
1 can (29 ounces)	3 garlic cloves,

tomato sauce
1 pound ground chicken breast (or turkey)
1/2 onion, chopped
1/3 cup fresh basil, chopped, reserving a few for garnish

minced
3/4 cup parmesan cheese, divided
4 red, orange, green, or yellow peppers
Salt and pepper

Directions:
Preheat the oven to 400F. Slice the top of the peppers off, remove the seeds and the seeds; set aside. Save the pepper tops.   Over medium flame or heat, put the oil in a skillet. Add the onion; sauté for 5 minutes, or until soft. Add the garlic; cook for 1 minute.   Season the ground chicken with the salt and the pepper; cook for about 10 to 12 minutes, stirring occasionally, until brown. While the chicken is cooking, mix the tomato sauce, the heavy cream, and the remaining garlic in another skillet; heat over low heat. Stir in the basil. Stir the cooked brown rice into the skillet of chicken. Add 1/2 cup of the parmesan cheese, about 1/2 cup of the tomato-cream mixture; toss to coat. Turn the heat off.   Divide the chicken mixture between 4 peppers, filling them to the top. Place the stuffed peppers in a baking dish that will allow them to stand; spoon a bit of the tomato-cream sauce over the top of the stuffed peppers. Pour the remaining sauce in the bottom of the dish; place the pepper tops back into the stuffed peppers. Bake for about 20 minutes, cover the dish with foil, and bake for 30 minutes more.   Serve with more parmesan and with basil garnishing, and mashed potato on the side.
Nutrition Info: Per Serving:660 cal., 33 g total fat (13 g sat fat), 145 mg chol., 1420 mg sodium, 1660 mg potassium, 58 g carb., 11 g fiber, 24 g sugar, and 34 g protein.

171. Beef Stuffed Bell Peppers
Servings: 6   Cooking Time: 1 Hour
Ingredients:
6 red bell peppers
1 pound ground beef
2 sweet onions, chopped
1 garlic cloves, minced
1 celery stalk, finely chopped
1 tablespoon pesto sauce

1 carrot, grated
2 tablespoons tomato paste
½ cup white rice
Salt and pepper to taste
1 cup tomato juice
1 ½ cups beef stock
1 thyme sprig

Directions:
Place the thyme sprig at the bottom of a pot.   Mix the beef, onions, garlic, carrot, celery, pesto sauce and tomato paste, as well as rice, salt and pepper in a bowl.   Cut the top of each bell pepper and remove the vines.   Stuff the bell peppers with the beef mixture and place them in the pot.   Pour in the tomato juice and stock and cover with a lid. Cook on low heat for 45 minutes.   Serve the bell peppers warm and fresh.
Nutrition Info: Per Serving:Calories:280 Fat:6.5g Protein:27.2g Carbohydrates:27.1g

172.Stuffed Eggplants
Servings: 4   Cooking Time: 35 Minutes
Ingredients:
2 eggplants, halved   2 cups kale, torn

lengthwise and 2/3 of the flesh scooped out
3 tablespoons olive oil
1 red onion, chopped
2 garlic cloves, minced
1 pint white mushrooms, sliced

2 cups quinoa, cooked
1 tablespoon thyme, chopped
Zest and juice of 1 lemon
Salt and black pepper to the taste
½ cup Greek yogurt
3 tablespoons parsley, chopped

Directions:
Rub the inside of each eggplant half with half of the oil and arrange them on a baking sheet lined with parchment paper.   Heat up a pan with the rest of the oil over medium heat, add the onion and the garlic and sauté for 5 minutes.   Add the mushrooms and cook for 5 minutes more.   Add the kale, salt, pepper, thyme, lemon zest and juice, stir, cook for 5 minutes more and take off the heat. Stuff the eggplant halves with the mushroom mix, introduce them in the oven and bake 400 degrees F for 20 minutes.   Divide the eggplants between plates, sprinkle the parsley and the yogurt on top and serve for lunch.
Nutrition Info:calories 512, fat 16.4, fiber 17.5, carbs 78, protein 17.2

173.Mushroom Pilaf
Servings: 4   Cooking Time: 50 Minutes
Ingredients:
2 tablespoons olive oil
1 shallot, chopped
2 garlic cloves, minced
1 pound button mushrooms

1 cup brown rice
2 cups chicken stock
1 bay leaf
1 thyme sprig
Salt and pepper to taste

Directions:
Heat the oil in a skillet and stir in the shallot and garlic. Cook for 2 minutes until softened and fragrant.   Add the mushrooms and rice and cook for 5 minutes.   Add the stock, bay leaf and thyme, as well as salt and pepper and continue cooking for 20 more minutes on low heat.   Serve the pilaf warm and fresh.
Nutrition Info: Per Serving:Calories:265 Fat:8.9g Protein:7.6g Carbohydrates:41.2g

174.Cream Cheese Artichoke Mix
Servings: 6   Cooking Time: 45 Minutes
Ingredients:
4 sheets matzo
½ cup artichoke hearts, canned
1 cup cream cheese
1 cup spinach, chopped
½ teaspoon salt

1 teaspoon ground black pepper
3 tablespoons fresh dill, chopped
3 eggs, beaten
1 teaspoon canola oil
½ cup cottage cheese

Directions:
In the bowl combine together cream cheese, spinach, salt, ground black pepper, dill, and cottage cheese.   Pour canola oil in the skillet, add artichoke hearts and roast them for 2-3 minutes over the medium heat. Stir them from time to time. Then add roasted artichoke hearts in the cheese mixture.   Add eggs and stir until homogenous. Place one sheet of matzo in the casserole mold.

Then spread it with cheese mixture generously. Cover the cheese layer with the second sheet of matzo. Repeat the steps till you use all ingredients. Then preheat oven to 360F. Bake matzo mina for 40 minutes. Cut the cooked meal into the servings.

Nutrition Info: Per Serving:calories 272, fat 17.3, fiber 4.3, carbs 20.2, protein 11.8

175. Caramelized Shallot Steaks

Servings: 6   Cooking Time: 45 Minutes

Ingredients:

Salt and pepper to taste	6 flank steaks
1 teaspoon dried oregano	6 shallots, sliced
1 teaspoon dried basil	4 tablespoons olive oil
	¼ cup dry white wine

Directions:

Season the steaks with salt, pepper, oregano and basil. Heat a grill pan over medium flame and place the steaks on the grill. Cook on each side for 6-7 minutes. Heat the oil in a skillet and stir in the shallots. Cook for 15 minutes, stirring often, until the shallots are caramelized. Add the wine and cook for another 5 minutes. Serve the steaks with shallots.

Nutrition Info: Per Serving:Calories:258 Fat:16.3g Protein:23.5g Carbohydrates:2.1g

176. Carrot And Potato Soup

Servings: 6   Cooking Time: 35 Minutes

Ingredients:

5 cups beef broth	1 teaspoon salt
4 carrots, peeled	1 tablespoon lemon juice
1 teaspoon dried thyme	1/3 cup fresh parsley, chopped
½ teaspoon ground cumin	1 chili pepper, chopped
1 ½ cup potatoes, chopped	1 tablespoon tomato paste
1 tablespoon olive oil	1 tablespoon sour cream
½ teaspoon ground black pepper	

Directions:

Line the baking tray with baking paper. Put sweet potatoes and carrot on the tray and sprinkle with olive oil and salt. Bake the vegetables for 25 minutes at 365F. Meanwhile, pour the beef broth in the pan and bring it to boil. Add dried thyme, ground cumin, chopped chili pepper, and tomato paste. When the vegetables are cooked, add them in the pan. Boil the vegetables until they are soft. Then blend the mixture with the help of the blender until smooth. Simmer it for 2 minutes and add lemon juice. Stir well. Then add sour cream and chopped parsley. Stir well. Simmer the soup for 3 minutes more.

Nutrition Info: Per Serving:calories 123, fat 4.1, fiber 2.9, carbs 16.4, protein 5.3

177. Macedonian Greens And Cheese Pie

Servings: 6   Cooking Time: 50 Minutes

Ingredients:

1 bunch chicory	200 g baby spinach
1 bunch rocket or arugula	250 g Greek feta, crumbled
1 bunch mint	4 eggs
1 bunch dill	50 g dried whole-wheat breadcrumbs
10 sheets whole-wheat filo pastry	6 green onions, trimmed
150 g halloumi, finely diced	Olive oil, to brush
150 g ricotta	

Directions:

Trim the rocket stalks and the chicory. Finely chop the green onions and the dill (include the dill stems). Strip the mint leaves. Pour water into a large-sized pan; bring to boil. Ready a bowl with iced water beside the stove. Add the chicory into the boiling water; blanch for 3 minutes and using a slotted spoon, transfer to the bowl with iced water. Repeat the process with the spinach and the rocket, blanching each for 1 minute; drain well. A handful at a time, tightly wring the greens to squeeze out the excess liquid, then pat dry with paper towel. Finely chop the blanched greens. Combine them with the eggs, herbs, feta, 30 g of the breadcrumbs, ricotta, and 3/4 of the halloumi; season. Preheat the oven to 180C. Grease a 5-cm deep 25cmx25 pie tin. Brush a filo sheet with the olive oil, place it in the pie tin, extending the edge of the filo outside the edge of the tin. Brush the remaining sheets of filo and add them to the pie tin, arranging them like wheel spokes. Sprinkle the remaining breadcrumbs over the base of the layered filo sheets. Top with the filling mixture. Loosely fold the filo sheets over to cover the filling, brush with oil, sprinkle with water, and scatter the halloumi over. Bake for 45 minutes. After 45 minutes, cover, and bake for additional 15 minutes, or until heated through.

Nutrition Info: Per Serving:374.8 Cal, 20 g total fat (12 g sat. fat), 22 g carb., 2 g fiber, 3 g sugar, 25g protein, and 1506.7 mg sodium.

178.   Chicken Stuffed Peppers

Servings: 6   Cooking Time: 0 Minutes

Ingredients:

1 cup Greek yogurt	1 bunch scallions, sliced
2 tablespoons mustard	¼ cup parsley, chopped
Salt and black pepper to the taste	1 cucumber, sliced
1 pound rotisserie chicken meat, cubed	3 red bell peppers, halved and deseeded
4 celery stalks, chopped	1 pint cherry tomatoes, quartered
2 tablespoons balsamic vinegar	

Directions:

In a bowl, mix the chicken with the celery and the rest of the ingredients except the bell peppers and toss well. Stuff the peppers halves with the chicken mix and serve for lunch.

Nutrition Info:calories 266, fat 12.2, fiber 4.5, carbs 15.7, protein 3.7

179. Turkey Fritters And Sauce

Servings: 4   Cooking Time: 30 Minutes

Ingredients:

2 garlic cloves, minced	Cooking spray
	For the sauce:
1 egg	1 cup Greek yogurt
1 red onion, chopped	1 cucumber, chopped

1 tablespoon olive oil
¼ teaspoon red pepper flakes
1 pound turkey meat, ground
½ teaspoon oregano, dried

1 tablespoon olive oil
¼ teaspoon garlic powder
2 tablespoons lemon juice
¼ cup parsley, chopped

Directions:
Heat up a pan with 1 tablespoon oil over medium heat, add the onion and the garlic, sauté for 5 minutes, cool down and transfer to a bowl.   Add the meat, turkey, oregano and pepper flakes, stir and shape medium fritters out of this mix.   Heat up another pan greased with cooking spray over medium-high heat, add the turkey fritters and brown for 5 minutes on each side.   Introduce the pan in the oven and bake the fritters at 375 degrees F for 15 minutes more.   Meanwhile, in a bowl, mix the yogurt with the cucumber, oil, garlic powder, lemon juice and parsley and whisk really well.   Divide the fritters between plates, spread the sauce all over and serve for lunch.
Nutrition Info:calories 364, fat 16.8, fiber 5.5, carbs 26.8, protein 23.4

180. Garlic Clove Roasted Chicken
Servings: 8   Cooking Time: 1 ½ Hours
Ingredients:
8 chicken legs
40 garlic cloves, crushed
1 shallot, sliced
½ cup white wine

1 bay leaf
1 thyme sprig
Salt and pepper to taste

Directions:
Season the chicken with salt and pepper. Combine it with the rest of the ingredients in a deep dish baking pan.   Cover the pan with aluminum foil and cook in the preheated oven at 350F for 1 hour.   Serve the chicken warm and fresh.
Nutrition Info: Per Serving:Calories:225 Fat:7.5g Protein:29.9g Carbohydrates:5.6g

181.Chickpeas, Spinach And Arugula Bowl
Servings: 5   Cooking Time: 25 Minutes
Ingredients:
1 cup chickpeas, canned, drained
½ teaspoon butter
½ teaspoon salt
½ teaspoon ground paprika
¾ teaspoon onion powder
6 oz quinoa, dried
12 oz chicken stock

2 tomatoes, chopped
1 cucumber, chopped
½ cup fresh spinach, chopped
½ cup arugula, chopped
½ cup lettuce chopped
1 tablespoon olive oil
4 teaspoons hummus

Directions:
Place chickpeas in the skillet. Add butter and salt. Roast the chickpeas for 5 minutes over the high heat. Stir them from time to time.   After this, place quinoa and chicken stock in the pan.   Cook the quinoa for 15 minutes over the medium heat. Then make the salad: mix up together tomatoes, cucumber, spinach, arugula, lettuce, and olive oil. Shake the salad gently.   Arrange roasted

chickpeas in every serving bowl.   Add salad and hummus.   Then add quinoa. Buddha bowl is cooked.
Nutrition Info: Per Serving:calories 330, fat 8.4, fiber 10.9, carbs 51.6, protein 14.1

182. Tuna Sandwiches
Servings: 4   Cooking Time: 10 Minutes
Ingredients:
1/3 cup sun-dried tomato packed in oil, drained
1/4 cup red bell pepper, finely chopped (optional)
1/4 cup red onions or 1/4 cup sweet Spanish onion, finely chopped
1/4 cup ripe green olives or 1/4 cup ripe olives, sliced
1/4 teaspoon black pepper, fresh ground
2 cans (6 ounce) tuna in water, drained, flaked

2 teaspoons capers (more to taste)
4 romaine lettuce or curly green lettuce leaves
4 teaspoons balsamic vinegar
4 teaspoons roasted red pepper
8 slices whole-grain bread (or 8 slices whole-wheat pita bread)
Olive oil
Optional:
3 tablespoons mayonnaise (or low-fat mayonnaise)

Directions:
Toast the bread, if desired.   In a small mixing bowl, mix the vinegar and the olive oil. Brush the oil mixture over 1 side of each bread slices or on the inside of the pita pockets.   Except for the lettuce, combine the remaining of the ingredients in a mixing bowl.   Place 1 lettuce leaf on the oiled side of 4 bread slices.   Top the leaves with the tuna mix; top with the remaining bread slices with the oiled side in.   If using pita, place 1 lettuce leave inside each pita slices, then fill with the tuna mixture; serve immediately.
Nutrition Info: Per Serving:338.1 Cal, 11.7 g total fat (2.1 g sat. fat), 28.5 g carb., 4.7 g sugar, 5.5 g fiber, 29.4 g protein, and 801.9 mg sodium.

183. Cream Cheese Tart
Servings: 6   Cooking Time: 20 Minutes
Ingredients:
1 cup wheat flour, whole grain
1/3 cup butter, softened
1 cup Mozzarella, shredded
3 tablespoons chives, chopped

½ teaspoon salt
1 tablespoon cream cheese
½ teaspoon ground paprika
4 eggs, beaten
1 teaspoon dried oregano

Directions:
In the mixer bowl combine together flour and salt. Add butter and blend the mixture until you get non-sticky dough or knead it with the help of the fingertips.   Roll up the dough and arrange it in the round tart mold.   Flatten it gently and bake for 10 minutes at 365F.   Meanwhile, mix up together eggs with Mozzarella cheese, cream cheese, and chives.   Remove the tart crust from the oven and chill for 5-10 minutes.   Then place the cheese mixture in the tart crust and flatten it well with the help of a spatula.   Bake the tart for 10 minutes. Use the kitchen torch to make the grilled tart

surface. Chill the cooked tart well and only after this slice it onto the servings.
Nutrition Info: Per Serving:calories 229, fat 14.8, fiber 0.8, carbs 16.7, protein 7.5

184. Cherry Tomato Caper Chicken

Servings: 4   Cooking Time: 1 Hour
Ingredients:

3 tablespoons olive oil	4 chicken breasts
4 garlic cloves, chopped	1 teaspoon capers, chopped
2 cups cherry tomatoes, halved	½ cup black olives, pitted and sliced
	1 thyme sprig

Directions:
Heat the oil in a skillet and add the chicken. Cook on high heat for 5 minutes on each side. Add the rest of the ingredients and season with salt and pepper. Cook in the preheated oven at 350F for 35 minutes. Serve the chicken and the sauce warm and fresh.
Nutrition Info: Per Serving:Calories:320 Fat:19.9g Protein:30.1g Carbohydrates:5.6g

185. Shrimp Pancakes

Servings: 4   Cooking Time: 10 Minutes
Ingredients:

4 eggs, beaten	1 teaspoon olive oil
4 teaspoons sour cream	1/3 cup Mozzarella, shredded
1 cup shrimps, peeled, boiled	½ teaspoon salt
1 teaspoon butter	1 teaspoon dried oregano

Directions:
In the mixing bowl, combine together sour cream, eggs, salt, and dried oregano. Place butter and olive oil in the crepe skillet and heat the ingredients up. Separate the egg liquid into 4 parts. Ladle the first part of the egg liquid in the skillet and flatten it in the shape of crepe. Sprinkle the egg crepe with ¼ part of shrimps and a small amount of Mozzarella. Roast the crepe for 2 minutes from one side and then flip it onto another. Cook the crepe for 30 seconds more. Repeat the same steps with all remaining ingredients.
Nutrition Info: Per Serving:calories 148, fat 8.5, fiber 0.2, carbs 1.5, protein 16.1

186. Herbed Chicken Stew

Servings: 6   Cooking Time: 1 Hour
Ingredients:

3 tablespoons olive oil	2 shallots, chopped
6 chicken legs	½ cup chopped parsley
4 garlic cloves, minced	2 tablespoons lemon juice
2 tablespoons pesto sauce	4 tablespoons vegetable stock
½ cup chopped cilantro	Salt and pepper to taste

Directions:
Heat the oil in a skillet and place the chicken in the hot oil. Cook on each side until golden brown then add the shallots, garlic and pesto sauce. Cook for 2 more minutes then add the rest of the ingredients. Season with salt and pepper and

continue cooking on low heat, covered with a lid, for 30 minutes. Serve the stew warm and fresh.
Nutrition Info: Per Serving:Calories:357 Fat:19.6g Protein:41.4g Carbohydrates:2.0g

187. Spiced Seared Scallops With Lemon Relish

Servings: 4   Cooking Time: 45 Minutes
Ingredients:

2 pounds scallops, cleaned	½ teaspoon ground coriander
½ teaspoon cumin powder	½ teaspoon smoked paprika
¼ teaspoon ground ginger	3 tablespoons olive oil
½ teaspoon salt	

Directions:
Pat the scallops dry with a paper towel. Sprinkle them with spices and salt. Heat the oil in a skillet and place half of the scallops in the hot oil. Cook for 1-2 minutes per side, just until the scallops look golden brown on the sides. Remove the scallops and place the remaining ones in the hot oil. Serve the scallops warm and fresh with your favorite side dish.
Nutrition Info: Per Serving:Calories:292 Fat:12.3g Protein:38.2g Carbohydrates:5.7g

188. White Bean Soup

Servings: 6   Cooking Time: 8 Hours
Ingredients:

1 cup celery, chopped	6 cups veggie stock
1 cup carrots, chopped	½ teaspoon basil, dried
1 yellow onion, chopped	½ teaspoon sage, dried
4 garlic cloves, minced	1 teaspoon thyme, dried
2 cup navy beans, dried	A pinch of salt and black pepper

Directions:
In your slow cooker, combine the beans with the stock and the rest of the ingredients, put the lid on and cook on Low for 8 hours. Divide the soup into bowls and serve right away.
Nutrition Info:calories 264, fat 17.5, fiber 4.5, carbs 23.7, protein 11.5

189. Coriander Pork And Chickpeas Stew

Servings: 4   Cooking Time: 8 Hours
Ingredients:

½ cup beef stock	2 and ½ pounds pork stew meat, cubed
1 tablespoon ginger, grated	1 red onion, chopped
1 teaspoon coriander, ground	4 garlic cloves, minced
2 teaspoons cumin, ground	½ cup apricots, cut into quarters
Salt and black pepper to the taste	15 ounces canned chickpeas, drained
28 ounces canned tomatoes, drained and chopped	1 tablespoon cilantro, chopped

Directions:

In your slow cooker, combine the meat with the stock, ginger and the rest of the ingredients except the cilantro and the chickpeas, put the lid on and cook on Low for 7 hours and 40 minutes. Add the cilantro and the chickpeas, cook the stew on Low for 20 minutes more, divide into bowls and serve.

Nutrition Info: calories 283, fat 11.9, fiber 4.5, carbs 28.8, protein 25.4

190. Crispy Pollock And Gazpacho

Servings: 4   Cooking Time: 15 Minutes

Ingredients:

4 tablespoons olive oil	85 g whole-wheat bread, torn into chunks
4 pieces Pollock fillets, skinless	2 garlic cloves, crushed
4 large tomatoes, cut into chunks	1/2 red onion, thinly sliced
3/4 cucumber, cut into chunks	1 yellow pepper, deseeded, cut into chunks
2 tablespoons sherry vinegar	

Directions:

Preheat the oven to 200C, gas to 6, or fan to 180C. Over a baking tray, scatter the chunks of bread. Toss with 1 tablespoon of the olive oil and bake for about 10 minutes, or until golden and crispy. Meanwhile, mix the cucumber, tomatoes, onion, pepper, crushed garlic, sherry vinegar, and 2 tablespoons of the olive oil; season well. Heat a non-stick large frying pan. Add the remaining 1 tablespoon of the olive oil and heat. When the oil is hot, add the fish; cook for about 4 minutes or until golden. Flip the fillet; cook for additional 1 to 2 minutes or until the fish cooked through. In a mixing bowl, quickly toss the salad and the croutons; divide among 4 plates and then serve with the fish.

Nutrition Info: Per Serving:296 Cal, 13 g total fat (2 g sat. fat), 19 g carb., 9 g sugar, 3 g fiber, 27 g protein, and 0.67 g sodium.

191. Falafel

Servings: 2   Cooking Time: 40 Minutes

Ingredients:

1 pound (about 2 cups) dry chickpeas or garbanzo beans (use dry, DO NOT use canned)	1 3/4 teaspoons salt
	1/4 teaspoon black pepper
	1/4 teaspoon cayenne pepper
1 1/2 tablespoons flour	2 teaspoons cumin
1 small onion, roughly chopped	3-5 cloves garlic, roasted, if desired
1 teaspoon ground coriander	Pinch ground cardamom
1/4 cup fresh parsley, chopped	Canola, grapeseed, peanut oil, or oil with high smoking point, for frying

Directions:

Pour the chickpeas into a large-sized bowl, cover with about 3-inch cold water, and soak overnight. The chickpeas will double to about 4-5 cups after soaking. Drain and then rinse well, pour into a food processor. Except for the oil for frying, add the remaining of the ingredients into the processor; pulse until the texture resembles a coarse meal. Periodically scrape the sides of the processor, pushing the mixture down the sides, process until the mixture resembles a texture that is between couscous and paste, making sure not to over process or they will turn into hummus. Transfer into a bowl. With a fork, stir the mixture, removing any large chickpeas that remained unprocessed. Cover the bowl with a plastic wrap; refrigerate for about 1 to 2 hours. Fill a skillet with 1 1/2-inch worth of oil. Slowly heat the oil over medium flame or heat. Meanwhile, scoop out 2 tablespoons worth of the falafel mixture; with wet hands form it into round ball or slider-shaped. You can make them smaller or larger if you want. They may stick together loosely, but when they start to fry, they will bind nicely. If the balls won't hold, add flour by the 1 tablespoon-worth until they hold. If they still don't hold, add 1-2 eggs. Test the hotness of your oil with 1 piece falafel in the center of the pan. If the oil is at the right temperature the falafel will brown 5-6 minutes total or 2-3 minutes each side. If it browns faster, the oil is too hot. Slightly cool the oil down and then test again. When you reach the right temperature, cook the falafel in 5-6 pieces batches until both sides are golden brown. With a slotted spoon, remove from the skillet, and drain on paper towels. Serve fresh and hot with hummus and then topped with tahini sauce.

Nutrition Info: Per Serving:60 cal., 1.5 g total fat (0 g sat fat), 0 mg chol., 135 mg sodium, 140 mg potassium, 10 g carb., 3 g fiber, 2 g sugar, and 3 g protein.

192. Prosciutto Balls

Servings: 4   Cooking Time: 10 Minutes

Ingredients:

8 Mozzarella balls, cherry size	4 oz bacon, sliced
1/4 teaspoon ground black pepper	3/4 teaspoon dried rosemary
	1 teaspoon butter

Directions:

Sprinkle the sliced bacon with ground black pepper and dried rosemary. Wrap every Mozzarella ball in the sliced bacon and secure them with toothpicks. Melt butter. Brush wrapped Mozzarella balls with butter. Line the tray with the baking paper and arrange Mozzarella balls in it. Bake the meal for 10 minutes at 365F.

Nutrition Info: Per Serving:calories 323, fat 26.8, fiber 0.1, carbs 0.6, protein 20.6

193. Chicken Skillet

Servings: 6   Cooking Time: 35 Minutes

Ingredients:

6 chicken thighs, bone-in and skin-on	1 red onion, chopped
Juice of 2 lemons	2 and 1/2 cups chicken stock
1 teaspoon oregano, dried	1 cup white rice
Salt and black pepper to the taste	1 tablespoon oregano, chopped
1 teaspoon garlic powder	1 cup green olives, pitted and sliced
2 garlic cloves, minced	1/3 cup parsley, chopped
2 tablespoons olive oil	1/2 cup feta cheese, crumbled

Directions:

Heat up a pan with the oil over medium heat, add the chicken thighs skin side down, cook for 4 minutes on each side and transfer to a plate.   Add the garlic and the onion to the pan, stir and sauté for 5 minutes.   Add the rice, salt, pepper, the stock, oregano, and lemon juice, stir, cook for 1-2 minutes more and take off the heat.   Add the chicken to the pan, introduce the pan in the oven and bake at 375 degrees F for 25 minutes.   Add the cheese, olives and the parsley, divide the whole mix between plates and serve for lunch.
Nutrition Info:calories 435, fat 18.5, fiber 13.6, carbs 27.8, protein 25.6

194.   Salmon Bowls

Servings: 4   Cooking Time: 40 Minutes
Ingredients:

2 cups farro	1 garlic cloves, minced
Juice of 2 lemons	
1/3 cup olive oil+ 2 tablespoons	¼ cup parsley, chopped
Salt and black pepper	¼ cup mint, chopped
1 cucumber, chopped	2 tablespoons mustard
¼ cup balsamic vinegar	4 salmon fillets, boneless

Directions:
Put water in a large pot, bring to a boil over medium-high heat, add salt and the farro, stir, simmer for 30 minutes, drain, transfer to a bowl, add the lemon juice, mustard, garlic, salt, pepper and 1/3 cup oil, toss and leave aside for now.   In another bowl, mash the cucumber with a fork, add the vinegar, salt, pepper, the parsley, dill and mint and whisk well.   Heat up a pan with the rest of the oil over medium heat, add the salmon fillets skin side down, cook for 5 minutes on each side, cool them down and break into pieces.   Add over the farro, add the cucumber dressing, toss and serve for lunch.
Nutrition Info:calories 281, fat 12.7, fiber 1.7, carbs 5.8, protein 36.5

195.   Chicken And Parmesan Pasta Pudding

Servings: 10   Cooking Time: 1 ¼ Hours
Ingredients:

3 chicken breasts, cubed	1 cup green peas
2 tablespoons olive oil	1 cup frozen sweet corn
1 teaspoon dried oregano	1 celery stalk, sliced
1 teaspoon dried basil	2 carrots, diced
8 oz. penne	1 cup heavy cream
	6 oz. mozzarella, crumbled

Directions:
Heat the oil in a skillet and add the chicken. Cook for a few minutes on all sides then add the oregano and basil. Cook for another 2 minutes then transfer in a deep dish baking pan.   Cook the penne in a large pot of salty water until al dente, not more than 8 minutes. Drain and place in the baking pan as well.   Stir in the peas, corn, celery and carrots and season with salt and pepper.   Drizzle in the cream and top with mozzarella cheese.   Bake in the preheated oven at 350F for 30 minutes. Serve the pudding warm and fresh.

Nutrition Info: Per Serving:Calories:266 Fat:13.2g Protein:17.7g Carbohydrates:19.8g

196.   Pan-fried Ling With Olive And Tomato

Servings: 4   Cooking Time: 10 Minutes
Ingredients:

800 g baby washed potatoes, steamed	2 truss tomatoes, cut into thin wedges
4 pink ling fillets, skinless	2 tablespoons Wattle Valley Chunky Basil with Cashew and Parmesan Dip
350 g tomato medley, sliced or halved	
3/4 cup Mediterranean mixed pitted olives, coarsely chopped	1/4 cup olive oil
	1/3 cup basil leaves
	1 tablespoon lemon juice
2 tablespoons olive oil spread or butter, divided (I Can't Believe It's Not Butter! ®)	1 tablespoon flat-leaf parsley, chopped

Directions:
Brush both sides of the fillets with 1 tablespoon of the olive oil. Over medium-high heat, heat a nonstick frying skillet or pan. Add the fish, cook per side for about 2 to 3 minutes or until just cooked through.   In a bowl, combine the olives, tomatoes, and basil. In another small bowl, combine the lemon juice, the dip, and the remaining olive oil. In another bowl, toss the potatoes with the spread and the basil. Drizzle the dip and lemon dressing over r the cooked fish; serve with the potatoes and the mixed olive-tomato.
Nutrition Info: Per Serving:543 cal., 30 g fat (9.5 g sat fat), 31.20 g carb., 7 g sugar, 6.3 g fiber, 33.30 g protein, and 623 mg sodium.

197.Mediterranean-style Fish And White-bean Puree

Servings: 4   Cooking Time: 5 Minutes
Ingredients:

4 pieces (about 120 g each) white fish fillets (red snapper or ocean perch)	15 ml olive oils
	30 ml olive oil
	1 tablespoon balsamic vinegar
1 1/2 tablespoons almond flour	1 garlic clove
Salt and pepper, to season	Salt and pepper, to season
1/2 cup Kalamata olives, chopped	2 cans (400 g each) cannellini beans, drained, and rinsed
1 tablespoons fresh oregano, chopped	1/2 cup ground almonds
2 tomatoes, vine-ripened, peeled, seeded, finely chopped	1 tablespoon lemon juice
	1 garlic clove
1 small fennel bulb, finely chopped, reserve fronds	125 ml olive oil
	1 tablespoons fresh oregano, chopped

Directions:
For the puree: Except for the olive oil and the oregano, process the rest of the ingredients in a food processor to combine. With the motor continuously running, add the olive oil in a steady, slow stream. Transfer into a bowl, stir the oregano, and cover with plastic wrap; set aside.   For the olive-tomato mix: In a bowl, place the olives,

fennel, oregano, tomatoes, and garlic. Chop the fennel fronds roughly; add into the olive mixture. Add the vinegar and the olive oil; season with the salt and the pepper and set aside.   For the fish: Season the flour with the salt and the pepper; toss the fish in the coat.   In a frying pan, heat the olive oil over medium heat. Add the fish, cook for about 1 to 2 minutes per side or until cooked through.   Place a spoonful of the bean puree into each serving plate. Place the fish on top of the puree. Divide the salsa between the plates; serve.

Nutrition Info: Per Serving:745 cal., 53 g fat (8 g sat fat), 33 g carb., 5 g sugar, 33 g protein, 65 mg chol., and 705.72 mg sodium.

198.   Spiced Tortilla

Servings: 4   Cooking Time: 20 Minutes

Ingredients:

8 eggs, beaten	300 g cherry tomato
500 g cooked potato, sliced	1 red chili, deseeded, shredded
2 teaspoon curry spice (we used cumin, coriander, and turmeric)	1 onion, sliced
	1 bunch coriander, finely chopped stalks, roughly chopped leaves
1 tablespoon sunflower oil	

Directions:

Preheat the broiler.   In a large oven-safe frying pan, heat the oil. When the oil is hot, add the onion and 1/2 of the red chili; cook for about 5 minutes or until softened.   Add the spices, cook for 1 minute. Add the tomatoes, the potatoes, and the coriander stalks. Stir to mix and distribute. Pour the eggs over the veggies; cook for about 8 to 10 minutes, or until almost set.   Transfer the pan into the broiler; broil for about 1 to 2 minutes until the top is set. Scatter the coriander leaves and the remaining 1/2 chili over the top.   Slice the tortilla into wedges; serve with green Mediterranean salad.

Nutrition Info: Per Serving:327 Cal, 17 g total fat (4 g sat. fat), 27 g carb., 5 g sugar, 3 g fiber, 19 g protein, and 0.69 g sodium.

199.   Yogurt Marinated Pork Chops

Servings: 6   Cooking Time: 2 Hours

Ingredients:

6 pork chops	1 mandarin, sliced
1 cup plain yogurt	1 red pepper, chopped
2 garlic cloves, chopped	Salt and pepper to taste

Directions:

Season the pork with salt and pepper and mix it with the remaining ingredients in a zip lock bag. Marinate for 1 ½ hours in the fridge.   Heat a grill pan over medium flame and cook the pork chops on each side until browned.   Serve the pork chops fresh and warm.

Nutrition Info: Per Serving:Calories:293 Fat:20.4g Protein:20.6g Carbohydrates:4.4g

200.   White Beans And Orange Soup

Servings: 4   Cooking Time: 37 Minutes

Ingredients:

1 yellow onion, chopped	3 orange slices, peeled
5 celery sticks, chopped	30 ounces canned white beans, drained
4 carrots, chopped	2 tablespoons tomato paste
1 cup olive oil	2 cups water
½ teaspoon oregano, dried	6 cups chicken stock
1 bay leaf	

Directions:

Heat up a pot with the oil over medium heat, add the onion, celery, carrots, the bay leaf and the oregano, stir and sauté for 5 minutes.   Add the orange slices and cook for 2 minutes more.   Add the rest of the ingredients, stir, bring to a simmer and cook over medium heat for 30 minutes. Ladle the soup into bowls and serve.

Nutrition Info:calories 273, fat 16.3, fiber 8.4, carbs 15.6, protein 7.4

201. Braised Beef In Oregano-tomato Sauce

Servings: 12   Cooking Time: 1 Hour And 30 Minutes

Ingredients:

2 onions, chopped	1 teaspoon salt
3 celery stalks, diced	3 pounds boneless
4 cloves garlic, minced	beef chuck roast, cut into 1-1/2-inch cubes
2 (28-ounce) cans Italian-style stewed tomatoes	1/2 cup chopped fresh parsley
1 cup dry red wine	1/4 cup vegetable oil
1 teaspoon dried oregano	3/4 teaspoon black pepper

Directions:

Place a pot on medium-high fire and heat for 2 minutes.   Add oil and heat for another 2 minutes. Add beef and brown on all sides.   Around 12 minutes.   Add onions, celery, and garlic, and sauté 5 minutes or until vegetables are tender. Add remaining ingredients and bring to a boil. Reduce heat to low, cover, and simmer for 60 minutes or until beef is fork tender.

Nutrition Info: Calories per Serving: 285; Carbs: 7.4g; Protein: 31.7g; Fats: 14.6g

202. Pork Chops And Herbed Tomato Sauce

Servings: 4   Cooking Time: 10 Minutes

Ingredients:

4 pork loin chops, boneless	¼ cup kalamata olives, pitted and halved
6 tomatoes, peeled and crushed	1 yellow onion, chopped
3 tablespoons parsley, chopped	1 garlic clove, minced
2 tablespoons olive oil	

Directions:

Heat up a pan with the oil over medium heat, add the pork chops, cook them for 3 minutes on each side and divide between plates.   Heat up the same pan again over medium heat, add the tomatoes, parsley and the rest of the ingredients, whisk, simmer for 4 minutes, drizzle over the chops and serve.

Nutrition Info: calories 334, fat 17, fiber 2, carbs 12, protein 34

203. Pita Chicken Burger With Spicy Yogurt

Servings: 4   Cooking Time: 15 Minutes

Ingredients:

½ cup chopped green onions	1 lb ground chicken
½ cup diced tomato	1 tbsp olive oil
½ cup plain low-fat yogurt	1/3 cup Italian seasoned breadcrumbs
½ tsp coarsely ground black pepper	2 cups shredded lettuce
1 ½ tsp chopped fresh oregano	2 large egg whites, lightly beaten
1 tbsp Greek or	2 tsps grated lemon
Moroccan seasoning blend	rind, divided
	4 pcs of 6-inch pitas, cut in half

Directions:

Mix thoroughly the ground chicken, 1 tsp lemon rind, egg whites, black pepper, Greek or Moroccan seasoning and green onions. Equally separate into eight parts and shaping each part into ¼ inch thick patty.   Put fire on medium high and place a large skillet. Fry the patties until browned or for two mins each side. Then slow the fire to medium, cover the skillet and continue cooking for another four minutes.   In a small bowl, mix thoroughly the oregano, yogurt and 1 tsp lemon rind.   To serve, spread the mixture on the pita, add cooked patty, 1 tbsp tomato and ¼ cup lettuce.

Nutrition Info: Calories per Serving: 434.3; Carbs: 44g; Protein: 30.6g; Fat: 15.1g

204. Beef Brisket And Veggies

Servings: 10   Cooking Time: 4 Hours

Ingredients:

3-pound beef brisket	1 teaspoon ground black pepper
1 carrot, peeled, chopped	1 bay leaf
1 onion, peeled	½ cup crushed tomatoes
1 garlic clove, peeled	3 cups of water
1 teaspoon peppercorns	1 celery stalk, chopped
1 teaspoon salt	

Directions:

Place the beef brisket in the saucepan.   Add carrot, onion, garlic clove, peppercorns, salt, ground black pepper, bay leaf, crushed tomatoes, celery stalk, and water.   Close the lid and bring the meat to boil.   Simmer the meal for 4 hours over the medium heat.   Serve the meat poached vegetables.

Nutrition Info: Per Serving: calories 321, fat 10.5, fiber 0.9, carbs 3, protein 50.4

205. Stewed Chicken Greek Style

Servings: 10   Cooking Time: 1 Hour And 15 Minutes

Ingredients:

½ cup red wine	10 small shallots, peeled
1 ½ cups chicken stock or more if needed	2 bay leaves
1 cup olive oil	2 cloves garlic, finely chopped
1 cup tomato sauce	2 tbsp chopped fresh parsley
1 pc, 4lbs whole chicken cut into pieces	2 tsps butter
1 pinch dried oregano or to taste	Salt and ground black pepper to taste

Directions:

Bring to a boil a large pot of lightly salted water. Mix in the shallots and let boil uncovered until tender for around three minutes. Then drain the shallots and dip in cold water until no longer warm. In another large pot over medium fire, heat butter and olive oil until bubbling and melted. Then sauté in the chicken and shallots for 15 minutes or until chicken is cooked and shallots are soft and

translucent. Then add the chopped garlic and cook for three mins more. Then add bay leaves, oregano, salt and pepper, parsley, tomato sauce and the red wine and let simmer for a minute before adding the chicken stock. Stir before covering and let cook for 50 minutes on medium-low fire or until chicken is tender.
Nutrition Info: Calories per Serving: 644.8; Carbs: 8.2g; Protein: 62.1g; Fat: 40.4g

206. Hot Pork Meatballs

Servings: 2   Cooking Time: 10 Minutes
Ingredients:

4 oz pork loin, grinded
½ teaspoon garlic powder
¼ teaspoon chili powder
1 tablespoon water
¼ teaspoon cayenne pepper
¼ teaspoon ground black pepper
¼ teaspoon white pepper
1 teaspoon olive oil

Directions:
Mix up together grinded meat, garlic powder, cayenne pepper, ground black pepper, white pepper, and water. With the help of the fingertips make the small meatballs. Heat up olive oil in the skillet. Arrange the kofte in the oil and cook them for 10 minutes totally. Flip the kofte on another side from time to time.
Nutrition Info: Per Serving:calories 162, fat 10.3, fiber 0.3, carbs 1, protein 15.7

207. Beef And Zucchini Skillet

Servings: 2   Cooking Time: 20 Minutes
Ingredients:

2 oz ground beef
½ onion, sliced
½ bell pepper, sliced
1 tablespoon butter
1 tablespoon tomato sauce
½ teaspoon salt
1 small zucchini, chopped
½ teaspoon dried oregano

Directions:
Place the ground beef in the skillet. Add salt, butter, and dried oregano. Mix up the meat mixture and cook it for 10 minutes. After this, transfer the cooked ground beef in the bowl. Place zucchini, bell pepper, and onion in the skillet (where the ground meat was cooking) and roast the vegetables for 7 minutes over the medium heat or until they are tender. Then add cooked ground beef and tomato sauce. Mix up well. Cook the beef toss for 2-3 minutes over the medium heat.
Nutrition Info: Per Serving:calories 182, fat 8.7, fiber 0.1, carbs 0.3, protein 24.1

208. Greek Chicken Stew

Servings: 8   Cooking Time: 1 Hour And 15minutes
Ingredients:

10 smalls shallots, peeled
1 cup olive oil
2 teaspoons butter
1 (4 pound) whole chicken, cut into pieces
2 cloves garlic, finely chopped
2 tablespoons chopped fresh parsley
salt and ground black pepper to taste
1 pinch dried oregano, or to taste
2 bay leaves
1 ½ cups chicken stock, or more if

½ cup red wine   needed
1 cup tomato sauce
Directions:
In a large pot, fill half full of water and bring to a boil. Lightly salt the water and once boiling add shallots and boil uncovered for 3 minutes. Drain and quickly place on an ice bath for 5 minutes. Drain well. In same pot, heat for 3 minutes and add oil and butter. Heat for 3 minutes. Add chicken and shallots. Cook 15 minutes. Add chopped garlic and cook for another 3 minutes or until garlic starts to turn golden. Add red wine and tomato sauce. Deglaze pot. Stir in bay leaves, oregano, pepper, salt, and parsley. Cook for 3 minutes. Stir in chicken stock. Cover and simmer for 40 minutes while occasionally stirring pot. Serve and enjoy while hot with a side of rice if desired.
Nutrition Info: Calories per Serving: 574; Carbs: 6.8g; Protein: 31.8g; Fats: 45.3g

209. Meatloaf

Servings: 6   Cooking Time: 35 Minutes
Ingredients:

2 lbs ground beef
2 eggs, lightly beaten
1/4 tsp dried basil
3 tbsp olive oil
1 1/2 tsp dried parsley
1/2 tsp dried sage
1 tsp oregano
2 tsp thyme
1 tsp rosemary
Pepper
Salt

Directions:
Pour 1 1/2 cups of water into the instant pot then place the trivet in the pot. Spray loaf pan with cooking spray. Add all ingredients into the mixing bowl and mix until well combined. Transfer meat mixture into the prepared loaf pan and place loaf pan on top of the trivet in the pot. Seal pot with lid and cook on high for 35 minutes. Once done, allow to release pressure naturally for 10 minutes then release remaining using quick release. Remove lid. Serve and enjoy.
Nutrition Info: Calories 365 Fat 18 g Carbohydrates 0.7 g Sugar 0.1 g Protein 47.8 g Cholesterol 190 mg

210. Tasty Lamb Ribs

Servings: 4   Cooking Time: 2 Hours
Ingredients:

2 garlic cloves, minced
¼ cup shallot, chopped
2 tablespoons fish sauce
2 tablespoons olive oil
1 and ½ tablespoons lemon juice
½ cup veggie stock
1 tablespoon coriander seeds, ground
1 tablespoon ginger, grated
Salt and black pepper to the taste
2 pounds lamb ribs

Directions:
In a roasting pan, combine the lamb with the garlic, shallots and the rest of the ingredients, toss, introduce in the oven at 300 degrees F and cook for 2 hours. Divide the lamb between plates and serve with a side salad.
Nutrition Info:calories 293, fat 9.1, fiber 9.6, carbs 16.7, protein 24.2

211. Peas And Ham Thick Soup

Servings: 4   Cooking Time: 30 Minutes

Ingredients:
Pepper and salt to taste
1 lb. ham, coarsely chopped
24 oz frozen sweet peas
4 cup ham stock

¼ cup white wine
1 carrot, chopped coarsely
1 onion, chopped coarsely
2 tbsp butter, divided

Directions:
On medium fireplace a medium pot and heat oil. Sauté for 6 minutes the onion or until soft and translucent. Add wine and cook for 4 minutes or until nearly evaporated. Add ham stock and bring to a simmer and simmer continuously while covered for 4 minutes. Add peas and cook for 7 minutes or until tender. Meanwhile, in a nonstick fry pan, cook to a browned crisp the ham in 1 tbsp butter, around 6 minutes. Remove from fire and set aside. When peas are soft, transfer to a blender and puree. Return to pot, continue cooking while seasoning with pepper, salt and ½ of crisped ham. Once soup is to your desired taste, turn off fire. Transfer to 4 serving bowls and garnish evenly with crisped ham.
Nutrition Info: Calories per Serving: 403; Carbs: 32.5g; Protein: 37.3g; Fat: 12.5g

---

212.	Bell Peppers On Chicken Breasts

Servings: 6   Cooking Time: 30 Minutes
Ingredients:
¼ tsp freshly ground black pepper
½ tsp salt
1 large red bell pepper, cut into ¼-inch strips
1 large yellow bell pepper, cut into ¼-inch strips
1 tsp chopped fresh oregano
2 1/3 cups coarsely chopped tomato

1 tbsp olive oil
2 tbsp finely chopped fresh flat-leaf parsley
20 Kalamata olives
3 cups onion sliced crosswise
6 4-oz skinless, boneless chicken breast halves, cut in half horizontally
Cooking spray

Directions:
On medium high fire, place a large nonstick fry pan and heat oil. Once oil is hot, sauté onions until soft and translucent, around 6 to 8 minutes. Add bell peppers and sauté for another 10 minutes or until tender. Add black pepper, salt and tomato. Cook until tomato juice has evaporated, around 7 minutes. Add olives, oregano and parsley, cook until heated through around 1 to 2 minutes. Transfer to a bowl and keep warm. Wipe pan with paper towel and grease with cooking spray. Return to fire and place chicken breasts. Cook for three minutes per side or until desired doneness is reached. If needed, cook chicken in batches. When cooking the last batch of chicken is done, add back the previous batch of chicken and the onion-bell pepper mixture and cook for a minute or two while tossing chicken to coat well in the onion-bell pepper mixture. Serve and enjoy.
Nutrition Info: Calories per Serving: 261.8; Carbs: 11.0g; Protein: 36.0g; Fat: 8.2g

---

213.	Yummy Turkey Meatballs

Servings: 4   Cooking Time: 25 Minutes
Ingredients:

¼ yellow onion, finely diced
1 14-oz can of artichoke hearts, diced
1 lb. ground turkey

1 tsp dried parsley
1 tsp oil
4 tbsp fresh basil, finely chopped
Pepper and salt to taste

Directions:
Grease a cookie sheet and preheat oven to 350⁰F. On medium fire, place a nonstick medium saucepan and sauté artichoke hearts and diced onions for 5 minutes or until onions are soft. Remove from fire and let cool. Meanwhile, in a big bowl, mix with hands parsley, basil and ground turkey. Season to taste. Once onion mixture has cooled add into the bowl and mix thoroughly. With an ice cream scooper, scoop ground turkey and form into balls, makes around 6 balls. Place on prepped cookie sheet, pop in the oven and bake until cooked through around 15-20 minutes. Remove from pan, serve and enjoy.
Nutrition Info: Calories per Serving: 328; Carbs: 11.8g; Protein: 33.5g; Fat: 16.3g

---

214.	Garlic Caper Beef Roast

Servings: 4   Cooking Time: 40 Minutes
Ingredients:
2 lbs beef roast, cubed
1 tbsp fresh parsley, chopped
1 tbsp capers, chopped
1 tbsp garlic, minced
1 cup chicken stock

1/2 tsp dried rosemary
1/2 tsp ground cumin
1 onion, chopped
1 tbsp olive oil
Pepper
Salt

Directions:
Add oil into the instant pot and set the pot on sauté mode. Add garlic and onion and sauté for 5 minutes. Add meat and cook until brown. Add remaining ingredients and stir well. Seal pot with lid and cook on high for 30 minutes. Once done, allow to release pressure naturally. Remove lid. Stir well and serve.
Nutrition Info: Calories 470 Fat 17.9 g Carbohydrates 3.9 g Sugar 1.4 g Protein 69.5 g Cholesterol 203 mg

---

215.	Olive Oil Drenched Lemon Chicken

Servings: 4   Cooking Time: 60 Minutes
Ingredients:
1 lemon, thinly sliced
1 red bell pepper, cut into 1-inch wide strips
1 red onion, cut into 1-inch wedges
1 tablespoon dried oregano
1/2 teaspoon coarsely ground black pepper
1/4 cup olive oil

2 tablespoons fresh lemon juice
2 tablespoons fresh lemon zest
3/4 teaspoon salt
4 large cloves garlic, pressed
4 skinless, boneless chicken breast halves
8 baby red potatoes, halved

Directions:
Preheat oven to 400⁰F. In a bowl, mix well pepper, salt, oregano, garlic, lemon zest, lemon juice, and olive oil. In a 9 x 13-inch casserole dish, evenly spread chicken in a single layer. Brush lemon juice mixture over chicken. In a bowl mix well lemon slices, red onion, bell pepper, and potatoes. Drizzle remaining olive oil sauce and toss

well to coat. Arrange vegetables and lemon slices around chicken breasts in baking dish.   Bake for 50 minutes; brush chicken and vegetables with pan drippings halfway through cooking time.   Let chicken rest for ten minutes before serving.
Nutrition Info: Calories per Serving: 517; Carbs: 65.1g; Protein: 30.8g; Fats: 16.7g

216.   Beef Spread

Servings: 4   Cooking Time: 25 Minutes
Ingredients:

8 oz beef liver	1 bay leaf
½ onion, peeled	½ teaspoon salt
½ carrot, peeled	1/3 cup water
½ teaspoon peppercorns	1 teaspoon ground black pepper

Directions:
Chop the beef liver and put it in the saucepan. Add onion, carrot, peppercorns, bay leaf, salt, and ground black pepper.   Add water and close the lid. Boil the beef liver for 25 minutes or until all ingredients are tender.   Transfer the cooked mixture in the blender and blend it until smooth. Then place the cooked pate in the serving bowl and flatten the surface of it.   Refrigerate the pate for 20-30 minutes before serving.
Nutrition Info: Per Serving:calories 109, fat 2.7, fiber 0.6, carbs 5.3, protein 15.3

217.Pork Chops And Relish

Servings: 6   Cooking Time: 14 Minutes
Ingredients:

6 pork chops, boneless	1 and ½ cups tomatoes, cubed
7 ounces marinated artichoke hearts, chopped and their liquid reserved	1 jalapeno pepper, chopped
A pinch of salt and black pepper	½ cup roasted bell peppers, chopped
1 teaspoon hot pepper sauce	½ cup black olives, pitted and sliced

Directions:
In a bowl, mix the chops with the pepper sauce, reserved liquid from the artichokes, cover and keep in the fridge for 15 minutes.   Heat up a grill over medium-high heat, add the pork chops and cook for 7 minutes on each side.   In a bowl, combine the artichokes with the peppers and the remaining ingredients, toss, divide on top of the chops and serve.
Nutrition Info:calories 215, fat 6, fiber 1, carbs 6, protein 35

218.   Tasty Beef Goulash

Servings: 2   Cooking Time: 30 Minutes
Ingredients:

1/2 lb beef stew meat, cubed	1/4 zucchini, chopped
1 tbsp olive oil	1/2 cabbage, sliced
1/2 onion, chopped	1 1/2 tbsp olive oil
1/2 cup sun-dried tomatoes, chopped	2 cups chicken broth
	Pepper
	Salt

Directions:
Add oil into the instant pot and set the pot on sauté mode.   Add onion and sauté for 3-5 minutes. Add tomatoes and cook for 5 minutes.   Add remaining ingredients and stir well.   Seal pot

with lid and cook on high for 20 minutes.   Once done, allow to release pressure naturally for 10 minutes then release remaining using quick release. Remove lid.   Stir well and serve.
Nutrition Info: Calories 389 Fat 15.8 g Carbohydrates 19.3 g Sugar 10.7 g Protein 43.2 g Cholesterol 101 mg

219.   Beef And Grape Sauce

Servings: 4   Cooking Time: 25 Minutes
Ingredients:

1-pound beef sirloin	1 teaspoon soy sauce
1 teaspoon molasses	¼ teaspoon fresh ginger, minced
1 tablespoon lemon zest, grated	1 cup grape juice
1 chili pepper, chopped	½ teaspoon salt
	1 tablespoon butter

Directions:
Sprinkle the beef sirloin with salt and minced ginger.   Heat up butter in the saucepan and add meat.   Roast it for 5 minutes from each side over the medium heat.   After this, add soy sauce, chili pepper, and grape juice.   Then add lemon zest and simmer the meat for 10 minutes.   Add molasses and mix up meat well.   Close the lid and cook meat for 5 minutes.   Serve the cooked beef with grape juice sauce.
Nutrition Info: Per Serving:calories 267, fat 10, fiber 0.2, carbs 7.4, protein 34.9

220.   Lamb And Tomato Sauce

Servings: 3   Cooking Time: 55 Minutes
Ingredients:

9 oz lamb shanks	1 teaspoon ground black pepper
1 onion, diced	
1 carrot, diced	1 ½ cup chicken stock
1 tablespoon olive oil	
1 teaspoon salt	1 tablespoon tomato paste

Directions:
Sprinkle the lamb shanks with salt and ground black pepper.   Heat up olive oil in the saucepan. Add lamb shanks and roast them for 5 minutes from each side.   Transfer meat in the plate. After this, add onion and carrot in the saucepan. Roast the vegetables for 3 minutes.   Add tomato paste and mix up well.   Then add chicken stock and bring the liquid to boil.   Add lamb shanks, stir well, and close the lid.   Cook the meat for 40 minutes over the medium-low heat.
Nutrition Info: Per Serving:calories 232, fat 11.3, fiber 1.7, carbs 7.3, protein 25.1

221.   Lamb And Sweet Onion Sauce

Servings: 4   Cooking Time: 40 Minutes
Ingredients:

2 pounds lamb meat, cubed	4 garlic cloves, minced
1 tablespoon sweet paprika	2 tablespoons olive oil
Salt and black pepper to the taste	1 pound sweet onion, chopped
1 and ½ cups veggie stock	1 cup balsamic vinegar

Directions:
Heat up a pot with the oil over medium heat, add the onion, vinegar, salt and pepper, stir and cook

for 10 minutes.   Add the meat and the rest of the ingredients, toss, bring to a simmer and cook over medium heat for 30 minutes.   Divide the mix between plates and serve.
Nutrition Info:calories 303, fat 12.3, fiber 7.1, carbs 15.2, protein 17.0

222.	Pork And Mustard Shallots Mix

Servings: 4   Cooking Time: 25 Minutes
Ingredients:

3 shallots, chopped	A pinch of salt and
1 pound pork loin, cut into strips	black pepper
½ cup veggie stock	2 teaspoons mustard
2 tablespoons olive oil	1 tablespoon parsley, chopped

Directions:
Heat up a pan with the oil over medium-high heat, add the shallots and sauté for 5 minutes.   Add the meat and cook for 10 minutes tossing it often. Add the rest of the ingredients, toss, cook for 10 minutes more, divide between plates and serve right away.
Nutrition Info:calories 296, fat 12.4, fiber 9.3, carbs 13.5, protein 22.5

223.	Rosemary Lamb

Servings: 4   Cooking Time: 6 Hours
Ingredients:

2 pounds lamb shoulder, cubed	3 garlic cloves, minced
1 tablespoon rosemary, chopped	4 bay leaves
½ cup lamb stock	Salt and black pepper to the taste

Directions:
In your slow cooker, combine the lamb with the rosemary and the rest of the ingredients, put the lid on and cook on High for 6 hours.   Divide the mix between palates and serve.
Nutrition Info:calories 292, fat 13.2, fiber 11.6, carbs 18.3, protein 14.2

224.	Mouth-watering Lamb Stew

Servings: 4   Cooking Time: 180 Minutes
Ingredients:

½ cup golden raisins	2 cups beef stock or lamb stock
1 cup dates, cut in half	Pepper and salt to taste
1 cup dried figs, cut in half	¼ tsp ground cloves
1 lb. lamb shoulder, trimmed of fat and cut into 2-inch cubes	½ tsp ground black pepper
1 onion, minced	1 tsp ground turmeric
1 tbsp fresh coriander, roughly chopped	1 tsp ground nutmeg
	1 tsp ground allspice
1 tbsp honey, optional	1 tsp ground cinnamon
1 tbsp olive oil	2 tsp ground mace
1 tbsp Ras el Hanout	2 tsp ground cardamom
2 cloves garlic, minced	2 tsp ground ginger
	½ tsp anise seeds'1/2 tsp ground cayenne pepper

Directions:

Preheat oven to 3000F.   In small bowl, add all Ras el Hanout ingredients and mix thoroughly. Just get what the ingredients need and store remaining in a tightly lidded spice jar.   On high fire, place a heavy bottomed medium pot and heat olive oil. Once hot, brown lamb pieces on each side for around 3 to 4 minutes.   Lower fire to medium high and add remaining ingredients, except for the coriander.   Mix well. Season with pepper and salt to taste. Cover pot and bring to a boil.   Once boiling, turn off fire, and pop pot into oven.   Bake uncovered for 2 to 2.5 hours or until meat is fork tender.   Once meat is tender, remove from oven. To serve, sprinkle fresh coriander, and enjoy.
Nutrition Info: Calories per Serving: 633.4; Carbs: 78.1g; Protein: 33.0g; Fat: 21.0g

225.	Beef With Tomatoes

Servings: 4   Cooking Time: 40 Minutes
Ingredients:

2 lb beef roast, sliced	1 cup beef stock
1 tbsp chives, chopped	1 tbsp oregano, chopped
1 tsp garlic, minced	1 cup tomatoes, chopped
1/2 tsp chili powder	
2 tbsp olive oil	Pepper
1 onion, chopped	Salt

Directions:
Add oil into the instant pot and set the pot on sauté mode.   Add garlic, onion, and chili powder and sauté for 5 minutes.   Add meat and cook for 5 minutes.   Add remaining ingredients and stir well.   Seal pot with lid and cook on high for 30 minutes.   Once done, allow to release pressure naturally for 10 minutes then release remaining using quick release. Remove lid.   Stir well and serve.
Nutrition Info: Calories 511 Fat 21.6 g Carbohydrates 5.6 g Sugar 2.5 g Protein 70.4 g Cholesterol 203 mg

226.	Chicken Thighs With Butternut Squash

Servings: 6   Cooking Time: 30 Minutes
Ingredients:

3 cups butternut squash, cubed	½ pound bacon
6 boneless chicken thighs	Extra coconut oil for frying
A sprig of fresh sage, chopped	Salt and pepper to taste

Directions:
Preheat the oven to 425F.   In a skillet, fry the bacon over medium heat until crisp. Set aside then crumble.   In the same skillet, sauté the butternut squash and season with salt and pepper to taste. Once the squash is cooked, remove from the skillet and set aside.   Using the same skillet, add coconut oil and cook the chicken thighs for 10 minutes on each side.   Season with salt and pepper and add the squash back.   Remove the skillet from the stove and bake in the oven for 15 minutes.   Garnish with bacon.
Nutrition Info: Calories per Serving: 315.3; Carbs: 11.3g; Protein: 25.0g; Fat: 18.9g

227.	Lamb And Peanuts Mix

Servings: 4   Cooking Time: 20 Minutes
Ingredients:

2 tablespoons lime juice
1 tablespoon balsamic vinegar
5 garlic cloves, minced
2 tablespoons olive oil

Salt and black pepper to the taste
1 and ½ pound lamb meat, cubed
3 tablespoons peanuts, toasted and chopped
2 scallions, chopped

Directions:
Heat up a pan with the oil over medium-high heat, add the meat, and cook for 4 minutes on each side. Add the scallions and the garlic and sauté for 2 minutes more.   Add the rest of the ingredients, toss cook for 10 minutes more, divide between plates and serve right away.
Nutrition Info:calories 300, fat 14.5, fiber 9.1, carbs 15.7, protein 17.5

228.   Grilled Chicken Breasts

Servings: 4   Cooking Time: 15 Minutes
Ingredients:
4 boneless skinless chicken breast halves
3 tablespoons lemon juice
3 tablespoons olive oil
3 tablespoons chopped fresh parsley

3 garlic cloves, crushed and minced
1 teaspoon paprika
1 /2 teaspoon dried oregano
1/2 teaspoon salt
1/2 teaspoon pepper

Directions:
In a large Ziplock bag, mix well oregano, paprika, garlic, parsley, olive oil, and lemon juice.   Pierce chicken with knife several times and sprinkle with salt and pepper.   Add chicken to bag and marinate 20 minutes or up to two days in the fridge. Remove chicken from bag and grill for 5 minutes per side in a 350oF preheated grill.   Remove chicken from grill and let it stand on a plate for 5 minutes before slicing.   Serve and enjoy with a side of rice or salad.
Nutrition Info: Calories per Serving: 485; Carbs: 2.7g; Protein: 72.8g; Fats: 19.3g

229.   Grilled Veggies And Chicken

Servings: 3   Cooking Time: 20 Minutes
Ingredients:
¼ teaspoon cayenne pepper
½ teaspoon garlic granules
½ teaspoon onion powder
1 cup organic tomatoes, blended
1 red onion
1 red pepper, chopped
1 tablespoon vinegar
1 teaspoon Italian seasoning

1 teaspoon rosemary
1 yellow squash, chopped
1 zucchini, chopped
1-pound organic chicken breast
2 cups fresh cherry tomatoes, halved
4 tablespoon extra-virgin olive oil
Pepper to taste
Salt to taste

Directions:
Marinade the chicken by mixing together 1 tablespoon of extra virgin olive oil, Italian seasoning, and rosemary. Season with salt the set aside for at least 2 hours.   In another bowl, make the salad by combining the red onion, fresh cherry tomatoes, red pepper, squash and zucchini. Add 1 tablespoon of extra virgin olive oil and season with salt and pepper to taste. Place inside a greased

tinfoil then set aside.   Prepare the grill and heat it to 350F. Cook the chicken breast and let it cook for 7 minutes on each side. Place the tinfoil with the veggies on the grill and cook it for five to 7 minutes. Meanwhile, make the vinaigrette my combining the cayenne pepper, onion powder, garlic granules, vinegar and blended organic tomatoes in a food processor. Add 2 tablespoon of extra virgin olive oil and season with salt and pepper to taste.
Nutrition Info: Calories per Serving: 363.6; Carbs: 14.2g; Protein: 45.2g; Fat: 14.0g

230.   Oregano-smoked Paprika Baked Chicken

Servings: 2   Cooking Time: 40 Minutes
Ingredients:
1 tbsp dried oregano
1 tsp freshly ground black pepper
1 tsp Himalayan salt
2 green onions, sliced
2 large boneless, skinless chicken breasts (about 400g/14oz each)

1 tsp smoked paprika
2 jalapeño peppers, seeded and sliced
2 medium tomatoes, diced
6 mini bell peppers of assorted colors, seeded and chopped
The juice of 1 lime

Directions:
Preheat oven to 450°F.   Mix all the spices in a small bowl. Rub all over chicken breasts.   Lightly grease an oven-proof dish with olive oil.   Place the chicken breasts in the dish and arrange the vegetables around it.   Cover with aluminum foil and bake for 35 minutes.   Set the oven to broil, remove the foil and cook under the broiler about 5 minutes, or until the chicken becomes golden brown.   Let the chicken rest for 5 minutes before slicing and serving.
Nutrition Info: Calories per Serving: 286; Carbs: 14.1g; Protein: 45.1g; Fats: 5.5g

231.   Cheddar Lamb And Zucchinis

Servings: 4   Cooking Time: 30 Minutes
Ingredients:
1 pound lamb meat, cubed
1 tablespoon avocado oil
2 cups zucchinis, chopped
½ cup red onion, chopped

Salt and black pepper to the taste
15 ounces canned roasted tomatoes, crushed
¾ cup cheddar cheese, shredded

Directions:
Heat up a pan with the oil over medium-high heat, add the meat and the onion and brown for 5 minutes.   Add the rest of the ingredients except the cheese, bring to a simmer and cook over medium heat for 20 minutes.   Add the cheese, cook everything for 5 minutes more, divide between plates and serve.
Nutrition Info:calories 306, fat 16.4, fiber 12.3, carbs 15.5, protein 18.5

232.   Fennel Pork

Servings: 4   Cooking Time: 2 Hours
Ingredients:
2 pork loin roast, trimmed, and boneless
Salt and black pepper to the taste

2 teaspoons fennel, ground
1 tablespoon fennel seeds
2 teaspoons red

3 garlic cloves, minced
pepper, crushed
¼ cup olive oil

Directions:
In a roasting pan, combine the pork with salt, pepper and the rest of the ingredients, toss, introduce in the oven and bake at 380 degrees F for 2 hours. Slice the roast, divide between plates and serve with a side salad.
Nutrition Info:calories 300, fat 4, fiber 2, carbs 6, protein 15

| 233. | Lamb And Feta Artichokes |

Servings: 6   Cooking Time: 8 Hours And 5 Minutes

Ingredients:
2 pounds lamb shoulder, boneless and roughly cubed
2 spring onions, chopped
1 tablespoon olive oil
3 garlic cloves, minced
1 tablespoon lemon juice
Salt and black pepper to the taste
1 and ½ cups veggie stock
6 ounces canned artichoke hearts, drained and quartered
½ cup feta cheese, crumbled
2 tablespoons parsley, chopped

Directions:
Heat up a pan with the oil over medium-high heat, add the lamb, brown 5 minutes and transfer to your slow cooker. Add the rest of the ingredients except the parsley and the cheese, put the lid on and cook on Low for 8 hours. Add the cheese and the parsley, divide the mix between plates and serve.
Nutrition Info:calories 330, fat 14.5, fiber 14.1, carbs 21.7, protein 17.5

| 234. | Lamb And Plums Mix |

Servings: 4   Cooking Time: 6 Hours And 10 Minutes

Ingredients:
4 lamb shanks
1 red onion, chopped
2 tablespoons olive oil
1 cup plums, pitted and halved
1 tablespoon sweet paprika
2 cups chicken stock
Salt and pepper to the taste

Directions:
Heat up a pan with the oil over medium-high heat, add the lamb, brown for 5 minutes on each side and transfer to your slow cooker. Add the rest of the ingredients, put the lid on and cook on High for 6 hours. Divide the mix between plates and serve right away.
Nutrition Info:calories 293, fat 13.2, fiber 9.7, carbs 15.7, protein 14.3

| 235. | Lamb And Mango Sauce |

Servings: 4   Cooking Time: 1 Hour

Ingredients:
2 cups Greek yogurt
1 cup mango, peeled and cubed
1 yellow onion, chopped
1/3 cup parsley,
½ teaspoon red pepper flakes
Salt and black pepper to the taste
2 tablespoons olive

chopped
1 pound lamb, cubed
oil
¼ teaspoon cinnamon powder

Directions:
Heat up a pan with the oil over medium-high heat, add the meat and brown for 5 minutes. Add the onion and sauté for 5 minutes more. Add the rest of the ingredients, toss, bring to a simmer and cook over medium heat for 45 minutes. Divide everything between plates and serve.
Nutrition Info:calories 300, fat 15.5, fiber 9.1, carbs 15.7, protein 15.5

| 236. | Pork Chops And Cherries Mix |

Servings: 4   Cooking Time: 12 Minutes

Ingredients:
4 pork chops, boneless
Salt and black pepper to the taste
½ cup cranberry juice
1 and ½ teaspoons spicy mustard
½ cup dark cherries, pitted and halved
Cooking spray

Directions:
Heat up a pan greased with the cooking spray over medium-high heat, add the pork chops, cook them for 5 minutes on each side and divide between plates. Heat up the same pan over medium heat, add the cranberry juice and the rest of the ingredients, whisk, bring to a simmer, cook for 2 minutes, drizzle over the pork chops and serve.
Nutrition Info:calories 262, fat 8, fiber 1, carbs 16, protein 30

| 237. | Lamb And Barley Mix |

Servings: 4   Cooking Time: 8 Hours And 10 Minutes

Ingredients:
2 tablespoons olive oil
1 cup barley soaked overnight, drained and rinsed
1 pound lamb meat, cubed
4 garlic cloves, minced
1 red onion, chopped
3 carrots, chopped
6 tablespoons dill, chopped
2 tablespoons tomato paste
3 cups veggie stock
A pinch of salt and black pepper

Directions:
Heat up a pan with the oil over medium-high heat, add the meat, brown for 5 minutes on each side and transfer to your slow cooker. Add the barley and the rest of the ingredients, put the lid on and cook on Low for 8 hours. Divide everything between plates and serve.
Nutrition Info:calories 292, fat 12.1, fiber 8.7, carbs 16.7, protein 7.2

| 238. | Cashew Beef Stir Fry |

Servings: 8   Cooking Time: 15 Minutes

Ingredients:
¼ cup coconut aminos
1 ½ pound ground beef
1 cup raw cashews
1 green bell pepper, julienned
1 red bell pepper, julienned
1 small onion, sliced
1 tablespoon garlic, minced
2 tablespoon ginger, grated
2 teaspoon coconut oil
Salt and pepper to taste

1 small can water
chestnut, sliced
Directions:
Heat a skillet over medium heat then add raw
cashews. Toast for a couple of minutes or until
slightly brown. Set aside.   In the same skillet,
add the coconut oil and sauté the ground beef for 5
minutes or until brown.   Add the garlic, ginger
and season with coconut aminos. Stir for one
minute before adding the onions, bell peppers and
water chestnuts. Cook until the vegetables are
almost soft.   Season with salt and pepper to taste.
Add the toasted cashews last.
Nutrition Info: Calories per Serving: 324.8; Carbs:
12.4g; Protein: 19.3g; Fat: 22.0g

---

239.   Cheesy Meat Bake

Servings: 4   Cooking Time: 40 Minutes
Ingredients:

6 oz pork butt, chopped	¼ cup carrot, grated
3 oz veal stew meat, chopped	2 oz Provolone cheese, grated
1 potato, peeled	¼ cup cream
¼ cup cauliflower, shredded	1 teaspoon butter
1 teaspoon tomato paste	1 teaspoon salt
	½ teaspoon chili flakes

Directions:
Melt butter in the saucepan and add all meat.
Sprinkle it with salt, chili flakes, and carrot.   Mix
up well and cook for 10 minutes.   Then add
tomato paste and mix up well.   Add shredded
cauliflower and roughly chopped potato.   Then
add cream and top it with cheese.   Cover the
saucepan with foil and transfer it in the preheated
to the 365F oven.   Bake the casserole for 30
minutes.
Nutrition Info: Per Serving:calories 211, fat 9,
fiber 1.3, carbs 9.5, protein 22.4

---

240.   Shrimp And Vegetable Rice

Servings: 1 Cup   Cooking Time: 48 Minutes
Ingredients:

3 TB. extra-virgin olive oil	1 cup green peas
1 medium yellow onion, finely chopped	4 cups water
1 TB. minced garlic	2 tsp. salt
2 medium carrots, shredded (1 cup)	10 strands saffron
	1 tsp. turmeric
	1/2 tsp. black pepper
	2 cups brown rice

Directions:
1/2 lb. medium raw shrimp (18 to 20), shells and
veins removed   In a large, 3-quart pot over
medium heat, heat extra-virgin olive oil. Add
yellow onion, and cook for 5 minutes.   Add garlic,
green peas, and carrots, and cook for 3 minutes.
Add water, salt, saffron, turmeric, and black pepper;
bring to a boil; and cook for about 3 minutes.
Add brown rice, cover, reduce heat to low, and cook
for 30 minutes.   Gently fold shrimp into rice,
cover, and cook for 10 minutes.   Remove from
heat, fluff with a fork, cover, and set aside for 10
minutes. Serve warm.

---

241.   Nutmeg Lamb Mix

Servings: 6   Cooking Time: 30 Minutes
Ingredients:

1 red onion, chopped	¾ cup celery, chopped
1 tablespoon olive oil	
1 garlic clove, minced	29 ounces canned tomatoes, drained and chopped
1 pound lamb meat, cubed	
Salt and black pepper to the taste	1 cup veggie stock
	½ teaspoon nutmeg, ground
	2 teaspoons parsley, chopped

Directions:
Heat up a pan with the oil over medium heat, add
the onion and the garlic and sauté for 5 minutes.
Add the meat and brown for 5 minutes more.
Add the rest of the ingredients, bring to a simmer
and cook over medium heat for 20 minutes.
Divide everything between plates and serve.
Nutrition Info:calories 284, fat 13.3, fiber 8.2,
carbs 14.5, protein 17.6

---

242.   Lamb And Zucchini Mix

Servings: 4   Cooking Time: 4 Hours
Ingredients:

2 pounds lamb stew meat, cubed	3 zucchinis, sliced
1 and ½ tablespoons avocado oil	1 tablespoon thyme, dried
1 brown onion, chopped	2 teaspoons sage, dried
3 garlic cloves, minced	1 cup chicken stock
	2 tablespoons tomato paste

Directions:
In a slow cooker, combine the lamb with the oil,
zucchinis and the rest of the ingredients, toss, put
the lid on and cook on High for 4 hours.   Divide
the mix between plates and serve right away.
Nutrition Info:calories 272, fat 14.5, fiber 10.1,
carbs 20.3, protein 13.3

---

243.   Pork And Green Beans Mix

Servings: 5   Cooking Time: 35 Minutes
Ingredients:

1 cup ground pork	½ teaspoon cayenne pepper
1 sweet pepper, chopped	
1 oz green beans, chopped	1 teaspoon dried oregano
½ onion, sliced	½ teaspoon dried basil
2 oz Parmesan, grated	
¼ cup chicken stock	1 teaspoon paprika
1 teaspoon olive oil	½ cup crushed tomatoes, canned

Directions:
Pour olive oil in the saucepan and heat it up.
Add ground pork and cook it for 2 minutes.
Then stir it carefully and sprinkle with cayenne
pepper, dried oregano, dried basil, and paprika.
Roast the meat for 5 minutes more and add green
beans, sweet pepper, and sliced onion.   Add
chicken stock and crushed tomatoes.   Mix up the
ground pork and close the lid.   Cook the meal for
20 minutes over the medium heat. Stir it from time
to time.   Then sprinkle the bolognese meat with
Parmesan and mix up well.   Cook the meal for 5
minutes more.
Nutrition Info: Per Serving:calories 257, fat 16.6,
fiber 1.9, carbs 6.2, protein 20.9

244. Artichoke Beef Roast

Servings: 6   Cooking Time: 45 Minutes

Ingredients:

2 lbs beef roast, cubed	1 tbsp capers, chopped
1 tbsp garlic, minced	10 oz can artichokes, drained and chopped
1 onion, chopped	2 cups chicken stock
1/2 tsp paprika	1 tbsp olive oil
1 tbsp parsley, chopped	Pepper
2 tomatoes, chopped	Salt

Directions:

Add oil into the instant pot and set the pot on sauté mode.   Add garlic and onion and sauté for 5 minutes.   Add meat and cook until brown. Add remaining ingredients and stir well.   Seal pot with lid and cook on high for 35 minutes. Once done, allow to release pressure naturally. Remove lid.   Serve and enjoy.

Nutrition Info: Calories 344 Fat 12.2 g Carbohydrates 9.2 g Sugar 2.6 g Protein 48.4 g Cholesterol 135 mg

245. Oregano And Pesto Lamb

Servings: 4   Cooking Time: 25 Minutes

Ingredients:

2 pounds pork shoulder, boneless and cubed	3 garlic cloves, minced
1/4 cup olive oil	2 teaspoons basil pesto
2 teaspoons oregano, dried	Salt and black pepper to the taste
1/4 cup lemon juice	

Directions:

Heat up a pan with the oil over medium-high heat, add the pork and brown for 5 minutes.   Add the rest of the ingredients, cook for 20 minutes more, tossing the mix from time to time, divide between plates and serve.

Nutrition Info:calories 297, fat 14.5, fiber 9.3, carbs 16.8, protein 22.2

246. Italian Beef Roast

Servings: 6   Cooking Time: 50 Minutes

Ingredients:

2 1/2 lbs beef roast, cut into chunks	2 tbsp olive oil
1 cup chicken broth	2 celery stalks, chopped
1 cup red wine	1 tsp garlic, minced
2 tbsp Italian seasoning	1 onion, sliced
1 bell pepper, chopped	Pepper
	Salt

Directions:

Add oil into the instant pot and set the pot on sauté mode.   Add the meat into the pot and sauté until brown.   Add onion, bell pepper, and celery and sauté for 5 minutes.   Add remaining ingredients and stir well.   Seal pot with lid and cook on high for 40 minutes.   Once done, allow to release pressure naturally. Remove lid.   Stir well and serve.

Nutrition Info: Calories 460 Fat 18.2 g Carbohydrates 5.3 g Sugar 2.7 g Protein 58.7 g Cholesterol 172 mg

247. Chili Pork Meatballs

Servings: 4   Cooking Time: 20 Minutes

Ingredients:

1 pound pork meat, ground	1 tablespoon ginger, grated
1/2 cup parsley, chopped	1 Thai chili, chopped
1 cup yellow onion, chopped	2 tablespoons olive oil
4 garlic cloves, minced	1 cup veggie stock
	2 tablespoons sweet paprika

Directions:

In a bowl, mix the pork with the other ingredients except the oil, stock and paprika, stir well and shape medium meatballs out of this mix.   Heat up a pan with the oil over medium-high heat, add the meatballs and cook for 4 minutes on each side. Add the stock and the paprika, toss gently, simmer everything over medium heat for 12 minutes more, divide into bowls and serve.

Nutrition Info:calories 224, fat 18, fiber 9.3, carbs 11.5, protein 14.4

248. Worcestershire Pork Chops

Servings: 3   Cooking Time: 15 Minutes

Ingredients:

2 tablespoons Worcestershire sauce	1 tablespoon lemon juice
8 oz pork loin chops	1 teaspoon olive oil

Directions:

Mix up together Worcestershire sauce, lemon juice, and olive oil.   Brush the pork loin chops with the sauce mixture from each side.   Preheat the grill to 395F.   Place the pork chops in the grill and cook them for 5 minutes.   Then flip the pork chops on another side and brush with remaining sauce mixture.   Grill the meat for 7-8 minutes more.

Nutrition Info: Per Serving:calories 267, fat 20.4, fiber 0, carbs 2.1, protein 17

249. Sage Tomato Beef

Servings: 4   Cooking Time: 40 Minutes

Ingredients:

2 lbs beef stew meat, cubed	1 onion, chopped
1/4 cup tomato paste	2 tbsp olive oil
1 tsp garlic, minced	1 tbsp sage, chopped
2 cups chicken stock	Pepper
	Salt

Directions:

Add oil into the instant pot and set the pot on sauté mode.   Add garlic and onion and sauté for 5 minutes.   Add meat and sauté for 5 minutes. Add remaining ingredients and stir well.   Seal pot with lid and cook on high for 30 minutes. Once done, allow to release pressure naturally. Remove lid.   Serve and enjoy.

Nutrition Info: Calories 515 Fat 21.5 g Carbohydrates 7 g Sugar 3.6 g Protein 70 g Cholesterol 203 mg

250. Square Meat Pies (sfeeha)

Servings: 1 Meat Pie   Cooking Time: 20 Minutes

Ingredients:

1 large yellow onion	11/4 tsp. salt
2 large tomatoes	1 tsp. seven spices
1 lb. ground beef	1 batch Multipurpose Dough (recipe in Chapter 12)
1/2 tsp. ground black pepper	

Directions:

Preheat the oven to 425ºF. In a food processor fitted with a chopping blade, pulse yellow onion and tomatoes for 30 seconds. Transfer tomato-onion mixture to a large bowl. Add beef, salt, black pepper, and seven spices, and mix well. Form Multipurpose Dough into 18 balls, and roll out to 4-inch circles. Spoon 2 tablespoons meat mixture onto center of each dough circle. Pinch together the two opposite sides of dough up to meat mixture, and pinch the opposite two sides together, forming a square. Place meat pies on a baking sheet, and bake for 20 minutes. Serve warm or at room temperature.

251. Lamb And Wine Sauce

Servings: 4   Cooking Time: 2 Hours And 40 Minutes

Ingredients:

2 tablespoons olive oil	2 cups dry red wine
2 pounds leg of lamb, trimmed and sliced	2 tablespoons tomato paste
3 garlic cloves, chopped	4 tablespoons avocado oil
2 yellow onions, chopped	1 teaspoon thyme, chopped
3 cups veggie stock	Salt and black pepper to the taste

Directions:

Heat up a pan with the oil over medium-high heat, add the meat, brown for 5 minutes on each side and transfer to a roasting pan. Heat up the pan again over medium heat, add the avocado oil, add the onions and garlic and sauté for 5 minutes. Add the remaining ingredients, stir, bring to a simmer and cook for 10 minutes. Pour the sauce over the meat, introduce the pan in the oven and bake at 370 degrees F for 2 hours and 20 minutes. Divide everything between plates and serve.

Nutrition Info:calories 273, fat 21, fiber 11.1, carbs 16.2, protein 18.3

252. Pork Meatloaf

Servings: 6   Cooking Time: 1 Hour And 20 Minutes

Ingredients:

1 red onion, chopped	2 eggs, whisked
Cooking spray	1/3 cup kalamata olives, pitted and chopped
2 garlic cloves, minced	
2 pounds pork stew, ground	4 tablespoons oregano, chopped
1 cup almond milk	Salt and black pepper to the taste
¼ cup feta cheese, crumbled	

Directions:

In a bowl, mix the meat with the onion, garlic and the other ingredients except the cooking spray, stir well, shape your meatloaf and put it in a loaf pan greased with cooking spray. Bake the meatloaf at 370 degrees F for 1 hour and 20 minutes. Serve the meatloaf warm.

Nutrition Info:calories 350, fat 23, fiber 1, carbs 17, protein 24

253. Lamb And Rice

Servings: 4   Cooking Time: 1 Hour And 10 Minutes

Ingredients:

1 tablespoon lime juice	1 ounce avocado oil
1 yellow onion, chopped	Salt and black pepper to the taste
1 pound lamb, cubed	2 cups veggie stock
2 garlic cloves, minced	1 cup brown rice
	A handful parsley, chopped

Directions:

Heat up a pan with the avocado oil over medium-high heat, add the onion, stir and sauté for 5 minutes. Add the meat and brown for 5 minutes more. Add the rest of the ingredients except the parsley, bring to a simmer and cook over medium heat for 1 hour. Add the parsley, toss, divide everything between plates and serve.

Nutrition Info:calories 302, fat 13.2, fiber 10.7, carbs 15.7, protein 14.3

254. Italian Beef

Servings: 4   Cooking Time: 35 Minutes

Ingredients:

1 lb ground beef	1/2 onion, chopped
1 tbsp olive oil	1 carrot, chopped
1/2 cup mozzarella cheese, shredded	14 oz can tomatoes, diced
1/2 cup tomato puree	Pepper
1 tsp basil	Salt
1 tsp oregano	

Directions:

Add oil into the instant pot and set the pot on sauté mode. Add onion and sauté for 2 minutes. Add meat and sauté until browned. Add remaining ingredients except for cheese and stir well. Seal pot with lid and cook on high for 35 minutes. Once done, release pressure using quick release. Remove lid. Add cheese and stir well and cook on sauté mode until cheese is melted. Serve and enjoy.

Nutrition Info: Calories 297 Fat 11.3 g Carbohydrates 11.1 g Sugar 6.2 g Protein 37.1 g Cholesterol 103 mg

255. Pork Chops And Peppercorns Mix

Servings: 4   Cooking Time: 20 Minutes

Ingredients:

1 cup red onion, sliced	¼ cup veggie stock
1 tablespoon black peppercorns, crushed	A pinch of salt and black pepper
5 garlic cloves, minced	2 tablespoons olive oil
	4 pork chops

Directions:

Heat up a pan with the oil over medium-high heat, add the pork chops and brown for 4 minutes on each side. Add the onion and the garlic and cook for 2 minutes more. Add the rest of the ingredients, cook everything for 10 minutes, tossing the mix from time to time, divide between plates and serve.

Nutrition Info:calories 232, fat 9.2, fiber 5.6, carbs 13.3, protein 24.2

256. Pork And Tomato Meatloaf

Servings: 8   Cooking Time: 55 Minutes

Ingredients:

2 cups ground pork	1 teaspoon salt
1 egg, beaten	1/3 onion, diced
¼ cup crushed	¼ cup black olives,

tomatoes
1 teaspoon ground black pepper
1 oz Swiss cheese, grated
1 teaspoon minced garlic

chopped
1 jalapeno pepper, chopped
1 teaspoon dried basil
Cooking spray

Directions:
Spray the loaf mold with cooking spray. Then combine together ground pork, egg, crushed tomatoes, salt, ground black pepper. Grated Swiss cheese, minced garlic, onion, olives, jalapeno pepper, and dried basil. Stir the mass until it is homogenous and transfer it in the prepared loaf mold. Flatten the surface of meatloaf well and cover with foil. Bake the meatloaf for 40 minutes at 375F. Then discard the foil and bake the meal for 15 minutes more. Chill the cooked meatloaf to the room temperature and then remove it from the loaf mold. Slice it on the servings.
Nutrition Info: Per Serving:calories 265, fat 18.3, fiber 0.6, carbs 1.9, protein 22.1

257. Beef And Eggplant Moussaka

Servings: 3   Cooking Time: 50 Minutes
Ingredients:

1 small eggplant, sliced
1 teaspoon olive oil
½ cup cream
1 egg, beaten
1 tablespoon wheat flour, whole grain
1 teaspoon cornstarch
3 oz Romano cheese, grated

½ cup ground beef
¼ teaspoon minced garlic
1 tablespoon Italian parsley, chopped
3 tablespoons tomato sauce
¾ teaspoon ground nutmeg

Directions:
Sprinkle the eggplants with olive oil and ground nutmeg and arrange in the casserole mold in one layer. After this, place the ground beef in the skillet. Add minced garlic, Italian parsley, and ground nutmeg. Then add tomato sauce and mix up the mixture well. Roast it for 10 minutes over the medium heat. Make the sauce: in the saucepan whisk together cream with egg. Bring the liquid to boil (simmer it constantly) and add wheat flour, cornstarch, and cheese. Stir well. Bring the liquid to boil and stir till cheese is melted. Remove the sauce from the heat. Put the cooked ground beef over the eggplants and flatten well. Then pour the cream sauce over the ground beef. Cover the meal with foil and secure the edges. Bake moussaka for 30 minutes at 365F.
Nutrition Info: Per Serving:calories 271, fat 16.1, fiber 5.9, carbs 15.4, protein 17.6

258. Hearty Meat And Potatoes

Servings: 2 Cups   Cooking Time: 30 Minutes
Ingredients:

1 lb. ground beef or lamb
1/4 cup extra-virgin olive oil
1 large yellow onion, chopped

5 large potatoes, peeled and cubed
11/2 tsp. salt
1 TB. seven spices
1/2 tsp. ground black pepper

Directions:
In a large, 3-quart pot over medium heat, brown beef for 5 minutes, breaking up chunks with a

wooden spoon. Add extra-virgin olive oil and yellow onion, and cook for 5 minutes. Toss in potatoes, salt, seven spices, and black pepper. Cover and cook for 10 minutes. Toss gently, and cook for 10 more minutes. Serve warm with a side of Greek yogurt.

259. Ita Sandwiches

Servings: 1 Pita Sandwich   Cooking Time: 20 Minutes
Ingredients:

1 lb. ground beef
1/2 tsp. ground black pepper

1 tsp. salt
1 tsp. seven spices
4 (6- or 7-in.) pitas

Directions:
Preheat the oven to 400ºF. In a medium bowl, combine beef, salt, black pepper, and seven spices. Lay out pitas on the counter, and divide beef mixture evenly among them, and spread beef to edge of pitas. Place pitas on a baking sheet, and bake for 20 minutes. Serve warm with Greek yogurt.

260. Easy Chicken With Capers Skillet

Servings: 4   Cooking Time: 35 Minutes
Ingredients:

4 boneless skinless chicken breast halves (6 ounces each)
1/4 teaspoon salt
3 tablespoons olive oil

1/4 teaspoon pepper
1-pint grape tomatoes
16 pitted Greek or ripe olives, sliced
3 tablespoons capers, drained

Directions:
Place a cast iron skillet on medium high fire and heat for 5 minutes. Meanwhile, season chicken with pepper and salt. Add oil to pan and heat for another minute. Add chicken and increase fire to high. Brown sides for 4 minutes per side. Lower fire to medium and add capers and tomatoes. Bake uncovered in a 4750F preheated oven for 12 minutes. Remove from oven and let it sit for 5 minutes before serving.
Nutrition Info: Calories per Serving: 336; Carbs: 6.0g; Protein: 36.0g; Fats: 18.0g

261. Lamb And Dill Apples

Servings: 4   Cooking Time: 25 Minutes
Ingredients:

3 green apples, cored, peeled and cubed
1 pound lamb stew meat, cubed
1 small bunch dill, chopped

Juice of 1 lemon
3 ounces heavy cream
2 tablespoon olive oil
Salt and black pepper to the taste

Directions:
Heat up a pan with the oil over medium-high heat, add the lamb and brown for 5 minutes. Add the rest of the ingredients, bring to a simmer and cook over medium heat for 20 minutes. Divide the mix between plates and serve.
Nutrition Info:calories 328, fat 16.7, fiber 10.5, carbs 21.6, protein 14.7

262. Tomatoes And Carrots Pork Mix

Servings: 4   Cooking Time: 7 Hours
Ingredients:

2 tablespoons olive oil
½ cup chicken stock
1 tablespoon ginger, grated
2 and ½ pounds pork stew meat, roughly cubed
Salt and black pepper to the taste
2 cups tomatoes, chopped
4 ounces carrots, chopped
1 tablespoon cilantro, chopped

Directions:
In your slow cooker, combine the oil with the stock, ginger and the rest of the ingredients, put the lid on and cook on Low for 7 hours. Divide the mix between plates and serve.
Nutrition Info:calories 303, fat 15, fiber 8.6, carbs 14.9, protein 10.8

263. Rosemary Pork Chops
Servings: 4   Cooking Time: 35 Minutes
Ingredients:
4 pork loin chops, boneless
Salt and black pepper to the taste
4 garlic cloves, minced
1 tablespoon rosemary, chopped
1 tablespoon olive oil

Directions:
In a roasting pan, combine the pork chops with the rest of the ingredients, toss, and bake at 425 degrees F for 10 minutes. Reduce the heat to 350 degrees F and cook the chops for 25 minutes more. Divide the chops between plates and serve with a side salad.
Nutrition Info:calories 161, fat 5, fiber 1, carbs 1, protein 25

264. Cauliflower Tomato Beef
Servings: 2   Cooking Time: 25 Minutes
Ingredients:
1/2 lb beef stew meat, chopped
1 tbsp balsamic vinegar
1 celery stalk, chopped
1/4 cup grape tomatoes, chopped
1 tsp paprika
1 onion, chopped
1 tbsp olive oil
1/4 cup cauliflower, chopped
Pepper
Salt

Directions:
Add oil into the instant pot and set the pot on sauté mode. Add meat and sauté for 5 minutes. Add remaining ingredients and stir well. Seal pot with lid and cook on high for 20 minutes. Once done, allow to release pressure naturally. Remove lid. Stir and serve.
Nutrition Info: Calories 306 Fat 14.3 g Carbohydrates 7.6 g Sugar 3.5 g Protein 35.7 g Cholesterol 101 mg

265. Pork And Sour Cream Mix
Servings: 4   Cooking Time: 40 Minutes
Ingredients:
1 and ½ pounds pork meat, boneless and cubed
1 red onion, chopped
1 tablespoon avocado oil
1 garlic clove, minced
½ cup chicken stock
2 tablespoons hot paprika
Salt and black pepper to the taste
1 and ½ cups sour cream
1 tablespoon cilantro, chopped

Directions:
Heat up a pot with the oil over medium heat, add the pork and brown for 5 minutes. Add the onion and the garlic and cook for 5 minutes more. Add the rest of the ingredients except the cilantro, bring to a simmer and cook over medium heat for 30 minutes. Add the cilantro, toss, divide between plates and serve.
Nutrition Info:calories 300, fat 9.5, fiber 4.5, carbs 15.5, protein 22

266. Cherry Stuffed Lamb
Servings: 2   Cooking Time: 40 Minutes
Ingredients:
9 oz lamb loin
1 oz pistachio, chopped
1 teaspoon cherries, pitted
¼ teaspoon dried thyme
½ teaspoon olive oil
1 teaspoon dried rosemary
1 garlic clove, minced
¼ teaspoon liquid honey

Directions:
Rub the lamb loin with dried thyme and rosemary. Then make a lengthwise cut in the meat. Mix up together pistachios, minced garlic, and cherries. Fill the meat with this mixture and secure the cut with the toothpick. Then brush the lamb loin with liquid honey and olive oil. Wrap the meat in the foil and bake at 365F for 40 minutes. When the meat is cooked, remove it from the foil. Let the meat chill for 10 minutes and then slice it.
Nutrition Info: Per Serving:calories 353, fat 20.4, fiber 1.8, carbs 6, protein 36.9

267. Honey Pork Strips
Servings: 4   Cooking Time: 8 Minutes
Ingredients:
10 oz pork chops
1 teaspoon liquid honey
1 teaspoon tomato sauce
1 teaspoon sunflower oil
½ teaspoon sage
½ teaspoon mustard

Directions:
Cut the pork chops on the strips and place in the bowl. Add liquid honey, tomato sauce, sunflower oil, sage, and mustard. Mix up the meat well and leave for 15-20 minutes to marinate. Meanwhile, preheat the grill to 385F. Arrange the pork strips in the grill and roast them for 4 minutes from each side. Sprinkle the meat with remaining honey liquid during to cooking to make the taste of meat juicier.
Nutrition Info: Per Serving:calories 245, fat 18.9, fiber 0.1, carbs 1.7, protein 16.1

268. Orange Lamb And Potatoes
Servings: 4   Cooking Time: 7 Hours
Ingredients:
1 pound small potatoes, peeled and cubed
2 cups stewed tomatoes, drained
3 and ½ pounds leg of lamb, boneless and cubed
Zest and juice of 1 orange
4 garlic cloves, minced
Salt and black pepper to the taste
½ cup basil, chopped

Directions:
In your slow cooker, combine the lamb with the potatoes and the rest of the ingredients, toss, put

the lid on and cook on Low for 7 hours.   Divide the mix between plates and serve hot.
Nutrition Info: calories 287, fat 9.5, fiber 7.3, carbs 14.8, protein 18.2

269.   Pork Kebabs

Servings: 6   Cooking Time: 14 Minutes
Ingredients:

1 yellow onion, chopped
1 pound pork meat, ground
3 tablespoons cilantro, chopped
1 tablespoon lime juice

1 garlic clove, minced
2 teaspoon oregano, dried
Salt and black pepper to the taste
A drizzle of olive oil

Directions:
In a bowl, mix the pork with the other ingredients except the oil, stir well and shape medium kebabs out of this mix.   Divide the kebabs on skewers, and brush them with a drizzle of oil.   Place the kebabs on your preheated grill and cook over medium heat for 7 minutes on each side.   Divide the kebabs between plates and serve with a side salad.
Nutrition Info: calories 229, fat 14, fiber 8.3, carbs 15.5, protein 12.4

270.   Vegetable Lover's Chicken Soup

Servings: 4   Cooking Time: 20 Minutes
Ingredients:

1 ½ cups baby spinach
2 tbsp orzo (tiny pasta)
¼ cup dry white wine
1 14oz low sodium chicken broth
2 plum tomatoes, chopped
1/8 tsp salt

½ tsp Italian seasoning
1 large shallot, chopped
1 small zucchini, diced
8-oz chicken tenders
1 tbsp extra virgin olive oil

Directions:
In a large saucepan, heat oil over medium heat and add the chicken. Stir occasionally for 8 minutes until browned. Transfer in a plate. Set aside.   In the same saucepan, add the zucchini, Italian seasoning, shallot and salt and stir often until the vegetables are softened, around 4 minutes.   Add the tomatoes, wine, broth and orzo and increase the heat to high to bring the mixture to boil. Reduce the heat and simmer.   Add the cooked chicken and stir in the spinach last.   Serve hot.
Nutrition Info: Calories per Serving: 207; Carbs: 14.8g; Protein: 12.2g; Fat: 11.4g

271. Lemony Lamb And Potatoes

Servings: 4   Cooking Time: 2 Hours And 10 Minutes
Ingredients:

2 pound lamb meat, cubed
2 tablespoons olive oil
2 springs rosemary, chopped
2 pounds baby potatoes, scrubbed and halved

2 tablespoons parsley, chopped
1 tablespoon lemon rind, grated
3 garlic cloves, minced
2 tablespoons lemon juice
1 cup veggie stock

Directions:
In a roasting pan, combine the meat with the oil and the rest of the ingredients, introduce in the oven and bake at 400 degrees F for 2 hours and 10 minutes.   Divide the mix between plates and serve.
Nutrition Info: calories 302, fat 15.2, fiber 10.6, carbs 23.3, protein 15.2

272.   Cumin Lamb Mix

Servings: 2   Cooking Time: 10 Minutes
Ingredients:

2 lamb chops (3.5 oz each)
1 tablespoon olive oil

1 teaspoon ground cumin
½ teaspoon salt

Directions:
Rub the lamb chops with ground cumin and salt. Then sprinkle them with olive oil.   Let the meat marinate for 10 minutes.   After this, preheat the skillet well.   Place the lamb chops in the skillet and roast them for 10 minutes. Flip the meat on another side from time to time to avoid burning.
Nutrition Info: Per Serving: calories 384, fat 33.2, fiber 0.1, carbs 0.5, protein 19.2

273.   Almond Lamb Chops

Servings: 4   Cooking Time: 20 Minutes
Ingredients:

1 teaspoon almond butter
2 teaspoons minced garlic
1 teaspoon butter, softened

½ teaspoon salt
½ teaspoon chili flakes
½ teaspoon ground paprika
12 oz lamb chop

Directions:
Churn together minced garlic, butter, salt, chili flakes, and ground paprika.   Carefully rub every lamb chop with the garlic mixture.   Toss almond butter in the skillet and melt it.   Place the lamb chops in the melted almond butter and roast them for 20 minutes (for 10 minutes from each side) over the medium-low heat.
Nutrition Info: Per Serving: calories 194, fat 9.5, fiber 0.5, carbs 1.4, protein 24.9

274.   Pork And Figs Mix

Servings: 4   Cooking Time: 40 Minutes
Ingredients:

3 tablespoons avocado oil
Salt and black pepper to the taste
1 cup red onions, chopped
1 cup figs, dried and chopped
1 tablespoon ginger, grated

1 and ½ pounds pork stew meat, roughly cubed
1 tablespoon garlic, minced
1 cup canned tomatoes, crushed
2 tablespoons parsley, chopped

Directions:
Heat up a pot with the oil over medium-high heat, add the meat and brown for 5 minutes.   Add the onions and sauté for 5 minutes more.   Add the rest of the ingredients, bring to a simmer and cook over medium heat for 30 minutes more.   Divide the mix between plates and serve.
Nutrition Info: calories 309, fat 16, fiber 10.4, carbs 21.1, protein 34.2

275. Lamb Chops

Servings: 1 Chop   Cooking Time: 6 Minutes

Ingredients:

6 (3/4-in.-thick) lamb chops	1 tsp. salt
2 TB. fresh rosemary, finely chopped	1 tsp. ground black pepper
3 TB. minced garlic	3 TB. extra-virgin olive oil

Directions:

In a large bowl, combine lamb chops, rosemary, garlic, salt, black pepper, and extra-virgin olive oil until chops are evenly coated. Let chops marinate at room temperature for at least 25 minutes. Preheat a grill to medium heat.   Place chops on the grill, and cook for 3 minutes per side for medium well.   Serve warm.

276. Chicken Quinoa Pilaf

Servings: 1 Cup   Cooking Time: 35 Minuutes

Ingredients:

2 (8-oz.) boneless, skinless chicken breasts, cut into 1/2-in. cubes	2 cups water
	2 tsp. salt
	1 TB. dried oregano
3 TB. extra-virgin olive oil	1 TB. turmeric
1 medium red onion, finely chopped	1 tsp. paprika
	1 tsp. ground black pepper
1 TB. minced garlic	2 cups red or yellow quinoa
1 (16-oz.) can diced tomatoes, with juice	1/2 cup fresh parsley, chopped

Directions:

In a large, 3-quart pot over medium heat, heat extra-virgin olive oil. Add chicken, and cook for 5 minutes.   Add red onion and garlic, stir, and cook for 5 minutes.   Add tomatoes with juice, water, salt, oregano, turmeric, paprika, and black pepper. Stir, and simmer for 5 minutes.   Add red quinoa, and stir. Cover, reduce heat to low, and cook for 20 minutes. Remove from heat.   Fluff with a fork, cover again, and let sit for 10 minutes.   Serve warm.

277. Greek Styled Lamb Chops

Servings: 4   Cooking Time: 4 Minutes

Ingredients:

¼ tsp black pepper	2 tbsp lemon juice
½ tsp salt	8 pcs of lamb loin chops, around 4 oz
1 tbsp bottled minced garlic	Cooking spray
1 tbsp dried oregano	

Directions:

Preheat broiler.   In a big bowl or dish, combine the black pepper, salt, minced garlic, lemon juice and oregano. Then rub it equally on all sides of the lamb chops.   Then coat a broiler pan with the cooking spray before placing the lamb chops on the pan and broiling until desired doneness is reached or for four minutes.

Nutrition Info: Calories per Serving: 131.9; Carbs: 2.6g; Protein: 17.1g; Fat: 5.9g

278. Bulgur And Chicken Skillet

Servings: 4   Cooking Time: 40 Minutes

Ingredients:

4 (6-oz.) skinless, boneless chicken breasts	1/2 cup uncooked bulgur
	2 teaspoons chopped
1 tablespoon olive oil, divided	fresh or 1/2 tsp. dried oregano
1 cup thinly sliced red onion	4 cups chopped fresh kale (about 2 1/2 oz.)
1 tablespoon thinly sliced garlic	1/2 cup thinly sliced bottled roasted red bell peppers
1 cup unsalted chicken stock	2 ounces feta cheese, crumbled (about 1/2 cup)
1 tablespoon coarsely chopped fresh dill	3/4 teaspoon kosher salt, divided
1/2 teaspoon freshly ground black pepper, divided	

Directions:

Place a cast iron skillet on medium high fire and heat for 5 minutes. Add oil and heat for 2 minutes. Season chicken with pepper and salt to taste. Brown chicken for 4 minutes per side and transfer to a plate.   In same skillet, sauté garlic and onion for 3 minutes. Stir in oregano and bulgur and toast for 2 minutes.   Stir in kale and bell pepper, cook for 2 minutes.   Pour in stock and season well with pepper and salt.   Return chicken to skillet and turn off fire. Pop in a preheated 400oF oven and bake for 15 minutes.   Remove form oven, fluff bulgur and turn over chicken. Let it stand for 5 minutes.   Serve and enjoy with a sprinkle of feta cheese.

Nutrition Info: Calories per Serving: 369; Carbs: 21.0g; Protein: 45.0g; Fats: 11.3g

279. Kibbeh With Yogurt

Servings: 1 Kibbeh   Cooking Time: 50 Minutes

Ingredients:

1/2 cup bulgur wheat, grind #1	1/2 tsp. ground cumin
4 cups water	1/2 tsp. ground cloves
1 large yellow onion, chopped	1/2 tsp. ground cinnamon
2 fresh basil leaves	1/2 tsp. dried sage
1 lb. lean ground chuck beef	1/4 cup long-grain rice
2 tsp. salt	1/2 lb. ground beef
1 tsp. ground black pepper	3 TB. extra-virgin olive oil
1/2 tsp. ground allspice	1/2 cup pine nuts
1/2 tsp. ground coriander	1 tsp. seven spices
	4 cups Greek yogurt
1/2 tsp. ground nutmeg	2 TB. minced garlic
	1 tsp. dried mint

Directions:

In a small bowl, soak bulgur wheat in 1 cup water for 30 minutes.   In a food processor fitted with a chopping blade, blend 1/2 of yellow onion and basil for 30 seconds. Add bulgur, and blend for 30 more seconds.   Add ground chuck, 11/2 teaspoons salt, black pepper, allspice, coriander, cumin, nutmeg, cloves, cinnamon, and sage, and blend for 1 minute. Transfer mixture to a large bowl, and knead for 3 minutes.   In a large pot, combine long-grain rice and remaining 3 cups water, and cook for 30 minutes.   In a medium skillet over medium heat, brown beef for 5 minutes, breaking up chunks with a wooden spoon.   Add remaining 1/2 of yellow onion, extra-virgin olive oil, remaining 1/2 teaspoon salt, pine nuts, and seven spices, and cook for 7 minutes. Set aside to cool.   Whisk Greek yogurt into cooked rice, add garlic and mint, reduce heat to low, and cook for 5 minutes. Form meat-bulgur mixture into 12 equal-size balls. Create a groove in center of each ball, fill with beef and onion mixture, and seal groove. Carefully drop balls into yogurt sauce, and cook for 15 minutes. Serve warm.

280. Mustard Chops With Apricot-basil Relish

Servings: 4   Cooking Time: 12 Minutes

Ingredients:

¼ cup basil, finely shredded	1 shallot, diced small
¼ cup olive oil	1 tsp ground cardamom
½ cup mustard	3 tbsp raspberry vinegar
¾ lb. fresh apricots, stone removed, and fruit diced	4 pork chops
	Pepper and salt

Directions:
Make sure that pork chops are defrosted well. Season with pepper and salt. Slather both sides of each pork chop with mustard. Preheat grill to medium-high fire.   In a medium bowl, mix cardamom, olive oil, vinegar, basil, shallot, and apricots. Toss to combine and season with pepper and salt, mixing once again.   Grill chops for 5 to 6 minutes per side. As you flip, baste with mustard. Serve pork chops with the Apricot-Basil relish and enjoy.
Nutrition Info: Calories per Serving: 486.5; Carbs: 7.3g; Protein: 42.1g; Fat: 32.1g

281. Pork And Peas

Servings: 4   Cooking Time: 20 Minutes

Ingredients:

4 ounces snow peas	¾ cup beef stock
2 tablespoons avocado oil	½ cup red onion, chopped
1 pound pork loin, boneless and cubed	Salt and white pepper to the taste

Directions:
Heat up a pan with the oil over medium-high heat, add the pork and brown for 5 minutes.   Add the peas and the rest of the ingredients, toss, bring to a simmer and cook over medium heat for 15 minutes. Divide the mix between plates and serve right away.
Nutrition Info:calories 332, fat 16.5, fiber 10.3, carbs 20.7, protein 26.5

282. Paprika And Feta Cheese On Chicken Skillet

Servings: 6   Cooking Time: 35 Minutes

Ingredients:

¼ cup black olives, sliced in circles	2 lb. free range organic boneless skinless chicken breasts
½ teaspoon coriander	
½ teaspoon paprika	2 tablespoons feta cheese
1 ½ cups diced tomatoes with the juice	2 tablespoons ghee or olive oil
1 cup yellow onion, chopped	Crushed red pepper to taste
1 teaspoon onion powder	Salt and black pepper to taste
2 garlic cloves, peeled	

and minced
Directions:
Preheat oven to 400oF.   Place a cast-iron pan on medium high fire and heat for 5 minutes. Add oil and heat for 2 minutes more.   Meanwhile in a large dish, mix well pepper, salt, crushed red pepper, paprika, coriander, and onion powder. Add chicken and coat well in seasoning.   Add chicken to pan and brown sides for 4 minutes per side. Increase fire to high.   Stir in garlic and onions. Lower fire to medium and mix well.   Pop pan in oven and bake for 15 minutes.   Remove from oven, turnover chicken and let it stand for 5 minutes before serving.
Nutrition Info: Calories per Serving: 232; Carbs: 5.0g; Protein: 33.0g; Fats: 8.0g

283. Jalapeno Beef Chili

Servings: 8   Cooking Time: 40 Minutes

Ingredients:

1 lb ground beef	1 lb ground pork
1 tsp garlic powder	4 tomatillos, chopped
1 jalapeno pepper, chopped	1/2 onion, chopped
	5 oz tomato paste
1 tbsp ground cumin	Pepper
1 tbsp chili powder	Salt

Directions:
Add oil into the instant pot and set the pot on sauté mode.   Add beef and pork and cook until brown. Add remaining ingredients and stir well.   Seal pot with lid and cook on high for 35 minutes. Once done, allow to release pressure naturally. Remove lid.   Stir well and serve.
Nutrition Info: Calories 217 Fat 6.1 g Carbohydrates 6.2 g Sugar 2.7 g Protein 33.4 g Cholesterol 92 mg

284. Kibbeh In A Pan

Servings: 1 Kibbeh   Cooking Time: 37 Minutes

Ingredients:

1/2 cup bulgur wheat, grind #1	2 tsp. salt
1 cup water	1/2 tsp. ground cumin
1 large yellow onion, chopped	1/2 tsp. ground nutmeg
2 fresh basil leaves	1/2 tsp. ground cloves
1 lb. lean ground chuck beef	1/2 tsp. ground cinnamon
1 tsp. ground black pepper	1/2 tsp. dried sage
1/2 tsp. ground allspice	1/2 lb. ground beef
1/2 tsp. ground coriander	4 TB. extra-virgin olive oil
	1/2 cup pine nuts
	1 tsp. seven spices

Directions:
In a small bowl, soak bulgur wheat in water for 30 minutes.   In a food processor fitted with a chopping blade, blend 1/2 of yellow onion and basil for 30 seconds. Add bulgur, and blend for 30 more seconds.   Add ground chuck, 11/2 teaspoons salt, black pepper, allspice, coriander, cumin, nutmeg, cloves, cinnamon, and sage, and blend for 1 minute. Transfer mixture to a large bowl, and knead for 3 minutes.   In a medium skillet over medium heat, brown beef for 5 minutes, breaking up chunks with a wooden spoon.   Add remaining 1/2 of yellow onion, 2 tablespoons extra-virgin olive oil, remaining 1/2 teaspoon salt, pine nuts, and seven spices, and cook for 7 minutes.   Preheat the oven

to 450°F. Grease an 8×8-inch baking dish with extra-virgin olive oil. Divide kibbeh dough in half, spread a layer of dough on bottom of the prepared baking dish, add a layer of sautéed vegetables, and top with remaining kibbeh dough. Paint top of kibbeh with remaining 2 tablespoons extra-virgin olive oil, and cut kibbeh into 12 equal-size pieces. Bake for 25 minutes. Let kibbeh rest for 15 minutes before serving.

285. Saffron Beef

Servings: 2   Cooking Time: 15 Minutes
Ingredients:

¾ teaspoon saffron	¼ teaspoon ground cinnamon
¾ teaspoon dried thyme	1 tablespoon butter
¾ teaspoon ground coriander	1/3 teaspoon salt
	9 oz beef sirloin

Directions:
Rub the beef sirloin with dried thyme, ground coriander, saffron, ground cinnamon, and salt. Leave the meat for at least 10 minutes to soak all the spices. Then preheat the grill to 395F. Place the beef sirloin in the grill and cook it for 5 minutes. Then spread the meat with butter carefully and cook for 10 minutes more. Flip it on another side from time to time.
Nutrition Info: Per Serving:calories 291, fat 13.8, fiber 0.3, carbs 0.6, protein 38.8

286. Cayenne Pork

Servings: 4   Cooking Time: 50 Minutes
Ingredients:

8 oz beef sirloin	1 teaspoon ground black pepper
1 poblano pepper, grinded	1 teaspoon salt
1 teaspoon minced garlic	½ teaspoon paprika
½ cup of water	1 teaspoon cayenne pepper
1 tablespoon butter	

Directions:
Toss the butter in the saucepan and melt it. Meanwhile rub the beef sirloin with minced garlic, salt, ground black pepper, paprika, and cayenne pepper. Put the meat in the hot butter and roast for 5 minutes from each side over the medium heat. After this, add water and poblano pepper. Cook the meat for 50 minutes over the medium heat. Then transfer the beef sirloin on the cutting board and shred it with the help of the fork.
Nutrition Info: Per Serving:calories 97, fat 5.5, fiber 0.5, carbs 3, protein 9.5

287. Basil And Shrimp Quinoa

Servings: 1 Cup   Cooking Time: 20 Minutes
Ingredients:

3 TB. extra-virgin olive oil	2 TB. minced garlic
1 cup fresh broccoli florets	11/2 tsp. salt
3 stalks asparagus, chopped (1 cup)	1 tsp. ground black pepper
4 cups chicken or vegetable broth	1 TB. lemon zest
	2 cups red quinoa
	1/2 cup fresh basil, chopped

Directions:
1/2 lb. medium raw shrimp (18 to 20), shells and veins removed   In a 2-quart pot over low heat, heat extra-virgin olive oil. Add garlic, and cook for

3 minutes.   Increase heat to medium, add broccoli and asparagus, and cook for 2 minutes. Add chicken broth, salt, black pepper, and lemon zest, and bring to a boil. Stir in red quinoa, cover, and cook for 15 minutes.   Fold in basil and shrimp, cover, and cook for 10 minutes.   Remove from heat, fluff with a fork, cover, and set aside for 10 minutes. Serve warm.

288. Ground Pork Salad

Servings: 8   Cooking Time: 15 Minutes
Ingredients:

1 cup ground pork	1 teaspoon butter
½ onion, diced	4 eggs, boiled
4 bacon slices	½ teaspoon salt
1 teaspoon sesame oil	1 teaspoon chili pepper
1 cup lettuce, chopped	¼ teaspoon liquid honey
1 tablespoon lemon juice	

Directions:
Make burgers: in the mixing bowl combine together ground pork, diced onion, salt, and chili pepper.   Make the medium size burgers.   Melt butter in the skillet and add prepared burgers. Roast them for 5 minutes from each side over the medium heat.   When the burgers are cooked, chill them little.   Place the bacon in the skillet and roast it until golden brown. Then chill the bacon and chop it roughly.   In the salad bowl combine together chopped bacon, sesame oil, lettuce, lemon juice, and honey. Mix up salad well. Peel the eggs and cut them on the halves. Arrange the eggs and burgers over the salad. Don't mix salad anymore.
Nutrition Info: Per Serving:calories 213, fat 15.4, fiber 0.1, carbs 1.5, protein 16.5

289. Beef And Dill Mushrooms

Servings: 3   Cooking Time: 35 Minutes
Ingredients:

1 cup cremini mushrooms, sliced	½ cup of water
4 oz beef loin, sliced onto the wedges	¼ cup cream
1 tablespoon olive oil	1 teaspoon tomato paste
1 teaspoon dried oregano	1 teaspoon ground black pepper
	1 teaspoon salt
	1 tablespoon fresh dill, chopped

Directions:
In the saucepan combine together olive oil and cremini mushrooms.   Add dried oregano, ground black pepper, salt, and dill. Mix up well.   Cook the mushrooms for 2-3 minutes and add sliced beef loin.   Cook the ingredients for 5 minutes over the medium heat.   After this, add cream, water, tomato paste, and mix up the meal well.   Simmer the beef stroganoff for 25 minutes over the medium heat.
Nutrition Info: Per Serving:calories 196, fat 11.8, fiber 0.8, carbs 3.3, protein 20.1

290. Beef Pitas

Servings: 4   Cooking Time: 15 Minutes
Ingredients:

1 ½ cup ground beef	1 teaspoon salt
½ red onion, diced	1 teaspoon fresh

1 teaspoon minced garlic
¼ cup fresh spinach, chopped
½ teaspoon chili pepper
1 teaspoon dried oregano

mint, chopped
4 tablespoons Plain yogurt
1 cucumber, grated
½ teaspoon dill
½ teaspoon garlic powder
4 pitta bread

Directions:
In the mixing bowl combine together ground beef, onion, minced garlic, spinach, salt, chili pepper, and dried oregano. Make the medium size balls from the meat mixture. Line the baking tray with baking paper and arrange the meatballs inside. Bake the meatballs for 15 minutes at 375F. Flip them on another side after 10 minutes of cooking. Meanwhile, make tzaziki: combine together fresh mint, yogurt, grated cucumber, dill, and garlic powder. Whisk the mixture for 1 minute. When the meatballs are cooked, place the over pitta bread and top with tzaziki.

Nutrition Info: Per Serving: calorie 253, fat 7.1, fiber 4, carbs 30.1, protein 16.3

291.	Lamb Burger On Arugula

Servings: 6   Cooking Time: 6 Minutes
Ingredients:
½ oz fresh mint, divided
1 tbsp salt
2 lbs. ground lamb
2 tbsp shelled and salted Pistachio nuts

3 oz dried apricots, diced
3 oz Feta crumbled – you can omit if you do not eat dairy
4 cups arugula

Directions:
In a bowl, with your hands blend feta, salt, ½ of fresh mint (diced), apricots and ground lamb. Then form into balls or patties with an ice cream scooper. Press ball in between palm of hands to flatten to half an inch. Do the same for remaining patties. In a nonstick thick pan on medium fire, place patties without oil and cook for 3 minutes per side or until lightly browned. Flip over once and cook the other side. Meanwhile, arrange 1 cup of arugula per plate. Total of 4 plates. Divide evenly and place cooked patties on top of arugula. In a food processor, process until finely chopped the remaining mint leaves and nuts. Sprinkle on top of patties, serve and enjoy.

Nutrition Info: Calories per Serving: 458.2; Carbs: 12.0g; Protein: 23.8g; Fat: 35.0g

292.	Flavorful Beef Bourguignon

Servings: 4   Cooking Time: 20 Minutes
Ingredients:
1 1/2 lbs beef chuck roast, cut into chunks
2/3 cup beef stock
2 tbsp fresh thyme
1 bay leaf
1 tsp garlic, minced
8 oz mushrooms, sliced

2 tbsp tomato paste
2/3 cup dry red wine
1 onion, sliced
4 carrots, cut into chunks
1 tbsp olive oil
Pepper
Salt

Directions:
Add oil into the instant pot and set the pot on sauté mode. Add meat and sauté until brown. Add onion and sauté until softened. Add remaining ingredients and stir well. Seal pot with lid and

cook on high for 12 minutes. Once done, allow to release pressure naturally. Remove lid. Stir well and serve.
Nutrition Info: Calories 744 Fat 51.3 g Carbohydrates 14.5 g Sugar 6.5 g Protein 48.1 g Cholesterol 175 mg

293.	Kefta Burgers

Servings: 1 Burger   Cooking Time: 10 Minutes
Ingredients:
1 lb. ground beef
1 cup fresh parsley, finely chopped
1 tsp. seven spices
11/2 tsp. salt
1 large yellow onion, finely sliced
1 TB. sumac
1/2 cup mayonnaise

3 TB. tahini paste
2 TB. balsamic vinegar
1/2 tsp. ground black pepper
4 (4-in.) pitas
1 medium tomato, sliced

Directions:
In a large bowl, combine beef, 1/2 cup parsley, seven spices, 1 teaspoon salt. Form mixture into 4 patties. In a medium bowl, combine remaining 1/2 cup parsley, yellow onion, and sumac. In a small bowl, whisk together mayonnaise, tahini paste, remaining 1/2 teaspoon salt, balsamic vinegar, and black pepper. Preheat a large skillet over medium-high heat. Place patties in the skillet, and cook for 5 minutes per side. To assemble burgers, open each pita into a pocket, and spread both sides with tahini mayonnaise. Add 1 burger patty, some parsley mixture, and a few tomato slices, and serve.

294.	Beef Dish

Servings: ¼ Pound   Cooking Time: 20 Minutes
Ingredients:
1 lb. skirt steak
2 TB. minced garlic
1/4 cup fresh lemon juice
2 TB. apple cider vinegar
3 TB. extra-virgin olive oil

1 tsp. salt
1/2 tsp. ground black pepper
1/4 tsp. ground cinnamon
1/4 tsp. ground cardamom
1 tsp. seven spices

Directions:
Using a sharp knife, cut skirt steak into thin, 1/4-inch strips. Place strips in a large bowl. Add garlic, lemon juice, apple cider vinegar, extra-virgin olive oil, salt, black pepper, cinnamon, cardamom, and seven spices, and mix well. Place steak in the refrigerator and marinate for at least 20 minutes and up to 24 hours. Preheat a large skillet over medium heat. Add meat and marinade, and cook for 20 minutes or until meat is tender and marinade has evaporated. Serve warm with pita bread and tahini sauce.

295.	Tasty Beef Stew

Servings: 4   Cooking Time: 30 Minutes
Ingredients:
2 1/2 lbs beef roast, cut into chunks
1 cup beef broth
1/2 cup balsamic vinegar
1 tbsp honey

1/2 tsp red pepper flakes
1 tbsp garlic, minced
Pepper
Salt

Directions:

Add all ingredients into the inner pot of instant pot and stir well. Seal pot with lid and cook on high for 30 minutes. Once done, allow to release pressure naturally. Remove lid. Stir well and serve.

Nutrition Info: Calories 562 Fat 18.1 g Carbohydrates 5.7 g Sugar 4.6 g Protein 87.4 g Cholesterol 253 mg

296. Pork And Sage Couscous

Servings: 4   Cooking Time: 7 Hours

Ingredients:

2 pounds pork loin boneless and sliced	¾ cup veggie stock
2 tablespoons olive oil	½ tablespoon garlic powder
½ tablespoon chili powder	Salt and black pepper to the taste
2 teaspoon sage, dried	2 cups couscous, cooked

Directions:
In a slow cooker, combine the pork with the stock, the oil and the other ingredients except the couscous, put the lid on and cook on Low for 7 hours. Divide the mix between plates, add the couscous on the side, sprinkle the sage on top and serve.

Nutrition Info:calories 272, fat 14.5, fiber 9.1, carbs 16.3, protein 14.3

297. Chicken Burgers With Brussel Sprouts Slaw

Servings: 4   Cooking Time: 15 Minutes

Ingredients:

¼ cup apple, diced	½ avocado, cubed
¼ cup green onion, diced	1/8 teaspoon red pepper flakes, optional
½ pound Brussels sprouts, shredded	1-pound cooked ground chicken
1 garlic clove, minced	3 slices bacon, cooked and diced
1 tablespoon Dijon mustard	Salt and pepper to taste
1/3 cup apple, sliced into strips	

Directions:
In a mixing bowl, combine together chicken, green onion, Dijon mustard, garlic, apple, bacon and pepper flakes. Season with salt and pepper to taste. Mix the ingredients then form 4 burger patties. Heat a grill pan over medium-high flame and grill the burgers. Cook for five minutes on side. Set aside. In another bowl, toss the Brussels sprouts and apples. In a small pan, heat coconut oil and add the Brussels sprouts mixture until everything is slightly wilted. Season with salt and pepper to taste. Serve burger patties with the Brussels sprouts slaw.

Nutrition Info: Calories per Serving: 325.1; Carbs: 11.5g; Protein: 32.2g; Fat: 16.7g

298. Beef And Potatoes With Tahini Sauce

Servings: 1/6 Casserole   Cooking Time: 35 Minutes

Ingredients:

1/2 large yellow onion	21/2 tsp. salt
1 lb. ground beef	2 cups plain Greek yogurt
1/2 tsp. ground black	3/4 cup tahini paste
pepper	11/2 cups water
6 small red potatoes, washed	1/4 cup fresh lemon juice
3 TB. extra-virgin olive oil	1 TB. minced garlic
	1/2 cup pine nuts

Directions:
Preheat the oven to 425ºF. In a food processor fitted with a chopping blade, blend yellow onion for 30 seconds. Transfer onion to a large bowl. Add beef, 1 teaspoon salt, black pepper, and mix well. Spread beef mixture evenly in the bottom of a 9-inch casserole dish, and bake for 20 minutes. Cut red potatoes into 1/4-inch-thick pieces, place in a bowl, and toss with 2 tablespoons extra-virgin olive oil and 1/2 teaspoon salt. Spread potatoes on a baking sheet, and bake for 20 minutes. In a large bowl, combine Greek yogurt, tahini paste, water, lemon juice, garlic, and remaining 1 teaspoon salt. Remove beef mixture and potatoes from the oven. Using a spatula, transfer potatoes to the casserole dish. Pour yogurt sauce over top, and bake for 15 more minutes. In a small pan over low heat, heat remaining 1 tablespoon extra-virgin olive oil. Add pine nuts, and toast for 1 or 2 minutes. Remove casserole dish from the oven, spoon pine nuts over top, and serve warm with brown rice.

299. Spicy Beef Chili Verde

Servings: 2   Cooking Time: 23 Minutes

Ingredients:

1/2 lb beef stew meat, cut into cubes	1 small onion, chopped
1/4 tsp chili powder	1/4 cup grape tomatoes, chopped
1 tbsp olive oil	1/4 cup tomatillos, chopped
1 cup chicken broth	
1 Serrano pepper, chopped	Pepper
1 tsp garlic, minced	Salt

Directions:
Add oil into the instant pot and set the pot on sauté mode. Add garlic and onion and sauté for 3 minutes. Add remaining ingredients and stir well. Seal pot with lid and cook on high for 20 minutes. Once done, allow to release pressure naturally. Remove lid. Stir well and serve.

Nutrition Info: Calories 317 Fat 15.1 g Carbohydrates 6.4 g Sugar 2.6 g Protein 37.8 g Cholesterol 101 mg

300. Lime And Mustard Lamb

Servings: 2   Cooking Time: 25 Minutes

Ingredients:

8 oz lamb ribs, trimmed	1 tablespoon lime juice
1 tablespoon olive oil	½ teaspoon lime zest, grated
¼ teaspoon mustard	½ teaspoon salt

Directions:
In the shallow bowl combine together olive oil, lime juice, lime zest, mustard, and salt. Rub the lamb ribs with the lime mixture well and place in the skillet. Roast the meat for 5 minutes from each side. Then add remaining lime mixture and close the lid. Cook the lamb ribs for 20 minutes over the medium heat. You can flip the ribs on another side during cooking.

Nutrition Info: Per Serving:calories 325, fat 22.2, fiber 0.1, carbs 0.2, protein 29.8

Poultry Recipes

301. Turkey And Salsa Verde

Servings: 4   Cooking Time: 50 Minutes

Ingredients:

1 big turkey breast, skinless, boneless and cubed

1 and ½ cups Salsa Verde

Salt and black pepper to the taste

1 tablespoon olive oil

1 and ½ cups feta cheese, crumbled

¼ cup cilantro, chopped

Directions:

In a roasting pan greased with the oil combine the turkey with the salsa, salt and pepper and bake 400 degrees F for 50 minutes.   Add the cheese and the cilantro, toss gently, divide everything between plates and serve.

Nutrition Info:calories 332, fat 15.4, fiber 10.5, carbs 22.1, protein 34.5

302. Chili Chicken Fillets

Servings: 8   Cooking Time: 7.5 Hours

Ingredients:

4 chicken fillets (5 oz each fillet)

8 bacon slices

1 teaspoon chili pepper

1 tablespoon olive oil

½ teaspoon salt

1 garlic clove, minced

Directions:

Cut every chicken fillet lengthwise.   In the shallow bowl mix up together chili pepper, olive oil, minced garlic, and salt.   Rub every chicken fillet with oil mixture and wrap in the sliced bacon. Transfer the prepared chicken fillets in the baking dish and cover with foil.   Bake the chicken fillets for 35 minutes at 365F.

Nutrition Info: Per Serving:calories 234, fat 15.2, fiber 0.5, carbs 8, protein 16.6

303. Chicken With Peas

Servings: 4   Cooking Time: 30 Minutes

Ingredients:

4 chicken fillets

1 teaspoon cayenne pepper

1 tablespoon mayonnaise

1 teaspoon salt

1 cup green peas

¼ cup of water

1 carrot, peeled, chopped

Directions:

Sprinkle the chicken fillet with cayenne pepper and salt.   Line the baking tray with foil and place chicken fillets in it.   Then brush the chicken with mayonnaise.   Add carrot and green peas.   Then add water and cover the ingredients with foil. Bake the chicken for 30 minutes at 355F.

Nutrition Info: Per Serving:calories 329 fat 12.3, fiber 2.3, carbs 7.9, protein 44.4

304. Chicken Wrap

Servings: 2   Cooking Time: 0 Minutes

Ingredients:

2 whole wheat tortilla flatbreads

6 chicken breast slices, skinless, boneless, cooked and shredded

A handful baby spinach

2 provolone cheese slices

4 tomato slices

10 kalamata olives, pitted and sliced

1 red onion, sliced

2 tablespoons roasted peppers, chopped

Directions:

Arrange the tortillas on a working surface, and divide the chicken and the other ingredients on each.   Roll the tortillas and serve them right away.

Nutrition Info:calories 190, fat 6.8, fiber 3.5, carbs 15.1, protein 6.6

305. Carrots And Tomatoes Chicken

Servings: 4   Cooking Time: 1 Hour And 10 Minutes

Ingredients:

2 pounds chicken breasts, skinless, boneless and halved

Salt and black pepper to the taste

3 garlic cloves, minced

3 tablespoons avocado oil

2 shallots, chopped

4 carrots, sliced

3 tomatoes, chopped

¼ cup chicken stock

1 tablespoon Italian seasoning

1 tablespoon parsley, chopped

Directions:

Heat up a pan with the oil over medium-high heat, add the chicken, garlic, salt and pepper and brown for 3 minutes on each side.   Add the rest of the ingredients except the parsley, bring to a simmer and cook over medium-low heat for 40 minutes. Add the parsley, divide the mix between plates and serve.

Nutrition Info:calories 309, fat 12.4, fiber 11.1, carbs 23.8, protein 15.3

306. Almond Chicken Bites

Servings: 8   Cooking Time: 5 Minutes

Ingredients:

1-pound chicken fillet

1 tablespoon potato starch

½ teaspoon salt

1 teaspoon paprika

2 tablespoons wheat flour, whole grain

1 egg, beaten

1 tablespoon almond butter

Directions:

Chop the chicken fillet on the small pieces and place in the bowl.   Add egg, salt, and potato starch. Mix up the chicken.   Then mix up wheat flour and paprika.   Then coat every chicken piece in wheat flour mixture.   Place almond butter in the skillet and heat it up.   Add chicken popcorn and roast it for 5 minutes over medium heat. Dry the chicken popcorn with the help of the paper towel.

Nutrition Info: Per Serving:calories 141, fat 5.9, fiber 0.4, carbs 3.3, protein 17.8

307. Chicken Wings And Dates Mix

Servings: 6   Cooking Time: 1 Hour

Ingredients:

12 chicken wings, halved

2 garlic cloves, minced

Juice of 1 lime

2 tablespoons

Zest of 1 lime

1 teaspoon cumin, ground

Salt and black pepper to the taste

avocado oil
1 cup dates, pitted and halved
½ cup chicken stock
1 tablespoon chives, chopped

Directions:
In a roasting pan, combine the chicken wings with the garlic, lime juice and the rest of the ingredients, toss, introduce in the oven and bake at 360 degrees F for 1 hour. Divide everything between plates and serve with a side salad.
Nutrition Info:calories 294, fat 19.4, fiber 11.8, carbs 21.4, protein 17.5

308. Turkey, Artichokes And Asparagus

Servings: 4   Cooking Time: 30 Minutes
Ingredients:
2 turkey breasts, boneless, skinless and halved
3 tablespoons olive oil
1 and ½ pounds asparagus, trimmed and halved
1 cup chicken stock
A pinch of salt and black pepper
1 cup canned artichoke hearts, drained
¼ cup kalamata olives, pitted and sliced
1 shallot, chopped
3 garlic cloves, minced
3 tablespoons dill, chopped

Directions:
Heat up a pan with the oil over medium-high heat, add the turkey and the garlic and brown for 4 minutes on each side. Add the asparagus, the stock and the rest of the ingredients except the dill, bring to a simmer and cook over medium heat for 20 minutes. Add the dill, divide the mix between plates and serve.
Nutrition Info:calories 291, fat 16, fiber 10.3, carbs 22.8, protein 34.5

309. Garlic Chicken And Endives

Servings: 4   Cooking Time: 15 Minutes
Ingredients:
1 pound chicken breasts, skinless, boneless and cubed
2 endives, sliced
2 tablespoons olive oil
4 garlic cloves, minced
½ cup chicken stock
2 tablespoons parmesan, grated
1 tablespoon parsley, chopped
Salt and black pepper to the taste

Directions:
Heat up a pan with the oil over medium-high heat, add the chicken and cook for 5 minutes. Add the endives, garlic, the stock, salt and pepper, stir, bring to a simmer and cook over medium-high heat for 10 minutes. Add the parmesan and the parsley, toss gently, divide everything between plates and serve.
Nutrition Info:calories 280, fat 9.2, fiber 10.8, carbs 21.6, protein 33.8

310. Butter Chicken Thighs

Servings: 4   Cooking Time: 30 Minutes
Ingredients:
1 teaspoon fennel seeds
1 garlic clove, peeled
1 tablespoon butter
1 teaspoon coconut
½ teaspoon salt
1 oz fennel bulb, chopped
1 oz shallot, chopped
oil
¼ teaspoon thyme
4 chicken thighs, skinless, boneless
1 teaspoon ground black pepper

Directions:
Rub the chicken thighs with ground black pepper. In the skillet mix up together butter and coconut oil. Add fennel seeds, garlic clove, thyme, salt, and shallot. Roast the mixture for 1 minute. Then add fennel bulb and chicken thighs. Roast the chicken thighs for 2 minutes from each side over the high heat. Then transfer the skillet with chicken in the oven and cook the meal for 20 minutes at 360F.
Nutrition Info: Per Serving:calories 324, fat 14.9, fiber 0.6, carbs 2.6, protein 42.7

311. Chicken And Olives Salsa

Servings: 4   Cooking Time: 25 Minutes
Ingredients:
2 tablespoon avocado oil
4 chicken breast halves, skinless and boneless
Salt and black pepper to the taste
1 tablespoon sweet paprika
1 red onion, chopped
1 tablespoon balsamic vinegar
2 tablespoons parsley, chopped
1 avocado, peeled, pitted and cubed
2 tablespoons black olives, pitted and chopped

Directions:
Heat up your grill over medium-high heat, add the chicken brushed with half of the oil and seasoned with paprika, salt and pepper, cook for 7 minutes on each side and divide between plates. Meanwhile, in a bowl, mix the onion with the rest of the ingredients and the remaining oil, toss, add on top of the chicken and serve.
Nutrition Info:calories 289, fat 12.4, fiber 9.1, carbs 23.8, protein 14.3

312. Slow Cooked Chicken And Capers Mix

Servings: 4   Cooking Time: 7 Hours
Ingredients:
2 chicken breasts, skinless, boneless and halved
2 cups canned tomatoes, crushed
2 garlic cloves, minced
2 cups chicken stock
1 yellow onion, chopped
2 tablespoons capers, drained
¼ cup rosemary, chopped
Salt and black pepper to the taste

Directions:
In your slow cooker, combine the chicken with the tomatoes, capers and the rest of the ingredients, put the lid on and cook on Low for 7 hours. Divide the mix between plates and serve.
Nutrition Info:calories 292, fat 9.4, fiber 11.8, carbs 25.1, protein 36.4

313. Chili Chicken Mix

Servings: 4   Cooking Time: 18 Minutes
Ingredients:
2 tablespoons olive oil
2 cups yellow onion, chopped
2 pounds chicken thighs, skinless and boneless
2 teaspoons oregano,

1 teaspoon onion powder
1 teaspoon smoked paprika
1 teaspoon chili pepper
½ teaspoon coriander seeds, ground

dried
2 teaspoon parsley flakes
30 ounces canned tomatoes, chopped
½ cup black olives, pitted and halved

Directions:
Set the instant pot on Sauté mode, add the oil, heat it up, add the onion, onion powder and the rest of the ingredients except the tomatoes, olives and the chicken, stir and sauté for 10 minutes. Add the chicken, tomatoes and the olives, put the lid on and cook on High for 8 minutes. Release the pressure naturally 10 minutes, divide the mix into bowls and serve.
Nutrition Info: calories 153, fat 8, fiber 2, carbs 9, protein 12

314. Ginger Duck Mix

Servings: 4   Cooking Time: 1 Hour And 50 Minutes
Ingredients:

4 duck legs, boneless
4 shallots, chopped
2 tablespoons olive oil
1 tablespoon ginger, grated

2 tablespoons rosemary, chopped
1 cup chicken stock
1 tablespoon chives, chopped

Directions:
In a roasting pan, combine the duck legs with the shallots and the rest of the ingredients except the chives, toss, introduce in the oven at 250 degrees F and bake for 1 hour and 30 minutes. Divide the mix between plates, sprinkle the chives on top and serve.
Nutrition Info: calories 299, fat 10.2, fiber 9.2, carbs 18.1, protein 17.3

315. Duck And Orange Warm Salad

Servings: 4   Cooking Time: 25 Minutes
Ingredients:

2 tablespoons balsamic vinegar
2 oranges, peeled and cut into segments
1 teaspoon orange zest, grated
1 tablespoons orange juice
2 tablespoons olive oil

3 shallot, minced
Salt and black pepper to the taste
2 duck breasts, boneless and skin scored
2 cups baby arugula
2 tablespoons chives, chopped

Directions:
Heat up a pan with the oil over medium-high heat, add the duck breasts skin side down and brown for 5 minutes. Flip the duck, add the shallot, and the other ingredients except the arugula, orange and the chives, and cook for 15 minutes more. Transfer the duck breasts to a cutting board, cool down, cut into strips and put in a salad bowl. Add the remaining ingredients, toss and serve warm.
Nutrition Info: calories 304, fat 15.4, fiber 12.6, carbs 25.1, protein 36.4

316. Turmeric Baked Chicken Breast

Servings: 2   Cooking Time: 40 Minutes
Ingredients:

8 oz chicken breast, skinless, boneless
2 tablespoons capers
1 teaspoon olive oil
½ teaspoon paprika

½ teaspoon ground turmeric
½ teaspoon salt
½ teaspoon minced garlic

Directions:
Make the lengthwise cut in the chicken breast. Rub the chicken with olive oil, paprika, capers, ground turmeric, salt, and minced garlic. Then fill the chicken cut with capers and secure it with the toothpicks. Bake the chicken breast for 40 minutes at 350F. Remove the toothpicks from the chicken breast and slice it.
Nutrition Info: Per Serving: calories 156, fat 5.4, fiber 0.6, carbs 1.3, protein 24.4

317. Chicken Tacos

Servings: 4   Cooking Time: 20 Minutes
Ingredients:

2 bread tortillas
1 teaspoon butter
2 teaspoons olive oil
6 oz chicken breast, skinless, boneless, sliced

1 teaspoon Taco seasoning
1/3 cup Cheddar cheese, shredded
1 bell pepper, cut on the wedges

Directions:
Pour 1 teaspoon of olive oil in the skillet and add chicken. Sprinkle the meat with Taco seasoning and mix up well. Roast chicken for 10 minutes over the medium heat. Stir it from time to time. Then transfer the cooked chicken in the plate. Add remaining olive oil in the skillet. Then add bell pepper and roast it for 5 minutes. Stir it all the time. Mix up together bell pepper with chicken. Toss butter in the skillet and melt it. Put 1 tortilla in the skillet. Put Cheddar cheese on the tortilla and flatten it. Then add chicken-pepper mixture and cover it with the second tortilla. Roast the quesadilla for 2 minutes from each side. Cut the cooked meal on the halves and transfer in the serving plates.
Nutrition Info: Per Serving: calories 194, fat 8.3, fiber 0.6, carbs 16.4, protein 13.2

318. Chicken And Butter Sauce

Servings: 5   Cooking Time: 30 Minutes
Ingredients:

1-pound chicken fillet
1/3 cup butter, softened

1 tablespoon rosemary
½ teaspoon thyme
1 teaspoon salt
½ lemon

Directions:
Churn together thyme, salt, and rosemary. Chop the chicken fillet roughly and mix up with churned butter mixture. Place the prepared chicken in the baking dish. Squeeze the lemon over the chicken. Chop the squeezed lemon and add in the baking dish. Cover the chicken with foil and bake it for 20 minutes at 365F. Then discard the foil and bake the chicken for 10 minutes more.

Nutrition Info: Per Serving:calories 285, fat 19.1, fiber 0.5, carbs 1, protein 26.5

319. Turkey And Cranberry Sauce

Servings: 4   Cooking Time: 50 Minutes
Ingredients:

1 cup chicken stock
2 tablespoons avocado oil
1 big turkey breast, skinless, boneless and sliced

½ cup cranberry sauce
1 yellow onion, roughly chopped
Salt and black pepper to the taste

Directions:
Heat up a pan with the avocado oil over medium-high heat, add the onion and sauté for 5 minutes.   Add the turkey and brown for 5 minutes more.   Add the rest of the ingredients, toss, introduce in the oven at 350 degrees F and cook for 40 minutes
Nutrition Info:calories 382, fat 12.6, fiber 9.6, carbs 26.6, protein 17.6

320. Coriander And Coconut Chicken

Servings: 4   Cooking Time: 30 Minutes
Ingredients:

2 tablespoons olive oil
Salt and black pepper to the taste
3 tablespoons coconut flesh, shredded
1 and ½ teaspoons orange extract
1 tablespoon ginger, grated

2 pounds chicken thighs, skinless, boneless and cubed
¼ cup orange juice
2 tablespoons coriander, chopped
1 cup chicken stock
¼ teaspoon red pepper flakes

Directions:
Heat up a pan with the oil over medium-high heat, add the chicken and brown for 4 minutes on each side.   Add salt, pepper and the rest of the ingredients, bring to a simmer and cook over medium heat for 20 minutes.   Divide the mix between plates and serve hot.
Nutrition Info:calories 297, fat 14.4, fiber 9.6, carbs 22, protein 25

321. Chicken Pilaf

Servings: 4   Cooking Time: 30 Minutes
Ingredients:

4 tablespoons avocado oil
2 pounds chicken breasts, skinless, boneless and cubed
½ cup yellow onion, chopped
4 garlic cloves, minced
8 ounces brown rice
4 cups chicken stock
½ cup kalamata olives, pitted

½ cup tomatoes, cubed
6 ounces baby spinach
½ cup feta cheese, crumbled
A pinch of salt and black pepper
1 tablespoon marjoram, chopped
1 tablespoon basil, chopped
Juice of ½ lemon

¼ cup pine nuts, toasted

Directions:

Heat up a pot with 1 tablespoon avocado oil over medium-high heat, add the chicken, some salt and pepper, brown for 5 minutes on each side and transfer to a bowl.   Heat up the pot again with the rest of the avocado oil over medium heat, add the onion and garlic and sauté for 3 minutes. Add the rice, the rest of the ingredients except the pine nuts, also return the chicken, toss, bring to a simmer and cook over medium heat for 20 minutes. Divide the mix between plates, top each serving with some pine nuts and serve.
Nutrition Info:calories 283, fat 12.5, fiber 8.2, carbs 21.5, protein 13.4

322. Chicken And Black Beans

Servings: 4   Cooking Time: 20 Minutes
Ingredients:

12 oz chicken breast, skinless, boneless, chopped
1 tablespoon taco seasoning
1 tablespoon nut oil
½ teaspoon cayenne pepper

½ teaspoon salt
½ teaspoon garlic, chopped
½ red onion, sliced
1/3 cup black beans, canned, rinsed
½ cup Mozzarella, shredded

Directions:
Rub the chopped chicken breast with taco seasoning, salt, and cayenne pepper.   Place the chicken in the skillet, add nut oil and roast it for 10 minutes over the medium heat. Mix up the chicken pieces from time to time to avoid burning.   After this, transfer the chicken in the plate.   Add sliced onion and garlic in the skillet. Roast the vegetables for 5 minutes. Stir them constantly. Then add black beans and stir well. Cook the ingredients for 2 minute more.   Add the chopped chicken and mix up well. Top the meal with Mozzarella cheese. Close the lid and cook the meal for 3 minutes.
Nutrition Info: Per Serving:calories 209, fat 6.4, fiber 2.8, carbs 13.7, 22.7

323. Coconut Chicken

Servings: 4   Cooking Time: 5 Minutes
Ingredients:

6 oz chicken fillet
¼ cup of sparkling water
3 tablespoons coconut flakes

1 egg
1 tablespoon coconut oil
1 teaspoon Greek Seasoning

Directions:
Cut the chicken fillet on small pieces (nuggets). Then crack the egg in the bowl and whisk it.   Mix up together egg and sparkling water.   Add Greek seasoning and stir gently.   Dip the chicken nuggets in the egg mixture and then coat in the coconut flakes.   Melt the coconut oil in the skillet and heat it up until it is shimmering.   Then add prepared chicken nuggets.   Roast them for 1 minute from each or until they are light brown. Dry the cooked chicken nuggets with the help of the paper towel and transfer in the serving plates.
Nutrition Info: Per Serving:calories 141, fat 8.9, fiber 0.3, carbs 1, protein 13.9

324. Ginger Chicken Drumsticks

Servings: 4   Cooking Time: 30 Minutes
Ingredients:

4 chicken drumsticks
1 apple, grated
1 tablespoon curry paste
1 teaspoon coconut oil

4 tablespoons milk
1 teaspoon chili flakes
½ teaspoon minced ginger

Directions:
Mix up together grated apple, curry paste, milk, chili flakes, and minced garlic. Put coconut oil in the skillet and melt it. Add apple mixture and stir well. Then add chicken drumsticks and mix up well. Roast the chicken for 2 minutes from each side. Then preheat oven to 360F. Place the skillet with chicken drumsticks in the oven and bake for 25 minutes.
Nutrition Info: Per Serving:calories 150, fat 6.4, fiber 1.4, carbs 9.7, protein 13.5

325. Parmesan Chicken

Servings: 3   Cooking Time: 30 Minutes
Ingredients:
1-pound chicken breast, skinless, boneless
2 oz Parmesan, grated
1 teaspoon dried oregano

½ teaspoon dried cilantro
1 tablespoon Panko bread crumbs
1 egg, beaten
1 teaspoon turmeric

Directions:
Cut the chicken breast on 3 servings. Then combine together Parmesan, oregano, cilantro, bread crumbs, and turmeric. Dip the chicken servings in the beaten egg carefully. Then coat every chicken piece in the cheese-bread crumbs mixture. Line the baking tray with the baking paper. Arrange the chicken pieces in the tray. Bake the chicken for 30 minutes at 365F.
Nutrition Info: Per Serving:calories 267, fat 9.5, fiber 0.5, carbs 3.2, protein 40.4

326. Pomegranate Chicken

Servings: 6   Cooking Time: 25 Minutes
Ingredients:
1-pound chicken breast, skinless, boneless
1 tablespoon za'atar
½ teaspoon salt

1 tablespoon pomegranate juice
1 tablespoon olive oil

Directions:
Rub the chicken breast with za'atar seasoning, salt, olive oil, and pomegranate juice. Marinate the chicken or 15 minutes and transfer in the skillet. Roast the chicken for 15 minutes over the medium heat. Then flip the chicken on another side and cook for 10 minutes more. Slice the chicken and place in the serving plates.
Nutrition Info: Per Serving:calories 107, fat 4.2, fiber 0, carbs 0.2, protein 16.1

327. Chicken With Artichokes And Beans

Servings: 4   Cooking Time: 40 Minutes
Ingredients:
2 tablespoons olive oil
2 chicken breasts, skinless, boneless and halved
Zest of 1 lemon,

Juice of 1 lemon
6 ounces canned artichokes hearts, drained
1 cup canned fava beans, drained and

grated
3 garlic cloves, crushed
Salt and black pepper to the taste
1 tablespoon thyme, chopped

rinsed
1 cup chicken stock
A pinch of cayenne pepper
Salt and black pepper to the taste

Directions:
Heat up a pan with the oil over medium-high heat, add chicken and brown for 5 minutes. Add lemon juice, lemon zest, salt, pepper and the rest of the ingredients, bring to a simmer and cook over medium heat for 35 minutes. Divide the mix between plates and serve right away.
Nutrition Info:calories 291, fat 14.9, fiber 10.5, carbs 23.8, protein 24.2

328. Chicken Pie

Servings: 6   Cooking Time: 50 Minutes
Ingredients:
¼ cup green peas, frozen
1 carrot, chopped
1 cup ground chicken
1 tablespoon butter, melted

5 oz puff pastry
¼ cup cream
1 teaspoon ground black pepper
1 oz Parmesan, grated

Directions:
Roll up the puff pastry and cut it on 2 parts. Place one puff pastry part in the non-sticky springform pan and flatten. Then mix up together green peas, chopped carrot, ground chicken, and ground black pepper. Place the chicken mixture in the puff pastry. Pour cream over mixture and sprinkle with Parmesan. Cover the mixture with second puff pastry half and secure the edges of it with the help of the fork. Brush the surface of the pie with melted butter and bake it for 50 minutes at 365F.
Nutrition Info: Per Serving:calories 223, fat 14.3, fiber 1, carbs 13.2, protein 10.5

329. Chicken And Semolina Meatballs

Servings: 8   Cooking Time: 10 Minutes
Ingredients:
1/3 cup carrot, grated
1 onion, diced
2 cups ground chicken
1 tablespoon semolina
1 egg, beaten
1 teaspoon dried oregano

½ teaspoon salt
1 teaspoon dried cilantro
1 teaspoon chili flakes
1 tablespoon coconut oil

Directions:
In the mixing bowl combine together grated carrot, diced onion, ground chicken, semolina, egg, salt, dried oregano, cilantro, and chili flakes. With the help of scooper make the meatballs. Heat up the coconut oil in the skillet. When it starts to shimmer, put meatballs in it. Cook the meatballs for 5 minutes from each side over the medium-low heat.
Nutrition Info: Per Serving:calories 102, fat 4.9, fiber 0.5, carbs 2.9, protein 11.2

330. Lemon Chicken Mix

Servings: 2   Cooking Time: 10 Minutes
Ingredients:

8 oz chicken breast, skinless, boneless
1 teaspoon Cajun seasoning
1 teaspoon olive oil
1 teaspoon balsamic vinegar
1 teaspoon lemon juice

Directions:
Cut the chicken breast on the halves and sprinkle with Cajun seasoning.   Then sprinkle the poultry with olive oil and lemon juice.   Then sprinkle the chicken breast with the balsamic vinegar. Preheat the grill to 385F.   Grill the chicken breast halves for 5 minutes from each side.   Slice Cajun chicken and place in the serving plate.

Nutrition Info: Per Serving: calories 150, fat 5.2, fiber 0, carbs 0.1, protein 24.1

331.	Turkey And Chickpeas

Servings: 4   Cooking Time: 5 Hours
Ingredients:
2 tablespoons avocado oil
1 big turkey breast, skinless, boneless and roughly cubed
Salt and black pepper to the taste
15 ounces canned chickpeas, drained and rinsed
1 red onion, chopped
15 ounces canned tomatoes, chopped
1 cup kalamata olives, pitted and halved
2 tablespoons lime juice
1 teaspoon oregano, dried

Directions:
Heat up a pan with the oil over medium-high heat, add the meat and the onion, brown for 5 minutes and transfer to a slow cooker.   Add the rest of the ingredients, put the lid on and cook on High for 5 hours.   Divide between plates and serve right away!

Nutrition Info: calories 352, fat 14.4, fiber 11.8, carbs 25.1, protein 26.4

332.	Cardamom Chicken And Apricot Sauce

Servings: 4   Cooking Time: 7 Hours
Ingredients:
Zest of ½ lemon, grated
2 teaspoons cardamom, ground
Salt and black pepper to the taste
2 chicken breasts, skinless, boneless and halved
2 tablespoons olive oil
Juice of ½ lemon
2 spring onions, chopped
2 tablespoons tomato paste
2 garlic cloves, minced
1 cup apricot juice
½ cup chicken stock
¼ cup cilantro, chopped

Directions:
In your slow cooker, combine the chicken with the lemon juice, lemon zest and the other ingredients except the cilantro, toss, put the lid on and cook on Low for 7 hours.   Divide the mix between plates, sprinkle the cilantro on top and serve.

Nutrition Info: calories 323, fat 12, fiber 11, carbs 23.8, protein 16.4

333.	Chicken And Artichokes

Servings: 4   Cooking Time: 20 Minutes
Ingredients:
2 pounds chicken
4 tablespoons olive

breast, skinless, boneless and sliced
A pinch of salt and black pepper
8 ounces canned roasted artichoke hearts, drained
oil
6 ounces sun-dried tomatoes, chopped
3 tablespoons capers, drained
2 tablespoons lemon juice

Directions:
Heat up a pan with half of the oil over medium-high heat, add the artichokes and the other ingredients except the chicken, stir and sauté for 10 minutes.   Transfer the mix to a bowl, heat up the pan again with the rest of the oil over medium-high heat, add the meat and cook for 4 minutes on each side.   Return the veggie mix to the pan, toss, cook everything for 2-3 minutes more, divide between plates and serve.

Nutrition Info: calories 552, fat 28, fiber 6, carbs 33, protein 43

334.	Buttery Chicken Spread

Servings: 6   Cooking Time: 20 Minutes
Ingredients:
8 oz chicken liver
3 tablespoon butter
1 white onion, chopped
1 bay leaf
1 teaspoon salt
½ teaspoon ground black pepper
½ cup of water

Directions:
Place the chicken liver in the saucepan.   Add onion, bay leaf, salt, ground black pepper, and water.   Mix up the mixture and close the lid. Cook the liver mixture for 20 minutes over the medium heat.   Then transfer it in the blender and blend until smooth.   Add butter and mix up until it is melted.   Pour the pate mixture in the pate ramekin and refrigerate for 2 hours.

Nutrition Info: Per Serving: calories 122, fat 8.3, fiber 0.5, carbs 2.3, protein 9.5

335.	Chicken And Spinach Cakes

Servings: 4   Cooking Time: 15 Minutes
Ingredients:
8 oz ground chicken
1 cup fresh spinach, blended
1 teaspoon minced onion
1 red bell pepper, grinded
½ teaspoon salt
1 egg, beaten
1 teaspoon ground black pepper
4 tablespoons Panko breadcrumbs

Directions:
In the mixing bowl mix up together ground chicken, blended spinach, minced garlic, salt, grinded bell pepper, egg, and ground black pepper.   When the chicken mixture is smooth, make 4 burgers from it and coat them in Panko breadcrumbs.   Place the burgers in the non-sticky baking dish or line the baking tray with baking paper.   Bake the burgers for 15 minutes at 365F.   Flip the chicken burgers on another side after 7 minutes of cooking.

Nutrition Info: Per Serving: calories 171, fat 5.7, fiber 1.7, carbs 10.5, protein 19.4

336.	Cream Cheese Chicken

Servings: 2   Cooking Time: 20 Minutes
Ingredients:
1 onion, chopped
1 sweet red pepper, roasted, chopped
1 tablespoon olive oil
½ teaspoon ground

1 cup spinach, chopped
½ cup cream
1 teaspoon cream cheese

black pepper
8 oz chicken breast, skinless, boneless, sliced

Directions:
Mix up together sliced chicken breast with ground black pepper and put in the saucepan.   Add olive oil and mix up.   Roast the chicken for 5 minutes over the medium-high heat. Stir it from time to time.   After this, add chopped sweet pepper, onion, and cream cheese.   Mix up well and bring to boil.   Add spinach and cream. Mix up well. Close the lid and cook chicken Alfredo for 10 minutes more over the medium heat.
Nutrition Info: Per Serving:calories 279, fat 14, fiber 2.5, carbs 12.4, protein 26.4

337.   Chicken And Lemongrass Sauce

Servings: 4   Cooking Time: 20 Minutes
Ingredients:
1 tablespoon dried dill
1 teaspoon butter, melted
½ teaspoon lemongrass
½ teaspoon cayenne pepper

1 teaspoon tomato sauce
3 tablespoons sour cream
1 teaspoon salt
10 oz chicken fillet, cubed

Directions:
Make the sauce: in the saucepan whisk together lemongrass, tomato sauce, sour cream, salt, and dried dill.   Bring the sauce to boil.   Meanwhile, pour melted butter in the skillet.   Add cubed chicken fillet and roast it for 5 minutes. Stir it from time to time.   Then place the chicken cubes in the hot sauce.   Close the lid and cook the meal for 10 minutes more over the low heat.
Nutrition Info: Per Serving:calories 166, fat 8.2, fiber 0.2, carbs 1.1, protein 21

338.   Spiced Chicken Meatballs

Servings: 4   Cooking Time: 20 Minutes
Ingredients:
1 pound chicken meat, ground
1 tablespoon pine nuts, toasted and chopped
1 egg, whisked
2 teaspoons turmeric powder
2 garlic cloves, minced

Salt and black pepper to the taste
1 and ¼ cups heavy cream
2 tablespoons olive oil
¼ cup parsley, chopped
1 tablespoon chives, chopped

Directions:
In a bowl, combine the chicken with the pine nuts and the rest of the ingredients except the oil and the cream, stir well and shape medium meatballs out of this mix.   Heat up a pan with the oil over medium-high heat, add the meatballs and cook them for 4 minutes on each side.   Add the cream, toss gently, cook everything over medium heat for 10 minutes more, divide between plates and serve.
Nutrition Info:calories 283, fat 9.2, fiber 12.8, carbs 24.4, protein 34.5

339.   Paprika Chicken Wings

Servings: 4   Cooking Time: 8 Minutes
Ingredients:
4 chicken wings, boneless
1 tablespoon honey
½ teaspoon paprika
¼ teaspoon cayenne pepper

¾ teaspoon ground black pepper
1 tablespoon lemon juice
½ teaspoon sunflower oil

Directions:
Make the honey marinade: whisk together honey, paprika, cayenne pepper, ground black pepper, lemon juice, and sunflower oil.   Then brush the chicken wings with marinade carefully.   Preheat the grill to 385F.   Place the chicken wings in the grill and cook them for 4 minutes from each side.
Nutrition Info: Per Serving:calories 26, fat 0.8, fiber 0.3, carbs 5.1, protein 0.3

340.   Chicken And Parsley Sauce

Servings: 4   Cooking Time: 25 Minutes
Ingredients:
1 cup ground chicken
2 oz Parmesan, grated
1 tablespoon olive oil
2 tablespoons fresh parsley, chopped
1 teaspoon chili pepper
1 teaspoon paprika

½ teaspoon dried oregano
¼ teaspoon garlic, minced
½ teaspoon dried thyme
1/3 cup crushed tomatoes

Directions:
Heat up olive oil in the skillet.   Add ground chicken and sprinkle it with chili pepper, paprika, dried oregano, dried thyme, and parsley. Mix up well.   Cook the chicken for 5 minutes and add crushed tomatoes. Mix up well.   Close the lid and simmer the chicken mixture for 10 minutes over the low heat.   Then add grated Parmesan and mix up.   Cook chicken bolognese for 5 minutes more over the medium heat.
Nutrition Info: Per Serving:calories 154, fat 9.3, fiber 1.1, carbs 3, protein 15.4

341.   Sage Turkey Mix

Servings: 4   Cooking Time: 40 Minutes
Ingredients:
1 big turkey breast, skinless, boneless and roughly cubed
Juice of 1 lemon
2 tablespoons avocado oil

1 red onion, chopped
2 tablespoons sage, chopped
1 garlic clove, minced
1 cup chicken stock

Directions:
Heat up a pan with the avocado oil over medium-high heat, add the turkey and brown for 3 minutes on each side.   Add the rest of the ingredients, bring to a simmer and cook over medium heat for 35 minutes.   Divide the mix between plates and serve with a side dish.
Nutrition Info:calories 382, fat 12.6, fiber 9.6, carbs 16.6, protein 33.2

342.   Chipotle Turkey And Tomatoes

Servings: 4   Cooking Time: 1 Hour

Ingredients:

2 pounds cherry tomatoes, halved

3 tablespoons olive oil

1 red onion, roughly chopped

1 big turkey breast, skinless, boneless and sliced

3 garlic cloves, chopped

3 red chili peppers, chopped

4 tablespoons chipotle paste

Zest of ½ lemon, grated

Juice of 1 lemon

Salt and black pepper to the taste

A handful coriander, chopped

Directions:

Heat up a pan with the oil over medium-high heat, add the turkey slices, cook for 4 minutes on each side and transfer to a roasting pan.   Heat up the pan again over medium-high heat, add the onion, garlic and chili peppers and sauté for 2 minutes. Add chipotle paste, sauté for 3 minutes more and pour over the turkey slices.   Toss the turkey slices with the chipotle mix, also add the rest of the ingredients except the coriander, introduce in the oven and bake at 400 degrees F for 45 minutes. Divide everything between plates, sprinkle the coriander on top and serve.

Nutrition Info: calories 264, fat 13.2, fiber 8.7, carbs 23.9, protein 33.2

343. Curry Chicken, Artichokes And Olives

Servings: 6   Cooking Time: 7 Hours

Ingredients:

2 pounds chicken breasts, boneless, skinless and cubed

12 ounces canned artichoke hearts, drained

1 cup chicken stock

1 red onion, chopped

1 cup kalamata olives, pitted and chopped

1 tablespoon white wine vinegar

1 tablespoon curry powder

2 teaspoons basil, dried

Salt and black pepper to the taste

¼ cup rosemary, chopped

Directions:

In your slow cooker, combine the chicken with the artichokes, olives and the rest of the ingredients, put the lid on and cook on Low for 7 hours. Divide the mix between plates and serve hot.

Nutrition Info: calories 275, fat 11.9, fiber 7.6, carbs 19.7, protein 18.7

344. Roasted Chicken

Servings: ¼ Chicken   Cooking Time: 1 Hour 15 Minutes

Ingredients:

1 (5-lb.) whole chicken

1 TB. extra-virgin olive oil

2 TB. minced garlic

1 tsp. salt

1 tsp. paprika

1 tsp. black pepper

1 tsp. ground coriander

1/2 tsp. ground cinnamon

1/2 large lemon, cut in 1/2

1 tsp. seven spices

1/2 large yellow onion, cut in 1/2

2 sprigs fresh rosemary

2 sprigs fresh thyme

2 sprigs fresh sage

2 large carrots, cut into 1-in. pieces

6 small red potatoes, washed and cut in 1/2

4 cloves garlic

Directions:

Preheat the oven to 450°F. Wash chicken and pat dry with paper towels. Place chicken in a roasting pan, and drizzle and then rub chicken with extra-virgin olive oil.   In a small bowl, combine garlic, salt, paprika, black pepper, coriander, seven spices, and cinnamon. Sprinkle and then rub entire chicken with spice mixture to coat.   Place 1/4 lemon, 1/4 yellow onion, 1 sprig rosemary, 1 sprig thyme, and 1 sprig sage in chicken cavity.   Place remaining rosemary, thyme, sage, lemon, and onion around chicken in the roasting pan. Add carrots, red potatoes, and garlic cloves to the roasting pan.   Roast for 15 minutes. Reduce temperature to 375°F, and roast for 1 more hour, basting chicken every 20 minutes.   Let chicken rest for 15 minutes before serving.

345. Curry Chicken Mix

Servings: 2   Cooking Time: 25 Minutes

Ingredients:

2 flatbread

7 oz chicken fillet

1 tablespoon yogurt

1 teaspoon minced garlic

1 teaspoon fresh parsley

½ teaspoon salt

½ teaspoon paprika

¼ teaspoon curry powder

1 tablespoon tomato sauce

Directions:

Make the marinade: mix up together yogurt, minced garlic, salt, paprika, and curry powder. Chop the chicken fillet on the medium cubes and put them in the marinade.   Mix up the chicken well and leave to marinate for at least 15 minutes. Then put the marinated chicken in the baking tray in one layer and bake it for 25 minutes at 350F. Flip the chicken on another side after 10 minutes of cooking.   Then put the cooked chicken on the flatbread and sprinkle with tomato sauce and parsley.

Nutrition Info: Per Serving: calories 290, fat 10.1, fiber 2.4, carbs 15.9, protein 32.5

346. Creamy Chicken

Servings: 4   Cooking Time: 35 Minutes

Ingredients:

1-pound chicken breast, skinless, boneless

3 oz Mozzarella, sliced

1 tomato, sliced

1 teaspoon Italian seasoning

½ teaspoon salt

1 tablespoon sour cream

1 teaspoon olive oil

Directions:

Make the cuts in the chicken breast in the shape of Hasselback.   Sprinkle the chicken with Italian seasoning, salt, and sour cream.   Massage the chicken breast gently.   Fill every chicken breast cut with sliced Mozzarella and sliced tomato. Arrange the chicken breast in the baking dish and sprinkle it with olive oil.   Bake the chicken Hasselback for 35 minutes at 355F.

Nutrition Info: Per Serving: calories 212, fat 8.8, fiber 0.2, carbs 1.6, protein 30.3

347. Chicken And Celery Quinoa Mix

Servings: 4   Cooking Time: 50 Minutes

Ingredients:

4 chicken things,
skinless and boneless
1 tablespoon olive oil
Salt and black pepper
to the taste
2 celery stalks,
chopped

2 spring onions,
chopped
2 cups chicken stock
½ cup cilantro,
chopped
½ cup quinoa
1 teaspoon lime zest,
grated

Directions:
Heat up a pot with the oil over medium-high heat,
add the chicken and brown for 4 minutes on each
side.   Add the onion and the celery, stir and sauté
everything for 5 minutes more.   Add the rest of
the ingredients, toss, bring to a simmer and cook
over medium-low heat for 35 minutes.   Divide
everything between plates and serve.
Nutrition Info:calories 241, fat 12.6, fiber 9.5,
carbs 15.6, protein 34.1

348.   Turmeric Chicken And Eggplant Mix

Servings: 4   Cooking Time: 30 Minutes
Ingredients:

2 cups eggplant,
cubed
Salt and black pepper
to the taste
2 tablespoons olive
oil
1 cup yellow onion,
chopped
2 tablespoons garlic,
minced
2 tablespoons hot
paprika

1 teaspoon turmeric
powder
1 and ½ tablespoons
oregano, chopped
1 cup chicken stock
1 pound chicken
breast, skinless,
boneless and cubed
1 cup half and half
1 tablespoon lemon
juice

Directions:
Heat up a pan with the oil over medium-high heat,
add the chicken and brown for 4 minutes on each
side.   Add the eggplant, onion and garlic and
sauté for 5 minutes more.   Add the rest of the
ingredients, bring to a simmer and cook over
medium heat for 16 minutes.   Divide the mix
between plates and serve.
Nutrition Info:calories 392, fat 11.6, fiber 8.3,
carbs 21.1, protein 24.2

349.   Honey Chicken

Servings: 5   Cooking Time: 25 Minutes
Ingredients:

5 chicken drumsticks
2 oz currant
½ teaspoon liquid
honey
1 teaspoon butter

1 teaspoon lime juice
½ teaspoon salt
¼ cup of water
½ teaspoon chili
pepper

Directions:
Mix up together chicken drumsticks with chili
pepper and salt.   Put butter in the skillet and heat
it up.   Add chicken drumsticks and cook them for
15 minutes or until they are cooked.   Meanwhile,
mash currant and mix it up with lime juice, liquid
honey, and water.   Pour the currant mixture over
the drumstick and close the lid.   Cook the meal
for 5 minutes over the medium heat.
Nutrition Info: Per Serving:calories 93, fat 3.4,
fiber 0.5, carbs 2.2, protein 12.8

350.   Chicken And Nutmeg Butter Sauce

Servings: 4   Cooking Time: 30 Minutes
Ingredients:

4 chicken thighs,
skinless, boneless
1 teaspoon ground
black pepper
½ teaspoon salt
¼ cup Cheddar
cheese, shredded
1 tablespoon cream
cheese

1 teaspoon paprika
½ teaspoon garlic
powder
1 teaspoon fresh dill,
chopped
1 tablespoon butter
1 teaspoon olive oil
½ teaspoon ground
nutmeg

Directions:
Grease the baking dish with butter.   Then heat up
olive oil in the skillet.   Meanwhile, rub the
chicken thighs with ground nutmeg, garlic powder,
paprika, and salt.   Add ground black pepper.
Roast the chicken thighs in the hot oil over the high
heat for 2 minutes from each side.   Then transfer
the chicken thighs in the prepared baking dish.
Mix up together Cheddar cheese, cream cheese, and
dill.   Top every chicken thigh with cheese
mixture and bake for 25 minutes at 365F.
Nutrition Info: Per Serving:calories 79, fat 7.5,
fiber 0.4, carbs 1.2, protein 2.4

351.   Cheddar Chicken Mix

Servings: 4   Cooking Time: 20 Minutes
Ingredients:

4 chicken fillets (4 oz
each fillet)
1 cup cherry tomatoes
1 tablespoon olive oil
1 tablespoon fresh
basil, chopped
½ teaspoon salt

½ teaspoon ground
black pepper
1 teaspoon balsamic
vinegar
1 teaspoon garlic
clove, diced
1 oz Cheddar cheese,
shredded

Directions:
Pour olive oil in the skillet and heat it up.
Sprinkle the chicken fillets with salt and ground
black pepper and put in the hot oil.   Roast the
chicken for 3 minutes from each side over the
medium heat.   Then cut the cherry tomatoes on
the halves and add in the olive oil.   Sprinkle the
vegetables with balsamic vinegar, garlic, and basil.
Mix up the ingredients well.   Sprinkle the
chicken with Cheddar cheese and close the lid.
Cook the chicken caprese for 10 minutes over the
medium heat.
Nutrition Info: Per Serving:calories 299, fat 17,
fiber 1.6, carbs 17.3, protein 21.3

352.   Chicken And Veggie Saute

Servings: 2   Cooking Time: 25 Minutes
Ingredients:

4 oz chicken fillet
4 tomatoes, peeled
1 bell pepper,
chopped
1 teaspoon olive oil

1 cup of water
1 teaspoon salt
1 chili pepper,
chopped
½ teaspoon saffron

Directions:
Pour water in the pan and bring it to boil.
Meanwhile, chop the chicken fillet.   Add the
chicken fillet in the boiling water and cook it for 10
minutes or until the chicken is tender.   After this,

put the chopped bell pepper and chili pepper in the skillet. Add olive oil and roast the vegetables for 3 minutes. Add chopped tomatoes and mix up well. Cook the vegetables for 2 minutes more. Then add salt and a ¾ cup of water from chicken. Add chopped chicken fillet and mix up. Cook the saute for 10 minutes over the medium heat.
Nutrition Info: Per Serving:calories 192, fat 7.2, fiber 3.8, carbs 14.4, protein 19.2

353. Thyme Chicken And Potatoes

Servings: 4   Cooking Time: 50 Minutes
Ingredients:

1 tablespoon olive oil
4 garlic cloves, minced
A pinch of salt and black pepper
2 pounds chicken breast, skinless, boneless and cubed

2 teaspoons thyme, dried
12 small red potatoes, halved
1 cup red onion, sliced
¾ cup chicken stock
2 tablespoons basil, chopped

Directions:
In a baking dish greased with the oil, add the potatoes, chicken and the rest of the ingredients, toss a bit, introduce in the oven and bake at 400 degrees F for 50 minutes. Divide between plates and serve.
Nutrition Info:calories 281, fat 9.2, fiber 10.9, carbs 21.6, protein 13.6

354. Creamy Chicken And Mushrooms

Servings: 4   Cooking Time: 30 Minutes
Ingredients:

1 red onion, chopped
1 tablespoon olive oil
2 garlic cloves, minced
Salt and black pepper to the taste
1 tablespoon thyme, chopped
1 and ½ cups chicken stock

2 carrots chopped
½ pound Bella mushrooms, sliced
1 cup heavy cream
2 chicken breasts, skinless, boneless and cubed
2 tablespoons chives, chopped
1 tablespoon parsley, chopped

Directions:
Heat up a Dutch oven with the oil over medium-high heat, add the onion and the garlic and sauté for 5 minutes. Add the chicken and the mushrooms, and sauté for 10 minutes more. Add the rest of the ingredients except the chives and the parsley, bring to a simmer and cook over medium heat for 15 minutes. Add the chives and parsley, divide the mix between plates and serve.
Nutrition Info:calories 275, fat 11.9, fiber 10.6, carbs 26.7, protein 23.7

355. Basil Turkey And Zucchinis

Servings: 4   Cooking Time: 1 Hour
Ingredients:

2 tablespoons avocado oil
1 pound turkey breast, skinless, boneless and sliced
Salt and black pepper to the taste

3 garlic cloves, minced
2 zucchinis, sliced
1 cup chicken stock
¼ cup heavy cream
2 tablespoons basil,
chopped

Directions:
Heat up a pot with the oil over medium-high heat, add the turkey and brown for 5 minutes on each side. Add the garlic and cook everything for 1 minute. Add the rest of the ingredients except the basil, toss gently, bring to a simmer and cook over medium-low heat for 50 minutes. Add the basil, toss, divide the mix between plates and serve.
Nutrition Info:calories 262, fat 9.8, fiber 12.2, carbs 25.8, protein 14.6

356. Herbed Almond Turkey

Servings: 4   Cooking Time: 40 Minutes
Ingredients:

1 big turkey breast, skinless, boneless and cubed
1 tablespoon olive oil
½ cup chicken stock
1 tablespoon basil, chopped
1 tablespoon rosemary, chopped

1 tablespoon oregano, chopped
1 tablespoon parsley, chopped
3 garlic cloves, minced
½ cup almonds, toasted and chopped
3 cups tomatoes, chopped

Directions:
Heat up a pan with the oil over medium-high heat, add the turkey and the garlic and brown for 5 minutes. Add the stock and the rest of the ingredients, bring to a simmer over medium heat and cook for 35 minutes. Divide the mix between plates and serve.
Nutrition Info:calories 297, fat 11.2, fiber 9.2, carbs 19.4, protein 23.6

357. Lime Chicken Thighs And Pomegranate Sauce

Servings: 2   Cooking Time: 10 Minutes
Ingredients:

1 tablespoon pomegranate molasses
8 oz chicken thighs (4 oz each chicken thigh)
½ teaspoon paprika
1 teaspoon cornstarch

½ teaspoon chili flakes
½ teaspoon ground black pepper
1 teaspoon olive oil
½ teaspoon lime juice

Directions:
In the shallow bowl mix up together ground black pepper, chili flakes, paprika, and cornstarch. Rub the chicken thighs with spice mixture. Heat up olive oil in the skillet. Add chicken thighs and roast them for 4 minutes from each side over the medium heat. When the chicken thighs are light brown, sprinkle them with pomegranate molasses and roast for 1 minute from each side.
Nutrition Info: Per Serving:calories 353, fat 21, fiber 0.4, carbs 9.3, protein 30.2

358. Mediterranean Meatloaf

Servings: 1/8 Loaf   Cooking Time: 45 Minutes
Ingredients:

2 lb. ground chicken
1/3 cup plain breadcrumbs
11/2 tsp. salt
1 tsp. garlic powder
1 tsp. ground black

1/2 tsp. dried thyme
2 TB. fresh Italian parsley, chopped
1 large egg
1 large carrot, shredded

pepper
1 tsp. paprika
1/2 tsp. dried oregano
2 TB. fresh basil, chopped

1 cup fresh or frozen green peas
1/2 cup sun-dried tomatoes, chopped
1 cup ketchup

Directions:
Preheat the oven to 400°F. Lightly coat all sides of a 9×5-inch loaf pan with olive oil spray. In a large bowl, combine chicken, breadcrumbs, salt, garlic powder, black pepper, paprika, oregano, thyme, basil, Italian parsley, egg, carrot, green peas, and sun-dried tomatoes. Transfer chicken mixture to the prepared pan, and even out top. Cover the pan with a piece of aluminum foil, and bake for 40 minutes. After 40 minutes have passed, pour ketchup over top of loaf and spread out evenly. Bake for 5 more minutes. Remove meatloaf from the oven, and let rest for 10 minutes before slicing and serving warm.

359. Lemon Chicken

Servings: 4   Cooking Time: 20 Minutes
Ingredients:
1-pound chicken breast, skinless, boneless
3 tablespoons lemon juice

1 tablespoon olive oil
1 teaspoon ground black pepper

Directions:
Cut the chicken breast on 4 pieces. Sprinkle every chicken piece with olive oil, lemon juice, and ground black pepper. Then place them in the skillet. Roast the chicken for 20 minutes over the medium heat. Flip the chicken pieces every 5 minutes.
Nutrition Info: Per Serving:calories 163, fat 6.5, fiber 0.2, carbs 0.6, protein 24.2

360. Chicken And Mushroom Mix

Servings: 2   Cooking Time: 20 Minutes
Ingredients:
9 oz chicken fillet, cubed
1/3 cup cream
¼ cup mushrooms, chopped
1 teaspoon butter
½ onion, diced

½ teaspoon ground black pepper
½ teaspoon salt
1 teaspoon hot pepper
1 teaspoon sunflower oil

Directions:
Sprinkle the chicken cubes with hot pepper and mix up. Pour sunflower oil in the skillet and roast chicken cubes for 5 minutes over the medium heat. Stir them from time to time. Toss butter in the separated skillet and melt it. Add mushrooms and sprinkle them with salt and ground black pepper. Add onion. Cook the vegetables for 10 minutes over the low heat. Stir them with the help of spatula every 3 minutes. Then add cream and bring to boil. Add roasted chicken cubes and mix up well. Close the lid and simmer the meal for 5 minutes.
Nutrition Info: Per Serving:calories 213, fat 10.7, fiber 0.5, carbs 3, protein 25.2

361. Chicken And Ginger Cucumbers Mix

Servings: 4   Cooking Time: 20 Minutes

Ingredients:
4 chicken breasts, boneless, skinless and cubed
Salt and black pepper to the taste
1 tablespoon ginger, grated
1 tablespoon garlic, minced
2 tablespoons balsamic vinegar

2 cucumbers, cubed
3 tablespoons olive oil
¼ teaspoon chili paste
½ cup chicken stock
½ tablespoon lime juice
1 tablespoon chives, chopped

Directions:
Heat up a pan with the oil over medium-high heat, add the chicken and brown for 3 minutes on each side. Add the cucumbers, salt, pepper and the rest of the ingredients except the chives, bring to a simmer and cook over medium heat for 15 minutes. Divide the mix between plates and serve with the chives sprinkled on top.
Nutrition Info:calories 288, fat 9.5, fiber 12.1, carbs 25.6, protein 28.6

362. Dill Chicken Stew

Servings: 2   Cooking Time: 25 Minutes
Ingredients:
1 ½ cup water
6 oz chicken fillet
1 chili pepper, chopped
1 onion, diced

1 teaspoon butter
½ teaspoon salt
½ teaspoon paprika
1 tablespoon fresh dill, chopped

Directions:
Pour water in the saucepan. Add chicken fillet and salt. Boil it for 15 minutes over the medium heat. Then remove the chicken fillet from water and shred it with the help of the fork. Return it back in the hot water. Melt butter in the skillet and add diced onion. Roast it until light brown and transfer in the shredded chicken. Add paprika, dill, chili pepper, and mix up. Close the lid and simmer Posole for 5 minutes. Ladle it in the serving bowls.
Nutrition Info: Per Serving:calories 207, fat 8.4, fiber 1.7, carbs 6.5, protein 25.7

363. Chicken Stuffed Zucchini

Servings: 2   Cooking Time: 30 Minutes
Ingredients:
1 zucchini
½ teaspoon chipotle pepper
½ teaspoon tomato sauce

½ cup ground chicken
1 oz Swiss cheese, shredded
½ teaspoon salt
4 tablespoons water

Directions:
Trim the zucchini and cut it on 2 halves. Remove the zucchini pulp. In the mixing bowl mix up together ground chicken, chipotle pepper, tomato sauce, and salt. Fill the zucchini with chicken mixture and top with Swiss cheese. Place the zucchini boats in the tray. Add water. Bake the boats for 30 minutes at 355F.
Nutrition Info: Per Serving:calories 137, fat 6.7, fiber 1.1, carbs 4.2, protein 15.2

364. Creamy Coriander Chicken

Servings: 4   Cooking Time: 55 Minutes
Ingredients:

2 chicken breasts, boneless, skinless and halved	2 spring onions, chopped
2 tablespoons avocado oil	2 garlic cloves, minced
½ teaspoon hot paprika	¼ cup heavy cream
1 cup chicken stock	A handful coriander, chopped
1 tablespoon almonds, chopped	Salt and black pepper to the taste

Directions:
Grease a roasting pan with the oil, add the chicken, paprika and the rest of the ingredients except the coriander and the heavy cream, toss, introduce in the oven and bake at 360 degrees F for 40 minutes. Add the cream and the coriander, toss, bake for 15 minutes more, divide between plates and serve.
Nutrition Info: calories 225, fat 8.9, fiber 10.2, carbs 20.8, protein 17.5

365. Chicken And Tomato Pan

Servings: 4   Cooking Time: 30 Minutes
Ingredients:

12 oz chicken fillet	1 yellow onion, diced
4 kalamata olives, chopped	1 tablespoon olive oil
4 tomatoes, chopped	½ cup of water

Directions:
Pour olive oil in the saucepan.   Add diced yellow onion and cook it for 5 minutes. Stir it from time to time.   After this, add olives and chopped tomatoes. Mix up well and cook vegetables for 5 minutes more. Meanwhile, chop the chicken fillet.   Add the chicken fillet in the tomato mixture and mix up.   Close the lid.   Simmer the chicken for 20 minutes over the medium heat.
Nutrition Info: Per Serving: calories 230, fat 10.6, fiber 2.2, carbs 7.6, protein 26

366. Smoked And Hot Turkey Mix

Servings: 4   Cooking Time: 40 Minutes
Ingredients:

1 big turkey breast, skinless, boneless and roughly cubed	1 red onion, sliced
1 tablespoon smoked paprika	2 tablespoons olive oil
2 chili peppers, chopped	½ cup chicken stock
Salt and black pepper to the taste	1 tablespoon parsley, chopped
	1 tablespoon cilantro, chopped

Directions:
Grease a roasting pan with the oil, add the turkey, onion, paprika and the rest of the ingredients, toss, introduce in the oven and bake at 425 degrees F for 40 minutes.   Divide the mix between plates and serve right away.
Nutrition Info: calories 310, fat 18.4, fiber 10.4, carbs 22.3, protein 33.4

367. Chicken With Artichokes

Servings: 3   Cooking Time: 30 Minutes
Ingredients:

1 can artichoke hearts, chopped	½ teaspoon ground thyme
12 oz chicken fillets (3 oz each fillet)	½ teaspoon white
1 teaspoon avocado oil	pepper
1/3 cup water	1/3 cup shallot, roughly chopped
	1 lemon, sliced

Directions:
Mix up together chicken fillets, artichoke hearts, avocado oil, ground thyme, white pepper, and shallot.   Line the baking tray with baking paper and place the chicken fillet mixture in it.   Then add sliced lemon and water.   Bake the meal for 30 minutes at 375F. Stir the ingredients during cooking to avoid burning.
Nutrition Info: Per Serving: calories 263, fat 8.8, fiber 3.7, carbs 10.9, protein 35.3

368. Brown Rice, Chicken And Scallions

Servings: 4   Cooking Time: 30 Minutes
Ingredients:

1 and ½ cups brown rice	6 scallions, chopped
3 cups chicken stock	Salt and black pepper to the taste
2 tablespoon balsamic vinegar	1 tablespoon sweet paprika
1 pound chicken breast, boneless, skinless and cubed	2 tablespoons avocado oil

Directions:
Heat up a pan with the oil over medium-high heat, add the chicken and brown for 5 minutes.   Add the scallions and sauté for 5 minutes more.   Add the rice and the rest of the ingredients, bring to a simmer and cook over medium heat for 20 minutes. Stir the mix, divide everything between plates and serve.
Nutrition Info: calories 300, fat 9.2, fiber 11.8, carbs 18.6, protein 23.8

369. Greek Chicken Bites

Servings: 6   Cooking Time: 20 Minutes
Ingredients:

1-pound chicken fillet	1 teaspoon sesame oil
1 tablespoon Greek seasoning	½ teaspoon salt
	1 teaspoon balsamic vinegar

Directions:
Cut the chicken fingers on small tenders (fingers) and sprinkle them with Greek seasoning, salt, and balsamic vinegar. Mix up well with the help of the fingertips.   Then sprinkle chicken with sesame oil and shake gently.   Line the baking tray with parchment.   Place the marinated chicken fingers in the tray in one layer.   Bake the chicken fingers for 20 minutes at 355F. Flip them on another side after 10 minutes of cooking.
Nutrition Info: Per Serving: calories 154, fat 6.4, fiber 0, carbs 0.8, protein 22

370. Chicken Kebabs

Servings: 4   Cooking Time: 20 Minutes
Ingredients:

1 red bell pepper, cut into squares	2 chicken breasts, skinless, boneless and cubed
1 red onion, roughly cut into squares	A pinch of salt and black pepper
2 teaspoons sweet paprika	¼ teaspoon cardamom, ground
1 teaspoon nutmeg, ground	Juice of 1 lemon
1 teaspoon Italian seasoning	3 garlic cloves, minced
¼ teaspoon smoked	

paprika   ½ cup olive oil

Directions:
In a bowl, combine the chicken with the onion, the bell pepper and the other ingredients, toss well, cover the bowl and keep in the fridge for 30 minutes.   Assemble skewers with chicken, peppers and the onions, place them on your preheated grill and cook over medium heat for 8 minutes on each side.   Divide the kebabs between plates and serve with a side salad.
Nutrition Info:calories 262, fat 14, fiber 2, carbs 14, protein 20

371. Chicken, Corn And Peppers

Servings: 4   Cooking Time: 1 Hour
Ingredients:

2 pounds chicken breast, skinless, boneless and cubed	1 red onion, chopped
2 tablespoons olive oil	¼ teaspoon cumin, ground
2 garlic cloves, minced	2 cups corn
2 red bell peppers, chopped	½ cup chicken stock
	1 teaspoon chili powder
	¼ cup cilantro, chopped

Directions:
Heat up a pot with the oil over medium-high heat, add the chicken and brown for 4 minutes on each side.   Add the onion and the garlic and sauté for 5 minutes more.   Add the rest of the ingredients, stir, bring to a simmer over medium heat and cook for 45 minutes.   Divide into bowls and serve.
Nutrition Info:calories 332, fat 16.1, fiber 8.4, carbs 25.4, protein 17.4

372. Spicy Cumin Chicken

Servings: 4   Cooking Time: 25 Minutes
Ingredients:

2 teaspoons chili powder	1 pound chicken breasts, skinless, boneless and halved
2 and ½ tablespoons olive oil	
Salt and black pepper to the taste	2 teaspoons sherry vinegar
1 and ½ teaspoons garlic powder	2 teaspoons hot sauce
1 tablespoon smoked paprika	2 teaspoons cumin, ground
½ cup chicken stock	½ cup black olives, pitted and sliced

Directions:
Heat up a pan with the oil over medium-high heat, add the chicken and brown for 3 minutes on each side.   Add the chili powder, salt, pepper, garlic powder and paprika, toss and cook for 4 minutes more.   Add the rest of the ingredients, toss, bring to a simmer and cook over medium heat for 15 minutes more.   Divide the mix between plates and serve.
Nutrition Info:calories 230, fat 18.4, fiber 9.4, carbs 15.3, protein 13.4

373. Chives Chicken And Radishes

Servings: 4   Cooking Time: 30 Minutes
Ingredients:

2 chicken breasts, skinless, boneless and cubed	1 cup chicken stock
	½ cup tomato sauce
Salt and black pepper to the taste	½ pound red radishes, cubed
1 tablespoon olive oil	2 tablespoon chives,

chopped

Directions:
Heat up a Dutch oven with the oil over medium-high heat, add the chicken and brown for 4 minutes on each side.   Add the rest of the ingredients except the chives, bring to a simmer and cook over medium heat for 20 minutes. Divide the mix between plates, sprinkle the chives on top and serve.
Nutrition Info:calories 277, fat 15, fiber 9.3, carbs 20.9, protein 33.2

374. Yogurt Chicken And Red Onion Mix

Servings: 4   Cooking Time: 30 Minutes
Ingredients:

2 pounds chicken breast, skinless, boneless and sliced	¼ cup Greek yogurt
	½ teaspoon onion powder
3 tablespoons olive oil	A pinch of salt and black pepper
2 garlic cloves, minced	4 red onions, sliced

Directions:
In a roasting pan, combine the chicken with the oil, the yogurt and the other ingredients, introduce in the oven at 375 degrees F and bake for 30 minutes. Divide chicken mix between plates and serve hot.
Nutrition Info:calories 278, fat 15, fiber 9.2, carbs 15.1, protein 23.3

375. Basil Chicken With Olives

Servings: 5   Cooking Time: 40 Minutes
Ingredients:

1.5-pound chicken breast, skinless, boneless	2 tablespoons sunflower oil
	1 tablespoon fresh basil, chopped
3 Kalamata olives, chopped	½ teaspoon chili flakes
1 teaspoon minced garlic	1 tablespoon lemon juice
1 teaspoon salt	
1 teaspoon ground black pepper	½ teaspoon honey
	¼ cup of water

Directions:
Combine together Kalamata olives, minced garlic, salt, ground black pepper, sunflower oil, basil, chili flakes, lemon juice, and honey.   Whisk the mixture until homogenous.   Chop the chicken breast roughly and arrange it in the baking dish. Pour olives mixture over the chicken.   Then mix up it with the help of the fingertips.   Add water and cover the baking dish with foil.   Pierce the foil with the help of the fork or knife to give the "air" for meat during cooking.   Bake the chicken for 40 minutes at 360F.
Nutrition Info: Per Serving:calories 213, fat 9.3, fiber 0.2, carbs 1.3, protein 29

376. Chicken Skewers (shish Tawook)

Servings: 1 Skewer   Cooking Time: 8 Minutes
Ingredients:

1 1/2 lb. boneless, skinless chicken breasts	2 TB. Greek yogurt
	2 TB. tomato paste
2 TB. minced garlic	1 TB. paprika
3 TB. fresh lemon juice	1/2 tsp. cayenne
	1 tsp. salt
3 TB. extra-virgin olive oil	1/2 tsp. ground black pepper

Directions:
Preheat a grill to medium heat. Cut chicken breast into 1-inch cubes and place in a large bowl. Add garlic, lemon juice, extra-virgin olive oil, Greek yogurt, tomato paste, paprika, cayenne, salt, and black pepper, and mix to combine. Skewer chicken, dividing equally among 5 skewers. Place chicken on the grill, and cook for 8 minutes, turning over every 2 minutes to grill all sides. Serve warm with hummus and pita bread.

377. Oregano Chicken And Zucchini Pan

Servings: 4   Cooking Time: 30 Minutes
Ingredients:

2 cups tomatoes, peeled and crushed	Salt and black pepper to the taste
1 and ½ pounds chicken breast, boneless, skinless and cubed	1 small yellow onion, sliced
2 tablespoons olive oil	2 garlic cloves, minced
2 zucchinis, sliced	2 tablespoons oregano, chopped
	1 cup chicken stock

Directions:
Heat up a pan with the oil over medium-high heat, add the chicken and brown for 3 minute son each side. Add the onion and the garlic and sauté for 4 minutes more. Add the rest of the ingredients except the oregano, bring to a simmer and cook over medium heat and cook for 20 minutes. Divide the mix between plates, sprinkle the oregano on top and serve.
Nutrition Info: calories 228, fat 9.5, fiber 9.1, carbs 15.6, protein 18.6

378. Stuffed Chicken

Servings: 2   Cooking Time: 35 Minutes
Ingredients:

10 oz chicken breast, skinless, boneless	1 teaspoon sour cream
2 tablespoons fresh cilantro, chopped	½ teaspoon salt
1 tomato, sliced	½ teaspoon sage
1 teaspoon fresh parsley, chopped	1 oz Mozzarella, sliced
	1 tablespoon pesto sauce

Directions:
Make the lengthwise cut in the chicken breast and fill it with fresh parsley, cilantro, sliced Mozzarella, and sliced tomatoes. Secure the chicken breast with toothpicks. After this, sprinkle the chicken with sage, salt, sour cream, and pesto sauce. Wrap the stuffed chicken breast in the foil and bake in the preheated to the 365F oven for 35 minutes.
Nutrition Info: Per Serving:calories 246, fat 9.8, fiber 0.6, carbs 2.5, protein 35.2

379. Chicken And Avocado Bowl

Servings: 3   Cooking Time: 15 Minutes
Ingredients:

3 chicken drumsticks	1 teaspoon olive oil
1 avocado, sliced	1 tablespoon lemon juice
½ cup cherry tomatoes	1 teaspoon sesame oil
2 bell peppers	½ teaspoon sesame seeds
1 teaspoon Italian herbs	

Directions:
Sprinkle the chicken drumsticks with lemon juice, Italian herbs, and olive oil and place them in the skillet. Roast the chicken drumsticks for 15 minutes. Flip them every 5 minutes. Meanwhile, cut the cherry tomatoes on the halves. Chop the bell peppers roughly. Place the vegetables in 3 serving plates. Add avocado and sprinkle the ingredients with sesame seeds and sesame oil. Add cooked roasted drumsticks.
Nutrition Info: Per Serving:calories 276, fat 19.3, fiber 6, carbs 13.2, protein 15.1

380. Chicken And Grapes Salad

Servings: 4   Cooking Time: 0 Minutes
Ingredients:

7 oz chicken breast, skinless, boneless, cooked	1 red onion, sliced
½ cup red grapes	½ cup Greek yogurt
1 oz celery stalk, chopped	½ teaspoon honey
	1 tablespoon fresh parsley, chopped
	1 cucumber, chopped

Directions:
Chop the chicken breast and place it in the salad bowl. Add red grapes, celery stalk, sliced red onion, parsley, and cucumber. Mix up the salad mixture. Then mix up together Greek yogurt and honey. Pour Greek yogurt mixture over the salad and stir well.
Nutrition Info: Per Serving:calories 116, fat 1.9, fiber 1.2, carbs 10.9, protein 14

381. Lime Turkey And Avocado Mix

Servings: 2   Cooking Time: 1 Hour And 10 Minutes
Ingredients:

2 tablespoons olive oil	Juice of 1 lime
1 turkey breast, boneless, skinless and halved	Zest of 1 lime, grated
	Salt and black pepper to the taste
2 ounces cherry tomatoes, halved	2 spring onions, chopped
A handful coriander, chopped	2 avocadoes, pitted, peeled and cubed

Directions:
In a roasting pan, combine the turkey with the oil and the rest of the ingredients, introduce in the oven and bake at 370 degrees F for 1 hour and 10 minutes. Divide between plates and serve.
Nutrition Info: calories 301, fat 8.9, fiber 10.2, carbs 19.8, protein 13.5

382. Coriander Chicken Drumsticks

Servings: 4   Cooking Time: 35 Minutes
Ingredients:

8 chicken drumsticks	½ teaspoon ground turmeric
1 lemon	1 teaspoon paprika
1 teaspoon minced garlic	1 teaspoon salt
1 teaspoon ground coriander	1 tablespoon olive oil
1/3 cup onion, chopped	1 teaspoon butter
	1/3 cup water

Directions:
Peel the lemon and chop the lemon pulp. Place it in the saucepan. Add minced garlic, ground coriander, onion, turmeric, paprika, salt, olive oil, and butter. Then add water and bring the mixture to boil. Mix it up. Add chicken drumsticks and close the lid. Simmer the chicken for 30 minutes over the medium-low heat.

Nutrition Info: Per Serving:calories 206, fat 9.9, fiber 0.9, carbs 3, protein 25.7

383. Turkey And Asparagus Mix

Servings: 4   Cooking Time: 30 Minutes

Ingredients:

1 bunch asparagus, trimmed and halved
1 big turkey breast, skinless, boneless and cut into strips
1 teaspoon basil, dried

2 tablespoons olive oil
A pinch of salt and black pepper
½ cup tomato sauce
1 tablespoon chives, chopped

Directions:

Heat up a pan with the oil over medium-high heat, add the turkey and brown for 4 minutes.   Add the asparagus and the rest of the ingredients except the chives, bring to a simmer and cook over medium heat for 25 minutes.   Add the chives, divide the mix between plates and serve.

Nutrition Info:calories 337, fat 21.2, fiber 10.2, carbs 21.4, protein 17.6

384. Braised Chicken

Servings: 1 Drumstick   Cooking Time: 52 Minutes

Ingredients:

6 chicken drumsticks, skin on
3 TB. extra-virgin olive oil
2 cups crimini mushrooms, cleaned
1 large yellow onion, chopped
12 cloves garlic

11/2 tsp. salt
1 tsp. ground black pepper
2 cups water
2 TB. tomato paste
1/3 cup tomato sauce
1 TB. brown sugar, packed
1/2 tsp. cayenne

Directions:

In a large, 3-quart pot over medium heat, brown chicken drumsticks for 10 minutes, rotating every 3 minutes. Remove chicken from the pot, and set aside.   In the pot, combine extra-virgin olive oil, crimini mushrooms, yellow onion, garlic, and salt. Cook for 7 minutes.   Add black pepper, water, tomato paste, tomato sauce, brown sugar, and cayenne, and simmer for 5 minutes.   Return chicken to the pot, reduce heat to low, cover, and simmer for 30 minutes.   Serve each drumstick with sauce and some vegetables.

385. Pesto Chicken Mix

Servings: 4   Cooking Time: 40 Minutes

Ingredients:

4 chicken breast halves, skinless and boneless
1 cup mozzarella, shredded

3 tomatoes, cubed
½ cup basil pesto
A pinch of salt and black pepper
Cooking spray

Directions:

Grease a baking dish lined with parchment paper with the cooking spray.   In a bowl, mix the chicken with salt, pepper and the pesto and rub well.   Place the chicken on the baking sheet, top with tomatoes and shredded mozzarella and bake at 400 degrees F for 40 minutes.   Divide the mix between plates and serve with a side salad.

Nutrition Info:calories 341, fat 20, fiber 1, carbs 4, protein 32

386. Chicken And Salsa Enchiladas

Servings: 5   Cooking Time: 15 Minutes

Ingredients:

10 oz chicken breast, boiled, shredded
1 teaspoon chipotle pepper
3 tablespoons green salsa
½ teaspoon minced garlic

5 corn tortillas
½ cup cream
¼ cup chicken stock
1 cup Mozzarella, shredded
1 teaspoon butter, softened

Directions:

Mix up together shredded chicken breast, chipotle pepper, green salsa, and minced garlic.   Then put the shredded chicken mixture in the center of every corn tortilla and roll them.   Spread the baking dish with softened butter from inside and arrange the rolled corn tortillas.   Then pour chicken stock and cream over the tortillas.   Top them with shredded Mozzarella.   Bake the enchiladas for 15 minutes at 365F.

Nutrition Info: Per Serving:calories 159, fat 5.3, fiber 1.6, carbs 12.3, protein 15.3

387. Paprika Chicken And Pineapple Mix

Servings: 4   Cooking Time: 15 Minutes

Ingredients:

2 cups pineapple, peeled and cubed
2 tablespoons olive oil
2 pounds chicken breasts, skinless, boneless and cubed

1 tablespoon smoked paprika
A pinch of salt and black pepper
1 tablespoon chives, chopped

Directions:

Heat up a pan with the oil over medium-high heat, add the chicken, salt and pepper and brown for 4 minutes on each side.   Add the rest of the ingredients, toss, cook for 7 minutes more, divide everything between plates and serve with a side salad.

Nutrition Info:calories 264, fat 13.2, fiber 8.3, carbs 25.1, protein 15.4

388. Chicken And Apples Mix

Servings: 4   Cooking Time: 40 Minutes

Ingredients:

½ cup chicken stock
1 red onion, sliced
2 green apples, cored and chopped
1 pound breast, skinless, boneless and cubed

½ cup tomato sauce
1 teaspoon thyme, chopped
1 and ½ tablespoons olive oil
1 tablespoon chives, chopped

Directions:

In a roasting pan, combine the chicken with the tomato sauce, apples and the rest of the ingredients except the chives, introduce the pan in the oven and bake at 425 degrees F for 40 minutes. Divide the mix between plates, sprinkle the chives on top and serve.

Nutrition Info:calories 292, fat 16.1, fiber 9.4, carbs 15.4, protein 16.4

389. Oregano Turkey And Peppers

Servings: 4   Cooking Time: 1 Hour

Ingredients:

2 red bell peppers, cut into strips
2 green bell peppers, cut into strips
1 red onion, chopped
4 garlic cloves,

2 cups chicken stock
1 big turkey breast, skinless, boneless and cut into strips
1 tablespoon oregano, chopped

minced
½ cup black olives, pitted and sliced

½ cup cilantro, chopped

Directions:
In a baking pan, combine the peppers with the turkey and the rest of the ingredients, toss, introduce in the oven at 400 degrees F and roast for 1 hour. Divide everything between plates and serve.
Nutrition Info:calories 229, fat 8.9, fiber 8.2, carbs 17.8, protein 33.6

390.   Tomato Chicken And Lentils

Servings: 8   Cooking Time: 1 Hour
Ingredients:

2 tablespoons olive oil
2 celery stalks, chopped
1 red onion, chopped
2 tablespoons tomato paste
2 garlic cloves, chopped

½ cup chicken stock
2 cups French lentils
1 pound chicken thighs, boneless and skinless
Salt and black pepper to the taste
1 tablespoon cilantro, chopped

Directions:
Heat up a Dutch oven with the oil over medium-high heat, add the onion and the garlic and sauté for 2 minutes. Add the chicken and brown for 3 minutes on each side. Add the rest of the ingredients except the cilantro, bring to a simmer and cook over medium-low heat for 45 minutes. Add the cilantro, stir, divide the mix into bowls and serve.
Nutrition Info:calories 249, fat 9.7, fiber 11.9, carbs 25.3, protein 24.3

391.   Chicken And Olives Tapenade

Servings: 4   Cooking Time: 25 Minutes
Ingredients:

2 chicken breasts, boneless, skinless and halved
1 cup black olives, pitted
Salt and black pepper to the taste
½ cup mixed parsley, chopped

½ cup olive oil
½ cup rosemary, chopped
Salt and black pepper to the taste
4 garlic cloves, minced
Juice of ½ lime

Directions:
In a blender, combine the olives with half of the oil and the rest of the ingredients except the chicken and pulse well. Heat up a pan with the rest of the oil over medium-high heat, add the chicken and brown for 4 minutes on each side. Add the olives mix, and cook for 20 minutes more tossing often.
Nutrition Info:calories 291, fat 12.9, fiber 8.5, carbs 15.8, protein 34.2

392.   Grilled Chicken On The Bone

Servings: 1 Drumstick And 1 Thigh   Cooking Time: 40 Minutes
Ingredients:

4 TB. minced garlic
1/2 cup fresh lemon juice
1/2 cup extra-virgin olive oil
1 TB. dried oregano
2 tsp. salt

1 tsp. ground black pepper
1 tsp. cayenne
1 tsp. paprika
4 chicken drumsticks
4 chicken thighs

Directions:

In a small bowl, whisk together garlic, lemon juice, extra-virgin olive oil, oregano, salt, black pepper, cayenne, and paprika. Place chicken drumsticks and chicken thighs in a large bowl, pour 1/2 of dressing over chicken, mix to coat evenly, and set in the refrigerator to marinate for 1 hour. Preheat the grill to medium-high heat. Place chicken evenly on the grill, and cook for 5 minutes per side. Reduce heat to medium-low, cover the grill, and cook chicken for 15 minutes per side or until juices run clear and internal temperature of chicken reads 175°F. Remove chicken from the grill, and let rest for 5 minutes before serving warm.

393.   Saffron Chicken Thighs And Green Beans

Servings: 4   Cooking Time: 25 Minutes
Ingredients:

2 pounds chicken thighs, boneless and skinless
2 teaspoons saffron powder
1 pound green beans, trimmed and halved

½ cup Greek yogurt
Salt and black pepper to the taste
1 tablespoon lime juice
1 tablespoon dill, chopped

Directions:
In a roasting pan, combine the chicken with the saffron, green beans and the rest of the ingredients, toss a bit, introduce in the oven and bake at 400 degrees F for 25 minutes. Divide everything between plates and serve.
Nutrition Info:calories 274, fat 12.3, fiber 5.3, carbs 20.4, protein 14.3

394.   Turkey, Leeks And Carrots

Servings: 4   Cooking Time: 1 Hour
Ingredients:

1 big turkey breast, skinless, boneless and cubed
2 tablespoons avocado oil
Salt and black pepper to the taste
1 tablespoon sweet paprika
½ cup chicken stock

1 leek, sliced
1 carrot, sliced
1 yellow onion, chopped
1 tablespoon lemon juice
1 teaspoon cumin, ground
1 tablespoon basil, chopped

Directions:
Heat up a pan with the oil over medium-high heat, add the turkey and brown for 4 minutes on each side. Add the leeks, carrot and the onion and sauté everything for 5 minutes more. Add the rest of the ingredients, bring to a simmer and cook over medium heat for 40 minutes. Divide the mix between plates and serve.
Nutrition Info:calories 249, fat 10.7, fiber 11.9, carbs 22.3, protein 17.3

395.   Sage And Nutmeg Chicken

Servings: 6   Cooking Time: 20 Minutes
Ingredients:

2-pound chicken breast, skinless, boneless
2 tablespoons lemon juice
1 teaspoon sage
½ teaspoon ground nutmeg
½ teaspoon dried oregano

1 teaspoon paprika
1 teaspoon onion powder
2 tablespoons olive oil
1 teaspoon chili flakes
1 teaspoon salt
1 teaspoon apple cider vinegar

Directions:

Make the marinade: whisk together apple cider vinegar, salt, chili flakes, olive oil, onion powder, paprika, dried oregano, ground nutmeg, sage, and lemon juice. Then rub the chicken with marinade carefully and leave for 25 minutes to marinate. Meanwhile, preheat grill to 385F. Place the marinated chicken breast in the grill and cook it for 10 minutes from each side. Cut the cooked chicken on the servings.

Nutrition Info: Per Serving: calories 218, fat 8.6, fiber 0.3, carbs 0.9, protein 32.2

396. Herbed Chicken

Servings: 4 Cooking Time: 40 Minutes

Ingredients:

- 2 chicken breasts, skinless, boneless and sliced
- 2 red onions, chopped
- 2 tablespoons olive oil
- 2 garlic cloves, minced
- 1 teaspoon oregano, dried
- ½ cup chicken stock
- 1 teaspoon basil, dried
- 1 teaspoon rosemary, dried
- 1 cup canned tomatoes, chopped
- Salt and black pepper to the taste

Directions:

Heat up a pot with the oil over medium-high heat, add the chicken and brown for 4 minutes on each side. Add the garlic and the onions and sauté for 5 minutes more. Add the rest of the ingredients, bring to a simmer and cook over medium heat for 25 minutes. Divide everything between plates and serve.

Nutrition Info: calories 251, fat 11.6, fiber 15.5, carbs 15.6, protein 9.1

397. Duck And Blackberries

Servings: 4 Cooking Time: 25 Minutes

Ingredients:

- 4 duck breasts, boneless and skin scored
- 2 tablespoons balsamic vinegar
- 1 cup chicken stock
- Salt and black pepper to the taste
- 4 ounces blackberries
- ¼ cup chicken stock
- 2 tablespoons avocado oil

Directions:

Heat up a pan with the avocado oil over medium-high heat, add duck breasts, skin side down and cook for 5 minutes. Flip the duck, add the rest of the ingredients, bring to a simmer and cook over medium heat for 20 minutes. Divide everything between plates and serve.

Nutrition Info: calories 239, fat 10.5, fiber 10.2, carbs 21.1, protein 33.3

398. Chicken And Onion Mix

Servings: 4 Cooking Time: 30 Minutes

Ingredients:

- 4 chicken steaks (4 oz each steak)
- ½ cup crushed tomatoes
- ¼ cup fresh cilantro
- 1 teaspoon olive oil
- 3 oz Parmesan, grated
- 3 tablespoon Panko breadcrumbs
- 1 garlic clove, diced
- ½ cup of water
- 1 onion, diced
- 2 eggs, beaten
- 1 teaspoon ground black pepper

Directions:

Pour olive oil in the saucepan. Add garlic and onion. Roast the vegetables for 3 minutes. Then add fresh cilantro, crushed tomatoes, and water. Simmer the mixture for 5 minutes. Meanwhile, mix up together ground black pepper and eggs. Dip the chicken steaks in the egg mixture. Then coat them in Panko breadcrumbs and again in the egg mixture. Coat the chicken steaks in grated Parmesan. Place the prepared chicken steaks in the crushed tomato mixture. Close the lid and cook chicken parm for 20 minutes. Flip the chicken steaks after 10 minutes of cooking. Serve the chicken parm with crushed tomatoes sauce.

Nutrition Info: Per Serving: calories 372, fat 21.2, fiber 2.5, carbs 12.3, protein 32.5

399. Cinnamon Duck Mix

Servings: 4 Cooking Time: 20 Minutes

Ingredients:

- 4 duck breasts, boneless and skin scored
- Salt and black pepper to the taste
- 1 teaspoon cinnamon powder
- 3 tablespoons chives, chopped
- ½ cup chicken stock
- 2 tablespoons parsley, chopped
- 1 tablespoon olive oil
- 3 tablespoons balsamic vinegar
- 2 red onions, chopped

Directions:

Heat up a pan with the oil over medium-high heat, add the duck skin side down and cook for 5 minutes. Add the cinnamon and the rest of the ingredients except the chives and cook for 5 minutes more. Flip the duck breasts again, bring the whole mix to a simmer and cook over medium heat for 10 minutes. Add the chives, divide everything between plates and serve.

Nutrition Info: calories 310, fat 13.5, fiber 9.2, carbs 16.7, protein 15.2

400. Lemony Turkey And Pine Nuts

Servings: 4 Cooking Time: 30 Minutes

Ingredients:

- 2 turkey breasts, boneless, skinless and halved
- A pinch of salt and black pepper
- 2 tablespoons avocado oil
- Juice of 2 lemons
- 1 tablespoon rosemary, chopped
- 3 garlic cloves, minced
- ¼ cup pine nuts, chopped
- 1 cup chicken stock

Directions:

Heat up a pan with the oil over medium-high heat, add the garlic and the turkey and brown for 4 minutes on each side. Add the rest of the ingredients, bring to a simmer and cook over medium heat for 20 minutes. Divide the mix between plates and serve with a side salad.

Nutrition Info: calories 293, fat 12.4, fiber 9.3, carbs 17.8, protein 24.5

401. Wrapped Plums

Servings: 8   Cooking Time: 0 Minutes

Ingredients:

2 ounces prosciutto, cut into 16 pieces
1 tablespoon chives, chopped
4 plums, quartered
A pinch of red pepper flakes, crushed

Directions:

Wrap each plum quarter in a prosciutto slice, arrange them all on a platter, sprinkle the chives and pepper flakes all over and serve.

Nutrition Info: calories 30, fat 1, fiber 0, carbs 4, protein 2

402. Tomato Cream Cheese Spread

Servings: 6   Cooking Time: 0 Minutes

Ingredients:

12 ounces cream cheese, soft
1 big tomato, cubed
¼ cup homemade mayonnaise
2 garlic clove, minced
2 tablespoons red onion, chopped
2 tablespoons lime juice
Salt and black pepper to the taste

Directions:

In your blender, mix the cream cheese with the tomato and the rest of the ingredients, pulse well, divide into small cups and serve cold.

Nutrition Info: calories 204, fat 6.7, fiber 1.4, carbs 7.3, protein 4.5

403. Italian Fries

Servings: 4   Cooking Time: 40 Minutes

Ingredients:

1/3 cup baby red potatoes
1 tablespoon Italian seasoning
3 tablespoons canola oil
1 teaspoon turmeric
½ teaspoon of sea salt
½ teaspoon dried rosemary
1 tablespoon dried dill

Directions:

Cut the red potatoes into the wedges and transfer in the big bowl.   After this, sprinkle the vegetables with Italian seasoning, canola oil, turmeric, sea salt, dried rosemary, and dried dill. Shake the potato wedges carefully.   Line the baking tray with baking paper.   Place the potatoes wedges in the tray. Flatten it well to make one layer.   Preheat the oven to 375F.   Place the tray with potatoes in the oven and bake for 40 minutes. Stir the potatoes with the help of the spatula from time to time.   The potato fries are cooked when they have crunchy edges.

Nutrition Info: Per Serving: calories 122, fat 11.6, fiber 0.5, carbs 4.5, protein 0.6

404. Tempeh Snack

Servings: 6   Cooking Time: 8 Minutes

Ingredients:

11 oz soy tempeh
½ teaspoon ground black pepper
1 teaspoon olive oil
¼ teaspoon garlic powder

Directions:

Cut soy tempeh into the sticks.   Sprinkle every tempeh stick with ground black pepper, garlic powder, and olive oil.   Preheat the grill to 375F. Place the tempeh sticks in the grill and cook them for 4 minutes from each side. The time of cooking depends on the tempeh sticks size.   The cooked tempeh sticks will have a light brown color.

Nutrition Info: Per Serving: calories 88, fat 2.5, fiber 3.6, carbs 10.2, protein 6.5

405. Avocado Dip

Servings: 8   Cooking Time: 0 Minutes

Ingredients:

½ cup heavy cream
1 green chili pepper, chopped
Salt and pepper to the taste
4 avocados, pitted, peeled and chopped
1 cup cilantro, chopped
¼ cup lime juice

Directions:

In a blender, combine the cream with the avocados and the rest of the ingredients and pulse well. Divide the mix into bowls and serve cold as a party dip.

Nutrition Info: calories 200, fat 14.5, fiber 3.8, carbs 8.1, protein 7.6

406. Feta And Roasted Red Pepper Bruschetta

Servings: 24   Cooking Time: 15 Minutes

Ingredients:

6 Kalamata olives, pitted, chopped
2 tablespoons green onion, minced
1/4 cup Parmesan cheese, grated, divided
1/4 cup extra-virgin olive oil brushing, or as needed
1/4 cup cherry tomatoes, thinly sliced
1 tablespoon extra-virgin olive oil
1 teaspoon lemon juice
1 tablespoon basil pesto
1 red bell pepper, halved, seeded
1 piece (12 inch) whole-wheat baguette, cut into 1/2-inch thick slices
1 package (4 ounce) feta cheese with basil and sun-dried tomatoes, crumbled
1 clove garlic, minced

Directions:

Preheat the oven broiler. Place the oven rack 6 inches from the source of heat.   Brush both sides of the baguette slices, with the 1/4 cup olive oil. Arrange the bread slices on a baking sheet; toast for about 1 minute each side, carefully watching to avoid burning. Remove the toasted slices, transferring into another baking sheet.   With the cut sides down, place the red peppers in a baking sheet; broil for about 8 to 10 minutes or until the skin is charred and blistered. Transfer the roasted peppers into a bowl; cover with plastic wrap. Let cool, remove the charred skin. Discard skin and chop the roasted peppers.   In a bowl, mix the roasted red peppers, cherry tomatoes, feta cheese, green onion, olives, pesto, 1 tablespoon olive oil, garlic, and lemon juice.   Top each bread with 1 tablespoon of the roasted pepper mix, sprinkle lightly with the Parmesan cheese.   Return the baking sheet with the topped bruschetta; broil for about 1-2 minutes or until the topping is lightly browned.

Nutrition Info: Per Serving:73 cal., 4.8 g total fat (1.4 sat. fat), 5 mg chol., 138 mg sodium, 5.3 g total carbs., 0.4 g fiber, 0.6 g sugar, and 2.1 g protein.

407. Meat-filled Phyllo (samboosek)

Servings: 1 Phyllo Pie   Cooking Time: 10 Minutes

Ingredients:

1 lb. ground beef or lamb	1 tsp. salt
1 medium yellow onion, finely chopped	1 pkg. frozen phyllo dough (12 sheets)
1 TB. seven spices	2/3 cup butter, melted

Directions:

In a medium skillet over medium heat, brown beef for 3 minutes, breaking up chunks with a wooden spoon.   Add yellow onion, seven spices, and salt, and cook for 5 to 7 minutes or until beef is browned and onions are translucent. Set aside, and let cool. Place first sheet of phyllo on your work surface, brush with melted butter, lay second sheet of phyllo on top, and brush with melted butter. Cut sheets into 3-inch-wide strips.   Spoon 2 tablespoons meat filling at end of each strip, and fold end strip to cover meat and form a triangle. Fold pointed end up and over to the opposite end, and you should see a triangle forming. Continue to fold up and then over until you come to the end of strip.   Place phyllo pies on a baking sheet, seal side down, and brush tops with butter. Repeat with remaining phyllo and filling.   Bake for 10 minutes or until golden brown.   Remove from the oven and set aside for 5 minutes before serving warm or at room temperature.

408. Tasty Black Bean Dip

Servings: 6   Cooking Time: 18 Minutes

Ingredients:

2 cups dry black beans, soaked overnight and drained	2 tbsp olive oil
	1 1/2 tbsp garlic, minced
1 1/2 cups cheese, shredded	1 medium onion, sliced
1 tsp dried oregano	4 cups vegetable stock
1 1/2 tsp chili powder	Pepper
2 cups tomatoes, chopped	Salt

Directions:

Add all ingredients except cheese into the instant pot.   Seal pot with lid and cook on high for 18 minutes.   Once done, allow to release pressure naturally. Remove lid. Drain excess water.   Add cheese and stir until cheese is melted.   Blend bean mixture using an immersion blender until smooth.   Serve and enjoy.

Nutrition Info: Calories 402 Fat 15.3 g Carbohydrates 46.6 g Sugar 4.4 g Protein 22.2 g Cholesterol 30 mg

409. Zucchini Cakes

Servings: 4   Cooking Time: 10 Minutes

Ingredients:

1 zucchini, grated	1/4 onion, minced
1/4 carrot, grated	1 teaspoon Italian seasonings
1 teaspoon minced garlic	

3 tablespoons coconut flour	1 egg, beaten
	1 teaspoon coconut oil

Directions:

In the mixing bowl combine together grated zucchini, carrot, minced onion, and garlic.   Add coconut flour, Italian seasoning, and egg.   Stir the mass until homogenous.   Heat up coconut oil in the skillet.   Place the small zucchini fritters in the hot oil. Make them with the help of the spoon. Roast the zucchini fritters for 4 minutes from each side.

Nutrition Info: Per Serving:calories 65, fat 3.3, fiber 3, carbs 6.3, protein 3.3

410. Parsley Nachos

Servings: 3   Cooking Time: 0 Minutes

Ingredients:

3 oz tortilla chips	2 kalamata olives, chopped
1/4 cup Greek yogurt	1 tablespoon paprika
1 tablespoon fresh parsley, chopped	1/4 teaspoon ground thyme
1/4 teaspoon minced garlic	

Directions:

In the mixing bowl mix up together Greek yogurt, parsley, minced garlic, olives, paprika, and thyme. Then add tortilla chips and mix up gently.   The snack should be served immediately.

Nutrition Info: Per Serving:calories 81, fat 1.6, fiber 2.2, carbs 14.1, protein 3.5

411. Plum Wraps

Servings: 4   Cooking Time: 10 Minutes

Ingredients:

4 plums	1/4 teaspoon olive oil
4 prosciutto slices	

Directions:

Preheat the oven to 375F.   Wrap every plum in prosciutto slice and secure with a toothpick (if needed).   Place the wrapped plums in the oven and bake for 10 minutes.

Nutrition Info: Per Serving:calories 62, fat 2.2, fiber 0.9, carbs 8, protein 4.3

412. Parmesan Chips

Servings: 4   Cooking Time: 20 Minutes

Ingredients:

1 zucchini	1/2 teaspoon paprika
2 oz Parmesan, grated	1 teaspoon olive oil

Directions:

Trim zucchini and slice it into the chips with the help of the vegetable slices.   Then mix up together Parmesan and paprika.   Sprinkle the zucchini chips with olive oil.   After this, dip every zucchini slice in the cheese mixture.   Place the zucchini chips in the lined baking tray and bake for 20 minutes at 375F.   Flip the zucchini sliced onto another side after 10 minutes of cooking.   Chill the cooked chips well.

Nutrition Info: Per Serving:calories 64, fat 4.3, fiber 0.6, carbs 2.3, protein 5.2

413. Chicken Bites

Servings: 6   Cooking Time: 5 Minutes

Ingredients:

1/2 cup coconut flakes	1 teaspoon salt
8 oz chicken fillet	1 tablespoon tomato

¼ cup Greek yogurt
1 teaspoon dried dill
1 teaspoon ground black pepper
sauce
1 teaspoon honey
4 tablespoons sunflower oil

Directions:
Chop the chicken fillet on the small cubes (popcorn cubes) Sprinkle them with dried dill, salt, and ground black pepper. Then add Greek yogurt and stir carefully. After this, pour sunflower oil in the skillet and heat it up. Coat chicken cubes in the coconut flakes and roast in the hot oil for 3-4 minutes or until the popcorn cubes are golden brown. Dry the popcorn chicken with the help of the paper towel. Make the sweet sauce: whisk together honey and tomato sauce. Serve the popcorn chicken hot or warm with sweet sauce.
Nutrition Info: Per Serving:calories 107, fat 5.2, fiber 0.8, carbs 2.8, protein 12.1

414. Chicken Kale Wraps

Servings: 4   Cooking Time: 10 Minutes
Ingredients:
4 kale leaves
4 oz chicken fillet
½ apple
1 tablespoon butter
¼ teaspoon chili pepper
¾ teaspoon salt
1 tablespoon lemon juice
¾ teaspoon dried thyme

Directions:
Chop the chicken fillet into the small cubes. Then mix up together chicken with chili pepper and salt. Heat up butter in the skillet. Add chicken cubes. Roast them for 4 minutes. Meanwhile, chop the apple into small cubes and add it in the chicken. Mix up well. Sprinkle the ingredients with lemon juice and dried thyme. Cook them for 5 minutes over the medium-high heat. Fill the kale leaves with the hot chicken mixture and wrap.
Nutrition Info: Per Serving:calories 106, fat 5.1, fiber 1.1, carbs 6.3, protein 9

415. Savory Pita Chips

Servings: 1 Cup   Cooking Time: 10 Minutes
Ingredients:
1/4 cup extra-virgin olive oil
3 pitas
1/4 cup zaatar

Directions:
Preheat the oven to 450°F. Cut pitas into 2-inch pieces, and place in a large bowl. Drizzle pitas with extra-virgin olive oil, sprinkle with zaatar, and toss to coat. Spread out pitas on a baking sheet, and bake for 8 to 10 minutes or until lightly browned and crunchy. Let pita chips cool before removing from the baking sheet. Store in an airtight container for up to 1 month.

416. Artichoke Skewers

Servings: 4   Cooking Time: 0 Minutes
Ingredients:
4 prosciutto slices
4 artichoke hearts, canned
4 kalamata olives
4 cherry tomatoes
¼ teaspoon cayenne pepper
¼ teaspoon sunflower oil

Directions:
Skewer prosciutto slices, artichoke hearts, kalamata olives, and cherry tomatoes on the wooden skewers.

Sprinkle antipasto skewers with sunflower oil and cayenne pepper.
Nutrition Info: Per Serving:calories 152, fat 3.7, fiber 10.8, carbs 23.2, protein 11.1

417.Kidney Bean Spread

Servings: 4   Cooking Time: 18 Minutes
Ingredients:
1 lb dry kidney beans, soaked overnight and drained
1 tsp garlic, minced
2 tbsp olive oil
1 tbsp fresh lemon juice
1 tbsp paprika
4 cups vegetable stock
1/2 cup onion, chopped
Pepper
Salt

Directions:
Add beans and stock into the instant pot. Seal pot with lid and cook on high for 18 minutes. Once done, allow to release pressure naturally. Remove lid. Drain beans well and reserve 1/2 cup stock. Transfer beans, reserve stock, and remaining ingredients into the food processor and process until smooth. Serve and enjoy.
Nutrition Info: Calories 461 Fat 8.6 g Carbohydrates 73 g Sugar 4 g Protein 26.4 g Cholesterol 0 mg

418. Mediterranean Polenta Cups Recipe

Servings: 24   Cooking Time: 5 Minutes
Ingredients:
1 cup yellow cornmeal
1 garlic clove, minced
1/2 teaspoon fresh thyme, minced or 1/4 teaspoon dried thyme
1/4 cup feta cheese, crumbled
1/2 teaspoon salt
1/4 teaspoon pepper
2 tablespoons fresh basil, chopped
4 cups water
4 plum tomatoes, finely chopped

Directions:
In a heavy, large saucepan, bring the water and the salt to a boil; reduce the heat to a gentle boil. Slowly whisk in the cornmeal; cook, stirring with a wooden spoon for about 15 to 20 minutes, or until the polenta is thick and pulls away cleanly from the sides of the pan. Remove from the heat; stir in the pepper and the thyme. Grease miniature muffin cups with cooking spray. Spoon a heaping tablespoon of the polenta mixture into each muffin cups. With the back of a spoon, make an indentation in the center of each; cover and chill until the mixture is set. Meanwhile, combine the feta cheese, tomatoes, garlic, and basil in a small-sized bowl. Unmold the chilled polenta cups; place them on an ungreased baking sheet. Tops each indentation with 1 heaping tablespoon of the feta mixture. Broil the cups 4 inches from the heat source for about 5 to 7 minutes, or until heated through.
Nutrition Info: Per Serving:26 cal, 1 mg chol., 62 mg sodium, 5 g carbs., 1 g fiber, and 1 g protein.

419. Tomato Triangles

Servings: 6   Cooking Time: 0 Minutes
Ingredients:
6 corn tortillas
1 tablespoon cream cheese
1 tablespoon ricotta
½ teaspoon minced garlic
1 tablespoon fresh

cheese

dill, chopped
2 tomatoes, sliced

Directions:
Cut every tortilla into 2 triangles.   Then mix up together cream cheese, ricotta cheese, minced garlic, and dill.   Spread 6 triangles with cream cheese mixture.   Then place sliced tomato on them and cover with remaining tortilla triangles.
Nutrition Info: Per Serving:calories 71, fat 1.6, fiber 2.1, carbs 12.8, protein 2.3

420. Chili Mango And Watermelon Salsa

Servings: 12   Cooking Time: 0 Minutes
Ingredients:
1 red tomato, chopped
Salt and black pepper to the taste
1 cup watermelon, seedless, peeled and cubed
1 red onion, chopped
2 mangos, peeled and chopped

2 chili peppers, chopped
¼ cup cilantro, chopped
3 tablespoons lime juice
Pita chips for serving

Directions:
In a bowl, mix the tomato with the watermelon, the onion and the rest of the ingredients except the pita chips and toss well.   Divide the mix into small cups and serve with pita chips on the side.
Nutrition Info:calories 62, fat 4.7, fiber 1.3, carbs 3.9, protein 2.3

421. Tomato Olive Salsa

Servings: 4   Cooking Time: 5 Minutes
Ingredients:
2 cups olives, pitted and chopped
1/4 cup fresh parsley, chopped
1/4 cup fresh basil, chopped
1 tbsp olive oil

2 tbsp green onion, chopped
1 cup grape tomatoes, halved
1 tbsp vinegar
Pepper
Salt

Directions:
Add all ingredients into the inner pot of instant pot and stir well.   Seal pot with lid and cook on high for 5 minutes.   Once done, allow to release pressure naturally for 5 minutes then release remaining using quick release. Remove lid.   Stir well and serve.
Nutrition Info: Calories 119 Fat 10.8 g Carbohydrates 6.5 g Sugar 1.3 g Protein 1.2 g Cholesterol 0 mg

422. Lavash Chips

Servings: 4   Cooking Time: 10 Minutes
Ingredients:
1 lavash sheet, whole grain
1 tablespoon canola oil

1 teaspoon paprika
½ teaspoon chili pepper
½ teaspoon salt

Directions:
In the shallow bowl whisk together canola oil, paprika, chili pepper, and salt.   Then chop lavash sheet roughly (in the shape of chips).   Sprinkle lavash chips with oil mixture and arrange in the tray to get one thin layer.   Bake the lavash chips for 10 minutes at 365F. Flip them on another side

from time to time to avoid burning.   Cool the cooked chips well.
Nutrition Info: Per Serving:calories 73, fat 4, fiber 0.7, carbs 8.4, protein 1.6

423. Homemade Salsa

Servings: 8   Cooking Time: 5 Minutes
Ingredients:
12 oz grape tomatoes, halved
1/4 cup fresh cilantro, chopped
1 fresh lime juice
28 oz tomatoes, crushed
1 tbsp garlic, minced

1 green bell pepper, chopped
1 red bell pepper, chopped
2 onions, chopped
6 whole tomatoes
Salt

Directions:
Add whole tomatoes into the instant pot and gently smash the tomatoes.   Add remaining ingredients except cilantro, lime juice, and salt and stir well. Seal pot with lid and cook on high for 5 minutes. Once done, allow to release pressure naturally for 10 minutes then release remaining using quick release. Remove lid.   Add cilantro, lime juice, and salt and stir well.   Serve and enjoy.
Nutrition Info: Calories 146 Fat 1.2 g Carbohydrates 33.2 g Sugar 4 g Protein 6.9 g Cholesterol 0 mg

424. Stuffed Zucchinis

Servings: 6   Cooking Time: 40 Minutes
Ingredients:
6 zucchinis, halved lengthwise and insides scooped out
2 garlic cloves, minced
2 tablespoons oregano, chopped

Juice of 2 lemons
Salt and black pepper to the taste
2 tablespoons olive oil
8 ounces feta cheese, crumbled

Directions:
Arrange the zucchini halves on a baking sheet lined with parchment paper, divide the cheese and the rest of the ingredients in each zucchini half and bake at 450 degrees F for 40 minutes.   Arrange the stuffed zucchinis on a platter and serve as an appetizer.
Nutrition Info:calories

425. Yogurt Dip

Servings: 6   Cooking Time: 0 Minutes
Ingredients:
2 cups Greek yogurt
2 tablespoons pistachios, toasted and chopped
A pinch of salt and white pepper
2 tablespoons mint, chopped

1 tablespoon kalamata olives, pitted and chopped
¼ cup za'atar spice
¼ cup pomegranate seeds
1/3 cup olive oil

Directions:
In a bowl, combine the yogurt with the pistachios and the rest of the ingredients, whisk well, divide into small cups and serve with pita chips on the side.
Nutrition Info:calories 294, fat 18, fiber 1, carbs 21, protein 10

426. Popcorn-pine Nut Mix

Servings: 10   Cooking Time: 10 Minutes

Ingredients:

1 tablespoon olive oil	1/4 cup popcorn,
1/2 cup pine nuts	white kernels,
1/2 teaspoon Italian	popped
seasoning	1/4 teaspoon salt
	2 tablespoons honey
	1/2 lemon zest

Directions:
Place the popped corn in a medium bowl. In a dry pan or skillet over low heat, toast the pine nuts, stirring frequently for about 4 to 5 minutes, until fragrant and some begin to brown; remove from the heat. Stir the oil in; add honey, the Italian seasoning, the lemon zest, and the salt. Stir to mix and pour over the popcorn; toss the ingredients to coat the popcorn kernels with the honey syrup. It's alright if most of the nuts sink in the bowl bottom. Let the mixture sit for about 2 minutes to allow the honey to cool and to get stickier. Transfer the bowl contents into a Servings: bowl so the nuts are on the top. Gently stir and serve.
Nutrition Info: Per Serving:80 cal, 6 g total fat (0.5 g sat. fat), 0 mg chol., 105 mg sodium, 60 mg pot., 5 total carbs., <1 g fiber, 4 g sugar, 2 g protein, 2% vitamin A, 8% vitamin C, 4% calcium, and 4% iron.

427. Scallions Dip

Servings: 8   Cooking Time: 0 Minutes
Ingredients:

6 scallions, chopped	1 tablespoon lemon
1 garlic clove, minced	juice
3 tablespoons olive	
oil	1 and ½ cups cream
Salt and black pepper	cheese, soft
to the taste	2 ounces prosciutto,
	cooked and crumbled

Directions:
In a bowl, mix the scallions with the garlic and the rest of the ingredients except the prosciutto and whisk well. Divide into bowls, sprinkle the prosciutto on top and serve as a party dip.
Nutrition Info:calories 144, fat 7.7, fiber 1.4, carbs 6.3, protein 5.5

428. Date Balls

Servings: 3   Cooking Time: 5 Minutes
Ingredients:

3 dates, pitted	½ teaspoon butter,
3 pistachio nuts	softened, salted

Directions:
Fill dates with butter and pistachio nuts. Bake the prepared dates for 5 minutes at 395F. Chill the cooked appetizer to the room temperature.
Nutrition Info: Per Serving:calories 42, fat 1.8, fiber 0.9, carbs 6.9, protein 0.7

429. Lavash Roll Ups

Servings: 2-4   Cooking Time: 10 Minutes
Ingredients:

2 lavash wraps	1/2 cup grape
(whole-wheat)	tomatoes, halved
1/4 cup roasted red	1 Medium cucumber,
peppers, sliced	sliced
1/4 cup black olives,	Fresh dill, for garnish
sliced	
1/2 cup hummus of	
choice	

Directions:

Lay out the lavash wraps on a clean surface. Evenly spread hummus over each piece. Layer the cucumbers across the wraps, about 1/2-inch from each other, leaving about 2-icnh empty space at the bottom of the wrap for rolling purposes. Place the roasted pepper slices around the cucumbers. Sprinkle with black olives and the tomatoes. Garnish with freshly chopped dill. Tightly roll each wrap, using the hummus at the end to almost glue the wrap into a roll. Slice each roll into 4 equal pieces. Secure each piece by sticking a toothpick through the center of each roll slice. Lay each on a serving bowl or tray; garnish more with fresh dill.
Nutrition Info: Per Serving:250 cal, 8 g total fat (0.5 g sat. fat), 0 mg chol., 440 mg sodium, 340 mg pot., 43 total carbs., 40 g fiber, 3 g sugar, 10 g protein, 15% vitamin A, 25% vitamin C, 6% calcium, and 8% iron.

430. Chickpeas And Eggplant Bowls

Servings: 4   Cooking Time: 10 Minutes
Ingredients:

2 eggplants, cut in	1 tablespoon olive oil
half lengthwise and	1 bunch parsley,
cubed	chopped
1 red onion, chopped	A pinch of salt and
Juice of 1 lime	black pepper
28 ounces canned	1 tablespoon balsamic
chickpeas, drained	vinegar
and rinsed	

Directions:
Spread the eggplant cubes on a baking sheet lined with parchment paper, drizzle half of the oil all over, season with salt and pepper and cook at 425 degrees F for 10 minutes. Cool the eggplant down, add the rest of the ingredients, toss, divide between appetizer plates and serve.
Nutrition Info:calories 263, fat 12, fiber 9.3, carbs 15.4, protein 7.5

431. Vinegar Beet Bites

Servings: 4   Cooking Time: 30 Minutes
Ingredients:

2 beets, sliced	1/3 cup balsamic
A pinch of sea salt	vinegar
and black pepper	1 cup olive oil

Directions:
Spread the beet slices on a baking sheet lined with parchment paper, add the rest of the ingredients, toss and bake at 350 degrees F for 30 minutes. Serve the beet bites cold as a snack.
Nutrition Info:calories 199, fat 5.4, fiber 3.5, carbs 8.5, protein 3.5

432. Baked Sweet-potato Fries

Servings: 6   Cooking Time: 25 Minutes
Ingredients:

1 1/2 teaspoons dried	1 teaspoon garlic
oregano	powder
1 teaspoon dried	3 large egg whites (a
thyme	scant 1/2 cup)
1/2 teaspoon salt	Vegetable oil, for the
2 large sweet	parchment
potatoes (about 2	For the
pounds), skins on,	Mediterranean spice:
scrubbed, cut into	Oregano
1/2-inch thick 4-inch	Thyme

long sticks   Garlic

Directions:
Place all of the Mediterranean spice ingredients in a small food processor or a spice grinder; briefly grind or process to blend.   Place the oven racks in the middle and upper position; preheat the oven to 450F.   Line 2 baking sheets with parchment paper; rub the paper with the oil.   Put the potatoes in a microwavable container, cover, and microwave for 2 minutes. Stir gently, cover, and microwave for about 1-2 minutes more or until the pieces are pliable; let rest for about 5 minutes covered. Pour into a platter.   In a large-sized bowl, whisk the eggs until frothy. Add the spice mix and whisk again to blend.   Working in batches, toss the sweet potatoes in the seasoned egg whites letting the excess liquid drip back into the bowl. Arrange the coated potatoes in a single layer on the prepared baking sheets.   Bake for 10 minutes; flip the pieces over using a spatula. Rotate the baking sheets from back to front and one to the other; bake for about 15 minutes or until dark golden brown. Serve immediately.
Nutrition Info: Per Serving:100 cal., 4 g total fat (0 g sat. fat), 0 mg chol., 60 mg sodium, 230 mg pot., 12 g total carbs., 2 g fiber, 2 g sugar, 3 g protein, 150% vitamin A, 2% vitamin C, 4% calcium, and 6% iron.

433.   Cucumber Rolls

Servings: 6   Cooking Time: 0 Minutes
Ingredients:

1 big cucumber, sliced lengthwise	8 ounces canned tuna, drained and mashed
1 tablespoon parsley, chopped	Salt and black pepper to the taste
1 teaspoon lime juice	

Directions:
Arrange cucumber slices on a working surface, divide the rest of the ingredients, and roll. Arrange all the rolls on a platter and serve as an appetizer.
Nutrition Info:calories 200, fat 6, fiber 3.4, carbs 7.6, protein 3.5

434.   Jalapeno Chickpea Hummus

Servings: 4   Cooking Time: 25 Minutes
Ingredients:

1 cup dry chickpeas, soaked overnight and drained	1/2 cup fresh cilantro 1 tbsp tahini 1/2 cup olive oil
1 tsp ground cumin	Pepper
1/4 cup jalapenos, diced	Salt

Directions:
Add chickpeas into the instant pot and cover with vegetable stock.   Seal pot with lid and cook on high for 25 minutes.   Once done, allow to release pressure naturally. Remove lid.   Drain chickpeas well and transfer into the food processor along with remaining ingredients and process until smooth. Serve and enjoy.
Nutrition Info: Calories 425 Fat 30.4 g Carbohydrates 31.8 g Sugar 5.6 g Protein 10.5 g Cholesterol 0 mg

435.   Healthy Spinach Dip

Servings: 4   Cooking Time: 8 Minutes
Ingredients:

14 oz spinach	2 tbsp olive oil
2 tbsp fresh lime juice	2 tbsp coconut cream
1 tbsp garlic, minced	Pepper
	Salt

Directions:
Add all ingredients except coconut cream into the instant pot and stir well.   Seal pot with lid and cook on low pressure for 8 minutes.   Once done, allow to release pressure naturally for 5 minutes then release remaining using quick release. Remove lid.   Add coconut cream and stir well and blend spinach mixture using a blender until smooth.   Serve and enjoy.
Nutrition Info: Calories 109 Fat 9.2 g Carbohydrates 6.6 g Sugar 1.1 g Protein 3.2 g Cholesterol 0 mg

436.   Marinated Cheese

Servings: 18   Cooking Time: 10 Minutes
Ingredients:

8 ounces cream cheese	2 garlic cloves, sliced
6 sprigs fresh thyme	1 teaspoon black pepper
3 sprigs fresh rosemary	1 lemon peel, cut into thin strips
1/2 cup sun-dried tomato vinaigrette dressing	

Directions:
Cut the cream cheese into 36 cubes. Place on a serving tray.   Combine the remaining ingredients together.   Pour the dressing over the cheese; toss lightly.   Refrigerate for at least 1 hour to marinate.
Nutrition Info: Per Serving:44 cal., 4.3 g total fat (2.4 sat. fat), 13.9 mg chol., 40.6 mg sodium, 0.7 g total carbs., 0 g fiber, 0.4 g sugar, and 0.8 g protein.

437.   Za'atar Fries

Servings: 5   Cooking Time: 35 Minutes
Ingredients:

1 teaspoon Za'atar spices	1 teaspoon salt
3 sweet potatoes	3 teaspoons sunflower oil
1 tablespoon dried dill	½ teaspoon paprika

Directions:
Pour water in the crockpot. Peel the sweet potatoes and cut them into the fries.   Line the baking tray with parchment.   Place the layer of the sweet potato in the tray.   Sprinkle the vegetables with dried dill, salt, and paprika.   Then sprinkle sweet potatoes with Za'atar and mix up well with the help of the fingertips.   Sprinkle the sweet potato fries with sunflower oil.   Preheat the oven to 375F. Bake the sweet potato fries for 35 minutes. Stir the fries every 10 minutes.
Nutrition Info: Per Serving:calories 28, fat 2.9, fiber 0.2, carbs 0.6, protein 0.2

438.   Tuna Salad

Servings: 2-4   Cooking Time: 10 Minutes
Ingredients:

1 can (5 ounce) albacore tuna, solid white	1 whole-wheat crackers (I used sleeve Ritz®)
1 to 2 tablespoons mayo or Greek yogurt	1/4 cup Kalamata olives, quartered

1/4 cup chickpeas, rinsed, drained (or preferred white beans)

1/4 cup roughly chopped marinated artichoke hearts

Directions:
Flake the tuna out of the can into medium-sized bowl. Add the chickpeas, olives, and artichoke hearts; toss to combine. Add mayo or Greek yogurt according to your taste; stir until well combined. Spoon the salad mixture onto crackers; serve.
Nutrition Info: Per Serving:130 cal., 5 g total fat (0.5 g sat. fat), 25 mg chol., 240 mg sodium, 240 mg pot., 8 g total carbs., 1 g fiber, <1 g sugar, 12 g protein, 2% vitamin A, 2% vitamin C, 4% calcium, and 6% iron.

439. Cheese Rolls

Servings: 1 Roll   Cooking Time: 5 Minutes
Ingredients:

1 cup ackawi cheese
1 cup shredded mozzarella cheese
2 TB. fresh parsley, finely chopped
1 large egg
1/2 tsp. ground black pepper

1 large egg yolk, beaten
2 TB. water
1 pkg. egg roll dough (20 count)
4 TB. extra-virgin olive oil

Directions:
In a large bowl, combine ackawi cheese, mozzarella cheese, parsley, egg, and black pepper. In a small bowl, whisk together egg yolk and water. Lay out 1 egg roll, place 2 tablespoons cheese mixture at one corner of egg roll, and brush opposite corner with egg yolk mixture. Fold over side of egg roll, with cheese, to the middle. Fold in left and right sides, and complete rolling egg roll, using egg-brushed side to seal. Set aside, seal side down, and repeat with remaining egg rolls and cheese mixture. In a skillet over low heat, heat 2 tablespoons extra-virgin olive oil. Add up to 4 cheese rolls, seal side down, and cook for 1 or 2 minutes per side or until browned. Repeat with remaining 2 tablespoons extra-virgin olive oil and egg rolls. Serve warm.

440. Olive, Pepperoni, And Mozzarella Bites

Servings: 2   Cooking Time: 10 Minutes
Ingredients:

1 pound block Mozzarella cheese
1 package pepperoni

1 can whole medium black olives

Directions:
Slice the block of mozzarella cheese into 1/2x1/2-inch cubes. Drain the olives from the liquid. With a toothpick, skewer the olive, pushing it 1/3 way up the toothpick. Fold a pepperoni into half or quarters and skewer after the olive. Finally, skewer a mozzarella cheese, not pushing all the way through the cube, about only half way through. Repeat with the remaining olives, pepperoni, and mozzarella cubes.
Nutrition Info: Per Serving:75 cal., 5.6 g total fat (2.5 g sat. fat), 14 mg chol., 221 mg sodium, 16 mg pot., 0.8 g total carbs., 0 g fiber, 0 g sugar, 5.6 g protein, 3% vitamin A, 0% vitamin C, 11% calcium, and 1% iron.

441. Eggplant Dip

Servings: 4   Cooking Time: 40 Minutes
Ingredients:

1 eggplant, poked with a fork
2 tablespoons tahini paste
2 tablespoons lemon juice
2 garlic cloves, minced

1 tablespoon olive oil
Salt and black pepper to the taste
1 tablespoon parsley, chopped

Directions:
Put the eggplant in a roasting pan, bake at 400 degrees F for 40 minutes, cool down, peel and transfer to your food processor. Add the rest of the ingredients except the parsley, pulse well, divide into small bowls and serve as an appetizer with the parsley sprinkled on top.
Nutrition Info:calories 121, fat 4.3, fiber 1, carbs 1.4, protein 4.3

442. Celery And Cucumber Snack

Servings: 4   Cooking Time: 0 Minutes
Ingredients:

6 oz celery stalk, roughly chopped
2 cucumbers, roughly chopped
1 teaspoon mustard

1 teaspoon honey
2 teaspoons lemon juice
1 tablespoon fresh cilantro, chopped

Directions:
Place celery stalk, cucumbers, and fresh cilantro in the big bowl. In the shallow bowl combine together mustard, honey, and lemon juice. Pour the liquid over the vegetables and shake them well. Transfer the vegetables in the jars and close with the lid. Store the vegetable snack jars up to 2 hours in the fridge.
Nutrition Info: Per Serving:calories 39, fat 0.5, fiber 1.6, carbs 8.5, protein 1.5

443. Oat Bites

Servings: 4   Cooking Time: 10 Minutes
Ingredients:

1 teaspoon honey
1 tablespoon rolled oats
1 tablespoon raisins, chopped

4 dates, pitted
¼ teaspoon ground cinnamon
1 teaspoon chia seeds, dried

Directions:
Mash the dates with the help of the fork until you get a mashed mixture. Then add honey, rolled oats, raisins, ground cinnamon, and chia seeds. Mix up the mixture with the help of the spoon until homogenous. Make the small balls and refrigerate them for at least 10-15 minutes.
Nutrition Info: Per Serving:calories 52, fat 0.9, fiber 1.8, carbs 11.4, protein 0.9

444. Eggplant Bites

Servings: 8   Cooking Time: 15 Minutes
Ingredients:

2 eggplants, cut into 20 slices
2 tablespoons olive oil
½ cup roasted peppers, chopped
½ cup kalamata

1 tablespoon lime juice
1 teaspoon red pepper flakes, crushed
Salt and black pepper to the taste

olives, pitted and chopped

2 tablespoons mint, chopped

Directions:
In a bowl, mix the roasted peppers with the olives, half of the oil and the rest of the ingredients except the eggplant slices and stir well. Brush eggplant slices with the rest of the olive oil on both sides, place them on the preheated grill over medium high heat, cook for 7 minutes on each side and transfer them to a platter. Top each eggplant slice with roasted peppers mix and serve.
Nutrition Info:calories 214, fat 10.6, fiber 5.8, carbs 15.4, protein 5.4

445. Creamy Pepper Spread

Servings: 4   Cooking Time: 15 Minutes
Ingredients:

1 lb red bell peppers, chopped and remove seeds
1 1/2 tbsp fresh basil
1 tbsp olive oil

1 tbsp fresh lime juice
1 tsp garlic, minced
Pepper
Salt

Directions:
Add all ingredients into the inner pot of instant pot and stir well. Seal pot with lid and cook on high for 15 minutes. Once done, allow to release pressure naturally for 10 minutes then release remaining using quick release. Remove lid. Transfer bell pepper mixture into the food processor and process until smooth. Serve and enjoy.
Nutrition Info: Calories 41 Fat 3.6 g Carbohydrates 3.5 g Sugar 1.7 g Protein 0.4 g Cholesterol 0 mg

446. Creamy Eggplant Dip

Servings: 4   Cooking Time: 20 Minutes
Ingredients:

1 eggplant
1/2 tsp paprika
1 tbsp olive oil
1 tbsp fresh lime juice

2 tbsp tahini
1 garlic clove
1 cup of water
Pepper
Salt

Directions:
Add water and eggplant into the instant pot. Seal pot with the lid and select manual and set timer for 20 minutes. Once done, release pressure using quick release. Remove lid. Drain eggplant and let it cool. Once the eggplant is cool then remove eggplant skin and transfer eggplant flesh into the food processor. Add remaining ingredients into the food processor and process until smooth. Serve and enjoy.
Nutrition Info: Calories 108 Fat 7.8 g Carbohydrates 9.7 g Sugar 3.7 g Protein 2.5 g Cholesterol 0 mg

447. Herbed Goat Cheese Dip

Servings: 4   Cooking Time: 0 Minutes
Ingredients:

¼ cup mixed parsley, chopped
¼ cup chives, chopped
8 ounces goat cheese, soft

Salt and black pepper to the taste
A drizzle of olive oil

Directions:
In your food processor mix the goat cheese with the parsley and the rest of the ingredients and pulse well. Divide into small bowls and serve as a party dip.
Nutrition Info:calories 245, fat 11.3, fiber 4.5, carbs 8.9, protein 11.2

448. Italian Wheatberry Cakes

Servings: 6   Cooking Time: 15 Minutes
Ingredients:

1 cup wheatberry, cooked
2 eggs
¼ cup ground chicken
1 tablespoon wheat flour, whole grain

1 teaspoon Italian seasoning
1 tablespoon olive oil
1 teaspoon salt

Directions:
In the mixing bowl mix up together wheatberry and ground chicken. Crack eggs in the mixture. Then add wheat flour, Italian seasoning, and salt. Mix up the mass with the help of the spoon until homogenous. Then make burgers and freeze them in the freezer for 20 minutes. Heat up olive oil in the skillet. Place frozen burgers in the hot oil and roast them for 4 minutes from each side over the high heat. Then cook burgers for 10 minutes more over the medium heat. Flip them onto another side from time to time.
Nutrition Info: Per Serving:calories 97, fat 5.7, fiber 1.5, carbs 9.2, protein 5.2

449. Healthy Kidney Bean Dip

Servings: 6   Cooking Time: 10 Minutes
Ingredients:

1 cup dry white kidney beans, soaked overnight and drained
1 tbsp fresh lemon juice
2 tbsp water
1/2 cup coconut yogurt

1 roasted garlic clove
1 tbsp olive oil
1/4 tsp cayenne
1 tsp dried parsley
Pepper
Salt

Directions:
Add soaked beans and 1 3/4 cups of water into the instant pot. Seal pot with lid and cook on high for 10 minutes. Once done, allow to release pressure naturally. Remove lid. Drain beans well and transfer them into the food processor. Add remaining ingredients into the food processor and process until smooth. Serve and enjoy.
Nutrition Info: Calories 136 Fat 3.2 g Carbohydrates 20 g Sugar 2.1 g Protein 7.7 g Cholesterol 0 mg

450. Lentils Spread

Servings: 12   Cooking Time: 0 Minutes
Ingredients:

1 garlic clove, minced
1 teaspoon oregano, dried
¼ teaspoon basil, dried
3 tablespoons olive oil

12 ounces canned lentils, drained and rinsed
1 tablespoon balsamic vinegar
Salt and black pepper to the taste

Directions:
In a blender, combine the lentils with the garlic and the rest of the ingredients, pulse well, divide into bowls and serve as an appetizer.

Nutrition Info: calories 287, fat 9.5, fiber 3.5, carbs 15.3, protein 9.3

451. Chickpeas Spread

Servings: 7   Cooking Time: 45 Minutes

Ingredients:

1 cup chickpeas, soaked
6 cups of water
½ cup lemon juice
3 tablespoon olive oil
1 teaspoon salt
1/3 teaspoon harissa

Directions:
Combine together chickpeas and water and boil for 45 minutes or until chickpeas are tender.   Then transfer chickpeas in the food processor.   Add 1 cup of chickpeas water and lemon juice.   After this, add salt and harissa.   Blend the hummus until it is smooth and fluffy.   Add olive oil and pulse it for 10 seconds more.   Transfer the cooked hummus in the bowl and store it in the fridge up to 2 days.
Nutrition Info: Per Serving: calories 160, fat 7.9, fiber 5. carbs 17.8, protein 5.7

452. Lime Yogurt Dip

Servings: 4   Cooking Time: 0 Minutes

Ingredients:

1 large cucumber, trimmed
3 oz Greek yogurt
1 teaspoon olive oil
3 tablespoons fresh dill, chopped
1 tablespoon lime juice
¾ teaspoon salt
1 garlic clove, minced

Directions:
Grate the cucumber and squeeze the juice from it. Then place the squeezed cucumber in the bowl. Add Greek yogurt, olive oil, dill, lime juice, salt, and minced garlic.   Mix up the mixture until homogenous.   Store tzaziki in the fridge up to 2 days.
Nutrition Info: Per Serving: calories 44, fat 1.8, fiber 0.7, carbs 5.1, protein 3.2

453. Almond Bowls

Servings: 5   Cooking Time: 15 Minutes

Ingredients:

1 cup almonds
3 tablespoons salt
2 cups of water

Directions:
Bring water to boil.   After this, add 2 tablespoons of salt in water and stir it.   When salt is dissolved, add almonds and let them soak for at least 1 hour. Meanwhile, line the tray with baking paper and preheat oven to 350F.   Dry the soaked almonds with a paper towel well and arrange them in one layer in the tray.   Sprinkle buts with remaining salt.   Bake the snack for 15 minutes. Mix it from time to time with the help of the spatula or spoon.
Nutrition Info: Per Serving: calories 110, fat 9.5, fiber 2.4, carbs 4.1, protein 4

454. Beet Spread

Servings: 4   Cooking Time: 35 Minutes

Ingredients:

1 tablespoon pumpkin puree
1 beet, peeled
1 teaspoon tahini paste
½ teaspoon sesame
1 teaspoon paprika
1 tablespoon olive oil
¼ cup water, boiled
1 tablespoon lime juice

seeds
½ teaspoon salt

Directions:
Place beet in the oven and bake it at 375F for 35 minutes.   Then chop it roughly and put in the food processor.   Blend the beet until smooth. After this, add tahini paste, pumpkin puree, paprika, olive oil, water, lime juice, and salt. Blend the hummus until smooth and fluffy. Then transfer the appetizer in the bowl and sprinkle with sesame seeds.
Nutrition Info: Per Serving: calories 99, fat 8.6, fiber 1.6, carbs 3.9, protein 2.1

455. Calamari Mediterranean

Servings: 2   Cooking Time: 10 Minutes

Ingredients:

1 tablespoon Italian parsley
1 teaspoon ancho chili, chopped
1 teaspoon cumin
1 teaspoon red pepper flakes
1/2 cup white wine
2 cups calamari
2 medium plum tomatoes, diced
2 tablespoons capers
2 tablespoons garlic cloves, roasted
2 tablespoons olive oil
2 tablespoons unsalted butter
3 tablespoons lime juice
Salt

Directions:
Heat a sauté pan. Add the oil, garlic, and the calamari; sauté for 1 minute. Add the capers, red pepper flakes, cumin, ancho chili and the diced tomatoes; cook for 1 minute.   Add the wine and the lime juice; simmer for 4 minutes.   Stir in the butter, parsley, and the salt; continue cooking until the sauce is thick.   Serve with whole-wheat French bread.
Nutrition Info: Per Serving: 308.8 cal., 25.7 g total fat (9.3 sat. fat), 30.5 mg chol., 267.8 mg sodium, 10.2 g total carbs., 1.7 g fiber, 2.8 g sugar, and 1.9 g protein.

456. Cheddar Dip

Servings: 6   Cooking Time: 10 Minutes

Ingredients:

¼ cup cilantro, chopped
1 chili pepper, chopped
1 cup Cheddar cheese
1 teaspoon garlic powder
¼ cup milk

Directions:
Bring the milk to boil.   Then add Cheddar cheese in the milk and simmer the mixture for 2 minutes. Stir it constantly.   After this, add cilantro, chili pepper, and garlic powder. Mix up the mixture well. If it doesn't get a smooth texture, use the hand blender to blend the mass.   It is recommended to serve the dip when it gets the room temperature.
Nutrition Info: Per Serving: calories 83, fat 6.5, fiber 0.1, carbs 1.2, protein 5.1

457. Olives And Cheese Stuffed Tomatoes

Servings: 24   Cooking Time: 0 Minutes

Ingredients:

2 tablespoons olive oil
¼ teaspoon red pepper flakes
½ cup feta cheese,
24 cherry tomatoes, top cut off and insides scooped out
2 tablespoons black olive paste

crumbled
¼ cup mint, torn

Directions:
In a bowl, mix the olives paste with the rest of the ingredients except the cherry tomatoes and whisk well. Stuff the cherry tomatoes with this mix, arrange them all on a platter and serve as an appetizer.
Nutrition Info:calories 136, fat 8.6, fiber 4.8, carbs 5.6, protein 5.1

458. Feta Cheese Log With Sun-dried Tomatoes And Kalamata Olives

Servings: 2   Cooking Time: 20 Minutes
Ingredients:
8 ounces feta cheese, crumbled
4 ounces cream cheese, softened
1/8-1/4 teaspoon cayenne pepper (depending on your taste)
1/4 cup chopped sun-dried tomato
1/4 cup chopped Kalamata olive
2 tablespoons extra-virgin olive oil
1/2 teaspoon dried Mediterranean oregano, crumbled
1 small garlic clove, minced
1/2 cup walnuts, toasted, chopped
1/4 cup fresh parsley, minced

Directions:
With a mixer, combine the feta cheese, cream cheese, and the olive oil on medium speed until well combined. Add the remaining ingredients and mix well. Shape the soft mixture into a 10-inch long log. Combine the parsley and the walnuts; roll the log over the mixture, pressing slightly to stick the parsley and the walnuts on the sides of the log. Wrap the log with plastic wrap; refrigerate for at least 5 hours to let the flavors blend. Remove the plastic wrap, lay the log on a parsley-lined serving platter. Serve with whole-wheat crackers and toasted whole-wheat slices of baguette.
Nutrition Info: Per Serving:1154 cal., 106.3 g total fat (43.9 sat. fat), 226.2 mg chol., 2395.3 mg sodium, 23 g total carbs., 5 g fiber, 13.5 g sugar, and 35.2 g protein.

459. Lemon Salmon Rolls

Servings: 6   Cooking Time: 0 Minutes
Ingredients:
6 wonton wrappers
7 oz salmon, grilled
6 lettuce leaves
1 carrot, peeled
1 cucumber, trimmed
1 tablespoon lemon juice
1 teaspoon olive oil
¼ teaspoon dried oregano

Directions:
Cut the carrot and cucumber onto the wedges. Then chop the grilled salmon. Arrange the salmon, carrot and cucumber wedges, and lettuce leaves on 6 wonton wraps. In the shallow bowl whisk together dried oregano, olive oil, and lemon juice. Sprinkle the roll mixture with oil dressing and wrap.
Nutrition Info: Per Serving:calories 90, fat 3.4, fiber 0.7, carbs 7.7, protein 7.7

460. Ginger And Cream Cheese Dip

Servings: 6   Cooking Time: 0 Minutes

Ingredients:
2 bunches cilantro, chopped
3 tablespoons balsamic vinegar
½ cup ginger, grated
½ cup olive oil
1 and ½ cups cream cheese, soft

Directions:
In your blender, mix the ginger with the rest of the ingredients and pulse well. Divide into small bowls and serve as a party dip.
Nutrition Info:calories 213, fat 4.9, fiber 4.1, carbs 8.8, protein 17.8

461. Lemon Endive Bites

Servings: 10   Cooking Time: 0 Minutes
Ingredients:
6 oz endive
2 pears, chopped
4 oz Blue cheese, crumbled
1 teaspoon olive oil
1 teaspoon lemon juice
¾ teaspoon ground cinnamon

Directions:
Separate endive into the spears (10 spears). In the bowl combine together chopped pears, olive oil, lemon juice, ground cinnamon, and Blue cheese. Fill the endive spears with cheese mixture.
Nutrition Info: Per Serving:calories 72, fat 3.8, fiber 1.9, carbs 7.4, protein 2.8

462. Perfect Italian Potatoes

Servings: 6   Cooking Time: 7 Minutes
Ingredients:
2 lbs baby potatoes, clean and cut in half
3/4 cup vegetable broth
6 oz Italian dry dressing mix

Directions:
Add all ingredients into the inner pot of instant pot and stir well. Seal pot with lid and cook on high for 7 minutes. Once done, allow to release pressure naturally for 3 minutes then release remaining using quick release. Remove lid. Stir well and serve.
Nutrition Info: Calories 149 Fat 0.3 g Carbohydrates 41.6 g Sugar 11.4 g Protein 4.5 g Cholesterol 0 mg

463. Feta Artichoke Dip

Servings: 8   Cooking Time: 30 Minutes
Ingredients:
8 ounces artichoke hearts, drained and quartered
¾ cup green olives, pitted and chopped
¾ cup basil, chopped
1 cup parmesan cheese, grated
5 ounces feta cheese, crumbled

Directions:
In your food processor, mix the artichokes with the basil and the rest of the ingredients, pulse well, and transfer to a baking dish. Introduce in the oven, bake at 375 degrees F for 30 minutes and serve as a party dip.
Nutrition Info:calories 186, fat 12.4, fiber 0.9, carbs 2.6, protein 1.5

464. Peach Skewers

Servings: 2   Cooking Time: 0 Minutes
Ingredients:

1 peach
4 Mozzarella balls, cherry size
½ teaspoon pistachio, chopped
1 teaspoon honey

Directions:
Cut the peach on 4 cubes. Then skewer peach cubes and Mozzarella balls on the skewers. Sprinkle them with honey and chopped pistachio.
Nutrition Info: Per Serving:calories 202, fat 14.3, fiber 1.2, carbs 10, protein 10.8

465. Chickpeas Salsa

Servings: 6   Cooking Time: 0 Minutes
Ingredients:
4 spring onions, chopped
15 ounces canned chickpeas, drained and rinsed
Salt and black pepper to the taste
1 cup baby spinach
2 tablespoons olive oil
2 tablespoons lemon juice
1 tablespoon cilantro, chopped

Directions:
In a bowl, mix the chickpeas with the spinach, spring onions and the rest of the ingredients, toss, divide into small cups and serve as a snack.
Nutrition Info:calories 224, fat 5.1, fiber 1, carbs 9.9, protein 15.1

466. Hummus Appetizer Bites

Servings: 1 Bite   Cooking Time: 10 Minutes
Ingredients:
11/4 cups all-purpose flour
1/2 tsp. salt
5 TB. cold butter
2 TB. vegetable shortening
1/4 cup ice water
1 batch Traditional Hummus (recipe in Chapter 11)
1 tsp. paprika
12 kalamata olives
12 fresh parsley leaves

Directions:
In a food processor fitted with a chopping blade, pulse 1 cup all-purpose flour and salt 5 times. Add cold butter and vegetable shortening, and pulse for 1 minute or until mixture resembles coarse meal. Continue to pulse while adding water for about 1 minute. Test dough; if it holds together when you pinch it, it doesn't require any additional moisture. If it does not come together, add another 3 tablespoons water. Remove dough from the food processor, place in a plastic bag, form into a flat disc, and refrigerate for 30 minutes. Preheat the oven to 425ºF. Remove dough from the plastic bag, and dust both sides with flour. Sprinkle your counter with flour. Using a rolling pin, roll out dough to 1/4 inch thickness. Using a 2-inch circle cookie cutter, cut out 12 circles of dough. Gently mold dough circles into a mini muffin tin, and using a fork, gently poke dough. Bake for 10 minutes. Remove from the oven, and set aside to cool. Spoon about 1 tablespoon Traditional Hummus on top of each cooled piecrust, sprinkle with paprika, and top with 1 kalamata olive and 1 parsley leaf each. Serve immediately or refrigerate.

467. Stuffed Avocado

Servings: 2   Cooking Time: 0 Minutes
Ingredients:
1 avocado, halved and pitted
1 and ½ tablespoon basil pesto

10 ounces canned tuna, drained
2 tablespoons sun-dried tomatoes, chopped
2 tablespoons black olives, pitted and chopped
Salt and black pepper to the taste
2 teaspoons pine nuts, toasted and chopped
1 tablespoon basil, chopped

Directions:
In a bowl, combine the tuna with the sun-dried tomatoes and the rest of the ingredients except the avocado and stir. Stuff the avocado halves with the tuna mix and serve as an appetizer.
Nutrition Info:calories 233, fat 9, fiber 3.5, carbs 11.4, protein 5.6

468. Grilled Polenta Vegetables Bites

Servings: 6-8   Cooking Time: 15 Minutes
Ingredients:
1 1/2 to 2 tablespoons olive oil
1 green bell pepper, chopped
1 tomato sliced
1 tube (18-ounce) Polenta, pre-cooked
1/2 teaspoon garlic powder
1/2 yellow onion, chopped into big chunks
2 jalapenos, sliced, de-seeded
2-3 slices Swiss cheese or your cheese of choice
5-6 pieces baby Bella mushrooms
Optional: Chopped parsley and black olives
Salt and pepper, to taste

Directions:
Preheat the grill. Meanwhile, slice the polenta into 1/4-1/2 slices. Brush both sides with the olive oil and set aside. Place the chopped vegetables into a mixing bowl, add the garlic, remaining oil, and season with salt and pepper to taste; toss lightly. Grill the polenta and the vegetables for about 15 to 20 minutes, turning at least once, until lightly browned. Remove from the grill and assemble the sandwiches with cheese, vegetables, and tomato slice. Top with the olives and parsley, if desired. Secure with toothpicks.
Nutrition Info: Per Serving:150 cal., 11 g total fat (3.5 sat. fat), 10 mg chol., 410 mg sodium, 360 mg pot., 16 g total carbs., 2 g fiber, 2 g sugar, 6 g protein, 15% vitamin A, 45% vitamin C, 10% calcium, and 6% iron.

469. Grapefruit Salad

Servings: 6   Cooking Time: 0 Minutes
Ingredients:
2 cups arugula
1 tablespoon honey
1 teaspoon mustard
1 teaspoon lemon juice
½ teaspoon olive oil
1 grapefruit, peeled
¾ cup walnuts, chopped

Directions:
Chop arugula roughly and place in the bowl. Add chopped walnuts. Then chop grapefruit and add it in the bowl too. Shake the salad well. After this, make salad dressing: whisk together mustard, honey, lemon juice, and olive oil. Pour the dressing over salad.
Nutrition Info: Per Serving:calories 122, fat 9.8, fiber 1.5, carbs 6.6, protein 4.2

470. Hummus With Ground Lamb

Servings: 8   Cooking Time: 15 Minutes

Ingredients:

12 ounces lamb meat, ground
½ cup pomegranate seeds
¼ cup parsley, chopped
10 ounces hummus
1 tablespoon olive oil
Pita chips for serving

Directions:

Heat up a pan with the oil over medium-high heat, add the meat, and brown for 15 minutes stirring often.   Spread the hummus on a platter, spread the ground lamb all over, also spread the pomegranate seeds and the parsley and sere with pita chips as a snack.

Nutrition Info:calories 133, fat 9.7, fiber 1.7, carbs 6.4, protein 5.4

471.Perfect Queso

Servings: 16   Cooking Time: 15 Minutes

Ingredients:

1 lb ground beef
32 oz Velveeta cheese, cut into cubes
10 oz can tomatoes, diced
1 1/2 tbsp taco seasoning
1 tsp chili powder
1 onion, diced
Pepper
Salt

Directions:

Set instant pot on sauté mode.   Add meat, onion, taco seasoning, chili powder, pepper, and salt into the pot and cook until meat is no longer pink. Add tomatoes and stir well. Top with cheese and do not stir.   Seal pot with lid and cook on high for 4 minutes.   Once done, release pressure using quick release. Remove lid.   Stir everything well and serve.

Nutrition Info: Calories 257 Fat 15.9 g Carbohydrates 10.2 g Sugar 4.9 g Protein 21 g Cholesterol 71 mg

472. Aromatic Artichokes

Servings: 1 Artichoke   Cooking Time: 45 Minutes

Ingredients:

4 artichokes
6 cups water
2 cloves garlic
1 bay leaf
1/3 cup fresh lemon juice
2 tsp. minced garlic
1/4 cup extra-virgin olive oil
1/2 tsp. salt
1/2 tsp. ground black pepper

Directions:

Using a pair of kitchen scissors, cut off the tips of artichoke leaves. With a sharp knife, cut 1 inch off top of artichokes. Pull off small leaves along base and stem, leaving only a 1-inch stem. Rinse artichokes in cold water.   In a steamer or large saucepan over medium-high heat, bring water, garlic cloves, and bay leaf to a simmer. Add steaming basket, place artichokes inside, cover, and steam for 40 minutes.   In a small bowl, whisk together minced garlic, lemon juice, extra-virgin olive oil, salt, and black pepper.   Transfer artichokes from the steamer to a serving dish, and spoon dressing over artichokes, being sure to get it between leaves.   Serve warm or cold.

473. Rosemary Olive Bread

Servings: 1 Pita   Cooking Time: 20 Minuutes

Ingredients:

11/2 TB. active dry yeast
11/2 cups warm water
1 tsp. sugar
1/4 cup plus 3 TB. extra-virgin olive oil
3 TB. fresh rosemary, roughly chopped
1 tsp. salt
10 kalamata olives, pitted and roughly chopped
1 tsp. ground black pepper
3 cups all-purpose flour

Directions:

In a large bowl, combine yeast, warm water, and sugar, and set aside for 5 minutes.   Add salt, 1/4 cup extra-virgin olive oil, rosemary, kalamata olives, black pepper, and 1 cup all-purpose flour, and stir to combine. Add another 1 cup all-purpose flour, and begin to knead dough. Add remaining 1 cup all-purpose flour, and knead for about 3 minutes or until dough comes together in a ball. If you're using an electric stand mixer, use the dough attachment to knead dough.   Remove dough from the bowl, and grease the bowl with 1 tablespoon extra-virgin olive oil. Return dough to the bowl, and turn over to coat dough in oil. Cover the bowl with plastic wrap and a thick towel, and set aside to rise for 2 hours.   Uncover the bowl, and gently pull dough together into a ball. Divide dough into 10 equal-size pieces, lightly dust with flour and cover with plastic wrap or a moist towel.   Flour your rolling pin and work surface. Roll out each dough ball to 1/4 inch thick, and place on a baking sheet. Let rolled-out dough sit for 10 minutes before cooking.   Preheat an iron or cast-iron skillet over medium-low heat, and brush lightly with extra-virgin olive oil. Add 1 rolled-out dough to the skillet, and cook for 2 or 3 minutes or until lightly browned. Flip over and cook for 2 more minutes. Transfer to a plate, and cover with a slightly damp towel. Brush the skillet with more extra-virgin olive oil before cooking next piece.   Store in an airtight container, and serve with a good extra-virgin olive oil and olives.

474. Parmesan Eggplant Bites

Servings: 8   Cooking Time: 30 Minutes

Ingredients:

2 eggs, beaten
3 oz Parmesan, grated
1 tablespoon coconut flakes
½ teaspoon ground paprika
1 teaspoon salt
2 eggplants, trimmed

Directions:

Slice the eggplants into the thin circles. Use the vegetable slicer for this step.   After this, sprinkle the vegetables with salt and mix up. Leave them for 5-10 minutes.   Then drain eggplant juice and sprinkle them with ground paprika.   Mix up together coconut flakes and Parmesan.   Dip every eggplant circle in the egg and then coat in Parmesan mixture.   Line the baking tray with parchment and place eggplants on it.   Bake the vegetables for 30 minutes at 360F. Flip the eggplants into another side after 12 minutes of cooking.

Nutrition Info: Per Serving:calories 87, fat 3.9, fiber 5, carbs 8.7, protein 6.2

475. Quinoa Bars

Servings: 15   Cooking Time: 25 Minutes

Ingredients:

1 cup rolled oats
7 oz almonds,

6 oz quinoa
5 tablespoons maple syrup
3 tablespoons peanut butter
chopped
1 teaspoon ground cinnamon
1 tablespoon coconut flakes

Directions:
In the bog bowl mix up together rolled oats, quinoa, almonds, and coconut flakes. Then add peanut butter and maple syrup. Stir the mixture carefully with the help of the spoon. Line the baking tray with parchment. Transfer the quinoa mixture in the tray and flatten it well. Bake granola for 25 minutes at 355F. Chill the cooked granola well and crack on the servings.
Nutrition Info: Per Serving:calories 177, fat 9.4, fiber 3.3, carbs 19.1, protein 5.9

476. Creamy Artichoke Dip

Servings: 8   Cooking Time: 5 Minutes
Ingredients:
28 oz can artichoke hearts, drain and quartered
1 1/2 cups parmesan cheese, shredded
1 cup sour cream
1 cup mayonnaise
3.5 oz can green chilies
1 cup of water
Pepper
Salt

Directions:
Add artichokes, water, and green chilis into the instant pot. Seal pot with the lid and select manual and set timer for 1 minute. Once done, release pressure using quick release. Remove lid. Drain excess water. Set instant pot on sauté mode. Add remaining ingredients and stir well and cook until cheese is melted. Serve and enjoy.
Nutrition Info: Calories 262 Fat 7.6 g Carbohydrates 14.4 g Sugar 2.8 g Protein 8.4 g Cholesterol 32 mg

477. Olive Eggplant Spread

Servings: 12   Cooking Time: 8 Minutes
Ingredients:
1 3/4 lbs eggplant, chopped
1/2 tbsp dried oregano
1/4 cup olives, pitted and chopped
1 tbsp tahini
1/4 cup fresh lime juice
1/2 cup water
2 garlic cloves
1/4 cup olive oil
Salt

Directions:
Add oil into the inner pot of instant pot and set the pot on sauté mode. Add eggplant and cook for 3-5 minutes. Turn off sauté mode. Add water and salt and stir well. Seal pot with lid and cook on high for 3 minutes. Once done, release pressure using quick release. Remove lid. Drain eggplant well and transfer into the food processor. Add remaining ingredients into the food processor and process until smooth. Serve and enjoy.
Nutrition Info: Calories 65 Fat 5.3 g Carbohydrates 4.7 g Sugar 2 g Protein 0.9 g Cholesterol 0 mg

478. Cucumber Bites

Servings: 12   Cooking Time: 0 Minutes
Ingredients:
1 English cucumber, sliced into 32 rounds
10 ounces hummus
16 cherry tomatoes,
1 tablespoon parsley, chopped
1 ounce feta cheese, crumbled
halved

Directions:
Spread the hummus on each cucumber round, divide the tomato halves on each, sprinkle the cheese and parsley on to and serve as an appetizer.
Nutrition Info:calories 162, fat 3.4, fiber 2, carbs 6.4, protein 2.4

479. Oregano Crackers

Servings: 8   Cooking Time: 15 Minutes
Ingredients:
½ cup wheat flour, whole grain
¼ cup Feta cheese, crumbled
¾ cup of water
1 teaspoon dried oregano
1 teaspoon salt
½ teaspoon sesame seeds

Directions:
Mix up together water and flour. Add dried oregano, salt, and Feta cheese. Knead the non-sticky dough. After this, roll up the dough into the thick sheet and cut the sheet on the crackers. Line the baking tray with baking paper. Arrange the uncooked crackers in the tray and bake for 14 minutes at 365F. After this, flip the crackers on another side and cook for 1 minute more. Chill the cooked crackers well.
Nutrition Info: Per Serving:calories 38, fat 1.1, fiber 0.3, carbs 5.6, protein 1.4

480. Tomato Salsa

Servings: 6   Cooking Time: 0 Minutes
Ingredients:
1 garlic clove, minced
4 tablespoons olive oil
5 tomatoes, cubed
1 tablespoon balsamic vinegar
¼ cup basil, chopped
1 tablespoon parsley, chopped
1 tablespoon chives, chopped
Salt and black pepper to the taste
Pita chips for serving

Directions:
In a bowl, mix the tomatoes with the garlic and the rest of the ingredients except the pita chips, stir, divide into small cups and serve with the pita chips on the side.
Nutrition Info:calories 160, fat 13.7, fiber 5.5, carbs 10.1, protein 2.2

481. Spicy Berry Dip

Servings: 4   Cooking Time: 15 Minutes
Ingredients:
10 oz cranberries
1/4 cup fresh orange juice
3/4 tsp paprika
1/2 tsp chili powder
1 tsp lemon zest
1 tbsp lemon juice

Directions:
Add all ingredients into the inner pot of instant pot and stir well. Seal pot with lid and cook on high for 15 minutes. Once done, allow to release pressure naturally for 5 minutes then release remaining using quick release. Remove lid. Blend cranberry mixture using a blender until getting the desired consistency. Serve and enjoy.
Nutrition Info: Calories 49 Fat 0.2 g Carbohydrates 8.6 g Sugar 4.1 g Protein 0.3 g Cholesterol 0 mg

482. Mozzarella Chips

Servings: 8   Cooking Time: 10 Minutes

Ingredients:

4 phyllo dough sheets 1 tablespoon olive oil
4 oz Mozzarella,
shredded

Directions:

Place 2 phyllo sheets in the pan and brush it with sprinkle it with Mozzarella. Then cover the cheese with 2 remaining phyllo sheets. Brush the top of Phyllo with olive oil and cut on 8 squares. Bake the chips for 10 minutes at 365F or until they are light brown.

Nutrition Info: Per Serving:calories 130, fat 5, fiber 0.5, carbs 15.5, protein 6.5

483. Salmon Rolls

Servings: 12 Cooking Time: 0 Minutes

Ingredients:

2 teaspoons lime   1 big long cucumber,
juice   thinly sliced
4 ounces cream   lengthwise
cheese, soft   2 teaspoons dill,
1 teaspoon lemon   chopped
zest, grated   4 ounces smoked
Salt and black pepper   salmon, cut into
to the taste   strips

Directions:

Arrange cucumber slices on a working surface and top each with a salmon strip. In a bowl, mix the rest of the ingredients, stir and spread over the salmon. Roll the salmon and cucumber strips, arrange them on a platter and serve as an appetizer.

Nutrition Info:calories 245, fat 15.5, fiber 4.8, carbs 16.8, protein 17.3

484. Cream Cheese Rolls

Servings: 2 Cooking Time: 0 Minutes

Ingredients:

1 lavash sheet   2 ham slices
1 tablespoon cream   1 tomato, sliced
cheese   3 lettuce leaves
1 bell pepper

Directions:

Spread lavash with cream cheese from one side. Then cut bell pepper on the wedges and arrange it over the cream cheese. Add sliced ham, tomato, and lettuce. Roll the lavash. Cut it on 2 servings and secure every lavash roll with a toothpick.

Nutrition Info: Per Serving:calories 169, fat 5.1, fiber 2.6, carbs 23.1, protein 8.9

485. Carrot Dip

Servings: 10 Cooking Time: 12 Minutes

Ingredients:

1 1/2 teaspoons   1 piece (2 inches)
ground coriander   fresh ginger root,
1 pound carrots,   peeled, thinly sliced
peeled, thinly sliced   3 cloves garlic, thinly
1/3 cup apricot   sliced
preserves   3/4 teaspoon salt,
1/8 teaspoon cayenne   divided
pepper   4 teaspoons toasted
2 tablespoons fresh   sesame oil
lemon juice   2 cups water

Directions:

Place the carrots, ginger, garlic, and 1/4 teaspoon salt in a large-sized saucepan. Add the water, cover, and bring to a boil. When boiling, reduce the heat,

simmer covered for about 10-12 minutes, or until the carrots are drained. Drain. Transfer the carrots to a food processor. Add the remaining 1/2 teaspoon salt and the rest of the ingredients; process until the mixture is smooth.

Nutrition Info: Per Serving:65 cal., 2.1 g total fat (0.3 sat. fat), 0 mg chol., 210 mg sodium, 12.1 g total carbs., 1.5 g fiber, 6.9 g sugar, and 0.6 g protein.

486. Walnuts Yogurt Dip

Servings: 8 Cooking Time: 0 Minutes

Ingredients:

3 garlic cloves,   ¼ cup dill, chopped
minced   ¼ cup walnuts,
2 cups Greek yogurt   chopped
1 tablespoon chives,   Salt and black pepper
chopped   to the taste

Directions:

In a bowl, mix the garlic with the yogurt and the rest of the ingredients, whisk well, divide into small cups and serve as a party dip.

Nutrition Info:calories 200, fat 6.5, fiber 4.6, carbs 15.5, protein 8.4

487. Rosemary Cauliflower Dip

Servings: 4 Cooking Time: 15 Minutes

Ingredients:

1 lb cauliflower   1 tbsp garlic, minced
florets   1 tbsp rosemary,
1 tbsp fresh parsley,   chopped
chopped   1 tbsp olive oil
1/2 cup heavy cream   1 onion, chopped
1/2 cup vegetable   Pepper
stock   Salt

Directions:

Add oil into the inner pot of instant pot and set the pot on sauté mode. Add onion and sauté for 5 minutes. Add remaining ingredients except for parsley and heavy cream and stir well. Seal pot with lid and cook on high for 10 minutes. Once done, allow to release pressure naturally for 10 minutes then release remaining using quick release. Remove lid. Add cream and stir well. Blend cauliflower mixture using immersion blender until smooth. Garnish with parsley and serve.

Nutrition Info: Calories 128 Fat 9.4 g Carbohydrates 10.4 g Sugar 4 g Protein 3.1 g Cholesterol 21 mg

488. Light & Creamy Garlic Hummus

Servings: 12 Cooking Time: 40 Minutes

Ingredients:

1 1/2 cups dry   1/2 cup tahini
chickpeas, rinsed   6 cups of water
2 1/2 tbsp fresh   Pepper
lemon juice   Salt
1 tbsp garlic, minced

Directions:

Add water and chickpeas into the instant pot. Seal pot with a lid and select manual and set timer for 40 minutes. Once done, allow to release pressure naturally. Remove lid. Drain chickpeas well and reserved 1/2 cup chickpeas liquid. Transfer chickpeas, reserved liquid, lemon juice, garlic, tahini, pepper, and salt into the food

processor and process until smooth. Serve and enjoy.
Nutrition Info: Calories 152 Fat 6.9 g Carbohydrates 17.6 g Sugar 2.8 g Protein 6.6 g Cholesterol 0 mg

489. Mediterranean-style Nachos Recipe

Servings: 12   Cooking Time: 15 Minutes
Ingredients:

6 pieces whole-wheat pita breads	1 teaspoon cornstarch
Cooking spray	2 cups Greek yogurt, plain
1/2 teaspoon ground cumin	2 tablespoons lemon juice
1/2 teaspoon ground coriander	1/4 teaspoon grated lemon peel
1/2 teaspoon paprika	1 teaspoon salt, divided
1/2 teaspoon pepper	
1/2 teaspoons salt	1/4 teaspoon pepper
1/2 cup hot water	1/2 cup pitted Greek olives, sliced
1/2 teaspoon beef stock concentrate	4 green onions, thinly sliced
1 pound ground lamb or beef	1/2 cup crumbled feta cheese
2 garlic cloves, minced	2 cups torn romaine lettuce
2 medium cucumbers, peeled, seeded, grated	2 medium tomatoes, seeded and chopped

Directions:
In a colander set over a bowl, toss the cucumbers with 1/2 teaspoon of the salt; let stand for 30 minutes, then squeeze and pat dry. Set aside. In a small-sized bowl, combine the coriander, cumin, 1/2 teaspoon pepper, paprika, and 1/2 teaspoon salt; set aside. Cut each pita bread into 8 wedges. Arrange them in a single layer on ungreased baking sheets. Sprits both sides of the wedges with cooking spray. Sprinkle with 3/4 teaspoon of the seasoning mix. Broil 3-4 inches from the heat source for about 3-4 minutes per side, or until golden brown. Transfer to wire racks, let cool. Whisk hot water and beef stock cube in a 1-cup liquid measuring cup until blended. In a large-sized skillet, cook the lamb, seasoning with the remaining seasoning mix, over medium heat until the meat is no longer pink. Add the garlic; cook for 1 minute. Drain. Stir in the cornstarch into the broth; mix until smooth. Gradually stir into the skillet; bring to a boil and cook, stirring, for 2 minutes or until thick. In a small-sized bowl, combine the cucumbers, yogurt, lemon peel, lemon juice, and the remaining salt and 1/4 teaspoon pepper. Arrange the pita wedges on a serving platter. Layer with the lettuce, lamb mixture, tomatoes, onions, olives, and cheese; serve immediately with the cucumber sauce.
Nutrition Info: Per Serving:232 cal, 6.7 g total fat (2.9 g sat. fat), 42 mg chol., 630 mg sodium, 412 mg pot., 24 total carbs., 3.3 g fiber, 4.1 g sugar, 20.2 g protein, 8% vitamin A, 12% vitamin C, 11% calcium, and 15% iron.

490. Baked Goat Cheese Caprese Salad

Servings: 4   Cooking Time: 15 Minutes
Ingredients:

1 (log 4 ounce) fresh goat cheese, halved	16 cherry tomatoes, diagonally cut into halves
1 pinch cayenne pepper, or to taste	2 tablespoons olive oil, divided
3 tablespoons basil chiffonade (thinly sliced fresh basil leaves), divided	Freshly ground black pepper, to taste

Directions:
Preheat the oven to 400F or 200C. Drizzle about 1 1/2 teaspoons olive oil into the bottom of 2 pieces 6-ounch ramekin. Sprinkle about 1 tablespoon of basil per ramekin. Place 1 goat half over each ramekin; surround with cherry tomato halves. Sprinkle with the black pepper and the cayenne. Spread the remaining basil on top of each. Place the ramekins on a baking sheet. Drizzle each serve with the remaining olive oil; bake for about 15 minutes or until bubbling. Serve warm.
Nutrition Info: Per Serving:178 cal., 15.5 g total fat (6.8 sat. fat), 22 mg chol., 152 mg sodium, 4.1 g total carbs., 0.9 g fiber, 0.7 g sugar, and 6.8 g protein.

491. Grilled Shrimp Kabobs

Servings: 4   Cooking Time: 4 Minutes
Ingredients:

1 1/2 cups whole-wheat dry breadcrumbs	1/4 cup olive oil
	2 tablespoons vegetable oil
1 clove garlic, finely minced or pressed	2 teaspoons dried parsley flakes
1 teaspoon dried basil leaves	Salt and pepper
2 pounds shrimp, peeled, deveined, leaving the tails on	16 skewers, soaked for at least 20 minutes in water or until ready to use if using wooden

Directions:
Rinse the shrimps and dry. Put the vegetable and the olive oil in a re-sealable plastic bag; add the shrimp and toss to coat with the oil mixture. Add the breadcrumbs, parsley, garlic, basil, salt, and pepper; toss to coat with the dry mix. Seal the bag, refrigerate for 1 hour. Thread the shrimps on the skewers. Grill on preheated grill for about 2 minutes each side or until golden, making sure not to overcook.
Nutrition Info: Per Serving: 502.7 cal., 24.8 g total fat (3.5 sat. fat), 285.8 mg chol., 1581.8 mg sodium, 31.7 g total carbs., 2 g fiber, 2.5 g sugar, and 36.4 g protein.

492. Red Pepper Tapenade

Servings: 4   Cooking Time: 0 Minutes
Ingredients:

7 ounces roasted red peppers, chopped	14 ounces canned artichokes, drained and chopped
1/2 cup parmesan, grated	1/4 cup capers, drained
1/3 cup parsley, chopped	
3 tablespoons olive oil	1 and 1/2 tablespoons lemon juice
	2 garlic cloves, minced

Directions:
In your blender, combine the red peppers with the parmesan and the rest of the ingredients and pulse well. Divide into cups and serve as a snack.

Nutrition Info:calories 200, fat 5.6, fiber 4.5, carbs 12.4, protein 4.6

493. Collard Green Chicken Roll Ups

Servings: 4   Cooking Time: 20 Minutes

Ingredients:

4 large collard greens
1/2 teaspoon hot sauce
1 tablespoon fresh cilantro, de-stemmed and chopped
1 small seedless cucumber cut into long match sticks

1/2 cup black olives, diced
1 pound of Foster Farms Simply Raised chicken
1 large avocado
Juice of 1/2 lime
Salt and pepper, to taste

Directions:

Place a large-sized grill pan over medium heat. Season both sides of the chicken with the salt and pepper. Place on the grill, cook until the meat is no longer pink and opaque all the way through. Remove from the heat.   Meanwhile, fill the bottom of a large skillet with few inches of water; bring to a boil over high heat. Ready a large-sized bowl filled with iced cubes and cold water near the stove.   Slice off the stems and the tough backbones from the collard greens using a paring knife.   Add one leaf at a time into the boiling water, blanching for about 30 to 45 seconds until they are pliable but not soft to fall apart when rolled. Remove from the boiling water and immediately add to the iced water, letting the water cool. Once cool, place the leaf on a paper towel or dish towel; dry well. Repeat the process with the remaining leaves.   Place the avocado in a bowl, add the cilantro, lime, hot sauce, and season with salt and pepper to taste; mash together to combine. Place a leaf on a clean, flat surface. Spread a dollop of the avocado mixture at the larger part of the collard greens. Top the avocado mixture with the chicken, cucumber, and olives.   Fold the top end of the collard over the filling; roll the leaf, tucking in the sides as you roll the bottom. Cut the rolls into halves; serve.

Nutrition Info: Per Serving:250 cal., 13 g total fat (2.5 g sat. fat), 75 mg chol., 450 mg sodium, 670 mg pot., 12 g total carbs., 6 g fiber, 2 g sugar, 25 g protein, 4% vitamin A, 20% vitamin C, 6% calcium, and15% iron.

494. Cauliflower Spread

Servings: 4   Cooking Time: 15 Minutes

Ingredients:

1 teaspoon tahini paste
3 tablespoons lemon juice
1/2 teaspoon minced garlic
1 teaspoon dried oregano

1 cup cauliflower
1/4 teaspoon cayenne pepper
1/2 teaspoon salt
1/4 teaspoon dried thyme
1 cup of water

Directions:

Pour water in the pan and add cauliflower.   Boil cauliflower for 15 minutes.   Then drain 1/2 part of liquid from cauliflower.   Transfer remaining liquid and cauliflower in the food processor.   Add tahini paste, lemon juice, minced garlic, dried oregano, cayenne pepper, salt, and dried thyme.

Blend the mixture until you get a smooth and fluffy mixture.   Store the cooked hummus in the fridge up to 3 days.

Nutrition Info: Per Serving:calories 19, fat 0.9, fiber 1, carbs 2.3, protein 0.9

495. Coriander Falafel

Servings: 8   Cooking Time: 10 Minutes

Ingredients:

1 bunch parsley leaves
1 yellow onion, chopped
5 garlic cloves, minced
1 teaspoon coriander, ground
A pinch of salt and black pepper
1/4 teaspoon cayenne pepper

1 cup canned garbanzo beans, drained and rinsed
1/4 teaspoon baking soda
1/4 teaspoon cumin powder
1 teaspoon lemon juice
3 tablespoons tapioca flour
Olive oil for frying

Directions:

In your food processor, combine the beans with the parsley, onion and the rest the ingredients except the oil and the flour and pulse well.   Transfer the mix to a bowl, add the flour, stir well, shape 16 balls out of this mix and flatten them a bit.   Heat up a pan with some oil over medium-high heat, add the falafels, cook them for 5 minutes on each side, transfer to paper towels, drain excess grease, arrange them on a platter and serve as an appetizer.

Nutrition Info:calories 112, fat 6.2, fiber 2, carbs 12.3, protein 3.1

496. Slow Cooked Cheesy Artichoke Dip

Servings: 6   Cooking Time: 60 Minutes

Ingredients:

10 oz can artichoke hearts, drained and chopped
4 cups spinach, chopped
8 oz cream cheese
3 tbsp sour cream
3/4 cup mozzarella cheese, shredded

1/4 cup mayonnaise
1/4 cup parmesan cheese, grated
3 garlic cloves, minced
1/2 tsp dried parsley
Pepper
Salt

Directions:

Add all ingredients into the inner pot of instant pot and stir well.   Seal the pot with the lid and select slow cook mode and set the timer for 60 minutes. Stir once while cooking.   Serve and enjoy.

Nutrition Info: Calories 226 Fat 19.3 g Carbohydrates 7.5 g Sugar 1.2 g Protein 6.8 g Cholesterol 51 mg

497. Marinated Chickpeas

Servings: 4   Cooking Time: 10 Minutes

Ingredients:

1 can (15 ounce) chickpeas (or garbanzo beans), drained, rinsed
1 tablespoon fresh oregano, chopped
1 tablespoon lemon juice

1 tablespoon lemon zest
1 teaspoon fresh parsley, chopped
1/4 teaspoon minced garlic
3 tablespoons olive oil

Sea salt, to taste
Directions:
Place the chickpeas in a bowl. Add the rest of the ingredients; toss to mix well. Marinate the chickpeas for 8 hours or overnight in the refrigerator.
Nutrition Info: Per Serving:176 cal., 11 g total fat (1.5 sat. fat), 0 mg chol., 290 mg sodium, 16.6 g total carbs., 3.3 g fiber, 0.2 g sugar, and 3.6 g protein.

498.   Easy Tomato Dip

Servings: 4   Cooking Time: 13 Minutes
Ingredients:

2 cups tomato puree	1 onion, chopped
1/2 tsp ground cumin	1 tbsp olive oil
1 tsp garlic, minced	Pepper
1/4 cup vinegar	Salt

Directions:
Add oil into the inner pot of instant pot and set the pot on sauté mode.   Add onion and sauté for 3 minutes.   Add remaining ingredients and stir well.   Seal pot with lid and cook on high for 10 minutes.   Once done, allow to release pressure naturally for 10 minutes then release remaining using quick release. Remove lid.   Blend tomato mixture using an immersion blender until smooth. Serve and enjoy.
Nutrition Info: Calories 94 Fat 3.9 g Carbohydrates 14.3 g Sugar 7.3 g Protein 2.5 g Cholesterol 0 mg

499.   Zucchini Pizza Rolls

Servings: 8   Cooking Time: 15 Minutes
Ingredients:

4 large zucchini, sliced lengthwise into 1/4-inch thick slices	1 tablespoon olive oil
1/2 cup sun-dried tomatoes, chopped	1 cup pizza sauce
1/2 cup black olives, chopped	Freshly ground black pepper
	Red pepper flakes (optional)
	Sea salt

Directions:
Preheat a grill or a broiler.   Brush each slice of zucchini lightly with the olive oil and season with salt and pepper; grill or broil for about 2 minutes each side, or until softened. Let cool slightly.   On 1/2 side of the zucchini slices, spread a thin layer of pizza sauce. Sprinkle the olives, sun-dried tomato, and if using, red pepper flakes over the sauce. Starting on the end with the pizza sauce, roll each slice. If necessary, secure with toothpicks.
Nutrition Info: Per Serving:20 cal., 1 g total fat (0 g sat. fat), 0 mg chol., 85 mg sodium, 140 mg pot., 2 g total carbs., <1 g fiber, 1 g sugar, <1 g protein, 10% vitamin A, 10% vitamin C, 2% calcium, and 2% iron.

500.   Creamy Spinach And Shallots Dip

Servings: 4   Cooking Time: 0 Minutes
Ingredients:

1 pound spinach, roughly chopped	¾ cup cream cheese, soft
2 shallots, chopped	Salt and black pepper to the taste
2 tablespoons mint, chopped	

Directions:
In a blender, combine the spinach with the shallots and the rest of the ingredients, and pulse well. Divide into small bowls and serve as a party dip.
Nutrition Info:calories 204, fat 11.5, fiber 3.1, carbs 4.2, protein 5.9

Fish And Seafood Recipes

501. Breaded And Spiced Halibut

Servings: 4   Cooking Time: 15 Minutes

Ingredients:

¼ cup chopped fresh chives

¼ cup chopped fresh dill

¼ tsp ground black pepper

¾ cup panko breadcrumbs

1 tsp sea salt

1 tbsp extra-virgin olive oil

1 tsp finely grated lemon zest

1/3 cup chopped fresh parsley

4 pieces of 6-oz halibut fillets

Directions:

Line a baking sheet with foil, grease with cooking spray and preheat oven to 4000F.   In a small bowl, mix black pepper, sea salt, lemon zest, olive oil, chives, dill, parsley and breadcrumbs. If needed add more salt to taste. Set aside.   Meanwhile, wash halibut fillets on cold tap water. Dry with paper towels and place on prepared baking sheet. Generously spoon crumb mixture onto halibut fillets. Ensure that fillets are covered with crumb mixture. Press down on crumb mixture onto each fillet.   Pop into the oven and bake for 10-15 minutes or until fish is flaky and crumb topping are already lightly browned.

Nutrition Info: Calories per serving: 336.4; Protein: 25.3g; Fat: 25.3g; Carbs: 4.1g

502. Cilantro Shrimp

Servings: 4   Cooking Time: 10 Minutes

Ingredients:

3 garlic cloves, diced

¼ cup fresh cilantro, chopped

1-pound shrimps

2 tablespoons butter

¼ cup milk

½ teaspoon salt

Directions:

Put butter in the skillet and bring it to boil.   Then add diced garlic and roast it for 3 minutes.   Add milk and salt. Bring the liquid to boil (it will take about 2 minutes).   After this, add shrimps and mix up well.   Cook the shrimps for 3 minutes over the medium heat.   Then add fresh cilantro. Close the lid and cook seafood for 5 minutes. Serve the cooked garlic shrimps with cilantro-garlic sauce.

Nutrition Info: Per Serving:calories 197, fat 8, fiber 0.1, carbs 3.3, protein 26.6

503. Garlicky Clams

Servings: 4   Cooking Time: 5 Minutes

Ingredients:

3 lbs clams, clean

4 garlic cloves

1/2 cup fresh lemon juice

1/4 cup olive oil

1 cup white wine

Pepper

Salt

Directions:

Add oil into the inner pot of instant pot and set the pot on sauté mode.   Add garlic and sauté for 1 minute.   Add wine and cook for 2 minutes. Add remaining ingredients and stir well.   Seal pot with lid and cook on high for 2 minutes. Once done, allow to release pressure naturally. Remove lid.   Serve and enjoy.

Nutrition Info: Calories 332 Fat 13.5 g Carbohydrates 40.5 g Sugar 12.4 g Protein 2.5 g Cholesterol 0 mg

504. Lemon Swordfish

Servings: 2   Cooking Time: 6 Minutes

Ingredients:

12 oz swordfish steaks (6 oz every fish steak)

1 teaspoon ground cumin

1 tablespoon lemon juice

¼ teaspoon salt

1 teaspoon olive oil

Directions:

Sprinkle the fish steaks with ground cumin and salt from each side.   Then drizzle the lemon juice over the steaks and massage them gently with the help of the fingertips.   Preheat the grill to 395F. Bruhs every fish steak with olive oil and place in the grill.   Cook the swordfish for 3 minutes from each side.

Nutrition Info: Per Serving:calories 289, fat 1.4, fiber 0.1, carbs 0.6, protein 43.4

505. Paprika Salmon And Green Beans

Servings: 3   Cooking Time: 20 Minutes

Ingredients:

¼ cup olive oil

½ tablespoon onion powder

½ teaspoon bouillon powder

½ teaspoon cayenne pepper

1 tablespoon smoked paprika

1-pound green beans

2 teaspoon minced garlic

3 tablespoon fresh herbs

6 ounces of salmon steak

Salt and pepper to taste

Directions:

Preheat the oven to 400F.   Grease a baking sheet and set aside.   Heat a skillet over medium low heat and add the olive oil. Sauté the garlic, smoked paprika, fresh herbs, cayenne pepper and onion powder. Stir for a minute then let the mixture sit for 5 minutes. Set aside.   Put the salmon steaks in a bowl and add salt and the paprika spice mixture. Rub to coat the salmon well.   Place the salmon on the baking sheet and cook for 18 minutes.   Meanwhile, blanch the green beans in boiling water with salt.   Serve the beans with the salmon.

Nutrition Info: Calories per Serving: 945.8; Fat: 66.6 g; Protein: 43.5 g; Carbs: 43.1 g

506. Cucumber-basil Salsa On Halibut Pouches

Servings: 4   Cooking Time: 17 Minutes

Ingredients:

1 lime, thinly sliced into 8 pieces

2 cups mustard greens, stems removed

4 – 5 radishes trimmed and quartered

4 4-oz skinless halibut filets

2 tsp olive oil

Pepper and salt to taste

1 ½ cups diced cucumber

1 ½ finely chopped fresh basil leaves

2 tsp fresh lime juice

4 large fresh basil leaves

Pepper and salt to taste

Cayenne pepper to taste – optional

Directions:
Preheat oven to 4000F.   Prepare parchment papers by making 4 pieces of 15 x 12-inch rectangles. Lengthwise, fold in half and unfold pieces on the table.   Season halibut fillets with pepper, salt and cayenne—if using cayenne.   Just to the right of the fold going lengthwise, place ½ cup of mustard greens. Add a basil leaf on center of mustard greens and topped with 1 lime slice. Around the greens, layer ¼ of the radishes. Drizzle with ½ tsp of oil, season with pepper and salt. Top it with a slice of halibut fillet.   Just as you would make a calzone, fold parchment paper over your filling and crimp the edges of the parchment paper beginning from one end to the other end. To seal the end of the crimped parchment paper, pinch it. Repeat process to remaining ingredients until you have 4 pieces of parchment papers filled with halibut and greens.   Place pouches in a baking pan and bake in the oven until halibut is flaky, around 15 to 17 minutes.   While waiting for halibut pouches to cook, make your salsa by mixing all salsa ingredients in a medium bowl.   Once halibut is cooked, remove from oven and make a tear on top. Be careful of the steam as it is very hot. Equally divide salsa and spoon ¼ of salsa on top of halibut through the slit you have created.   Serve and enjoy.
Nutrition Info: Calories per serving: 335.4; Protein: 20.2g; Fat: 16.3g; Carbs: 22.1g

507.   Sardine Meatballs

Servings: 4   Cooking Time: 10 Minutes
Ingredients:

11 oz sardines, canned, drained	2 tablespoon wheat flour, whole grain
1/3 cup shallot, chopped	1 egg, beaten
1 teaspoon chili flakes	1 tablespoon chives, chopped
½ teaspoon salt	1 teaspoon olive oil
	1 teaspoon butter

Directions:
Put the butter in the skillet and melt it.   Add shallot and cook it until translucent.   After this, transfer the shallot in the mixing bowl.   Add sardines, chili flakes, salt, flour, egg, chives, and mix up until smooth with the help of the fork. Make the medium size cakes and place them in the skillet.   Add olive oil.   Roast the fish cakes for 3 minutes from each side over the medium heat. Dry the cooked fish cakes with the paper towel if needed and transfer in the serving plates.
Nutrition Info: Per Serving:calories 221, fat 12.2, fiber 0.1, carbs 5.4, protein 21.3

508.   Basil Tilapia

Servings: 3   Cooking Time: 20 Minutes
Ingredients:

12 oz tilapia fillet	1 cup fresh basil
2 oz Parmesan, grated	1 tablespoon pine nuts
1 tablespoon olive oil	1 garlic clove, peeled
½ teaspoon ground black pepper	¾ teaspoon white pepper
3 tablespoons	

avocado oil

Directions:
Make pesto sauce: blend the avocado oil, fresh basil, pine nuts, garlic clove, and white pepper until smooth.   After this, cut the tilapia fillet on 3 servings.   Sprinkle every fish serving with olive oil and ground black pepper.   Roast the fillets over the medium heat for 2 minutes from each side. Meanwhile, line the baking tray with baking paper. Arrange the roasted tilapia fillets in the tray. Then top them with pesto and Parmesan.   Bake the fish for 15 minutes at 365F.
Nutrition Info: Per Serving:calories 321, fat 17, fiber 1.2, carbs 4.4, protein 37.4

509.   Honey Halibut

Servings: 5   Cooking Time: 15 Minutes
Ingredients:

1-pound halibut	½ teaspoon lime juice
1 teaspoon lime zest	
½ teaspoon honey	
1 teaspoon olive oil	¼ teaspoon salt
	¼ teaspoon chili flakes

Directions:
Cut the fish on the sticks and sprinkle with salt and chili flakes.   Whisk together lime zest, honey, olive oil, and lime juice.   Brush the halibut sticks with the honey mixture from each side.   Line the baking tray with baking paper and place the fish inside.   Bake the halibut for 15 minutes at 375F. Flip the fish on another side after 7 minutes of cooking.
Nutrition Info: Per Serving:calories 254, fat 19, fiber 0, carbs 0.7, protein 18.8

510.   Stuffed Mackerel

Servings: 5   Cooking Time: 30 Minutes
Ingredients:

4 teaspoons capers, drained	½ teaspoon salt
1-pound whole mackerel, peeled, trimmed	1 tablespoon lime juice
1 teaspoon garlic powder	¼ teaspoon chili flakes
½ teaspoon ground coriander	½ white onion, sliced
	4 teaspoons butter
	3 tablespoons water

Directions:
Rub the fish with salt, garlic powder, and chili flakes.   Then sprinkle it with lime juice.   Line the baking tray with parchment and arrange the fish inside.   Fill the mackerel with capers and butter.   Then sprinkle fish with water.   Cover the fish with foil and secure the edges.   Bake the mackerel for 30 minutes at 365F.
Nutrition Info: Per Serving:calories 262, fat 17.5, fiber 0.4, carbs 1.8, protein 25.5

511. Healthy Carrot & Shrimp

Servings: 4   Cooking Time: 6 Minutes
Ingredients:

1 lb shrimp, peeled and deveined	1 tbsp olive oil
1 tbsp chives, chopped	1 cup fish stock
1 onion, chopped	1 cup carrots, sliced
	Pepper
	Salt

Directions:
Add oil into the inner pot of instant pot and set the pot on sauté mode. Add onion and sauté for 2 minutes. Add shrimp and stir well. Add remaining ingredients and stir well. Seal pot with lid and cook on high for 4 minutes. Once done, release pressure using quick release. Remove lid. Serve and enjoy.
Nutrition Info: Calories 197 Fat 5.9 g Carbohydrates 7 g Sugar 2.5 g Protein 27.7 g Cholesterol 239 mg

512. Tomato Cod Mix

Servings: 2   Cooking Time: 5.5 Hours
Ingredients:

1 teaspoon tomato paste	1 white onion, sliced
1 teaspoon garlic, diced	1/3 cup chicken stock
1 jalapeno pepper, chopped	7 oz Spanish cod fillet
	1 teaspoon paprika
	1 teaspoon salt

Directions:
Pour chicken stock in the saucepan. Add tomato paste and mix up the liquid until homogenous. Add garlic, onion, jalapeno pepper, paprika, and salt. Bring the liquid to boil and then simmer it. Chop the cod fillet and add it in the tomato liquid. Close the lid and simmer the fish for 10 minutes over the low heat. Serve the fish in the bowls with tomato sauce.
Nutrition Info: Per Serving:calories 113, fat 1.2, fiber 1.9, carbs 7.2, protein 18.9

513. Garlic Mussels

Servings: 4   Cooking Time: 10 Minutes
Ingredients:

1-pound mussels	1 teaspoon ground coriander
1 chili pepper, chopped	½ teaspoon salt
1 cup chicken stock	1 cup fresh parsley, chopped
½ cup milk	4 tablespoons lemon juice
1 teaspoon olive oil	
1 teaspoon minced garlic	

Directions:
Pour milk in the saucepan. Add chili pepper, chicken stock, olive oil, minced garlic, ground coriander, salt, and lemon juice. Bring the liquid to boil and add mussels. Boil the mussel for 4 minutes or until they will open shells. Then add chopped parsley and mix up the meal well. Remove it from the heat.
Nutrition Info: Per Serving:calories 136, fat 4.7, fiber 0.6, carbs 7.5, protein 15.3

514. Mahi Mahi And Pomegranate Sauce

Servings: 4   Cooking Time: 10 Minutes
Ingredients:

1 and ½ cups chicken stock	4 tablespoons tahini paste
1 tablespoon olive oil	Seeds from 1 pomegranate
4 mahi mahi fillets, boneless	1 tablespoon parsley, chopped
Juice of 1 lime	

Directions:
Heat up a pan with the oil over medium-high heat, add the fish and cook for 3 minutes on each side. Add the rest of the ingredients, flip the fish again,

cook for 4 minutes more, divide everything between plates and serve.
Nutrition Info:calories 224, fat 11.1, fiber 5.5, carbs 16.7, protein 11.4

515. Honey Balsamic Salmon

Servings: 2   Cooking Time: 3 Minutes
Ingredients:

2 salmon fillets	2 tbsp honey
1/4 tsp red pepper flakes	1 cup of water
2 tbsp balsamic vinegar	Pepper
	Salt

Directions:
Pour water into the instant pot and place trivet in the pot. In a small bowl, mix together honey, red pepper flakes, and vinegar. Brush fish fillets with honey mixture and place on top of the trivet. Seal pot with lid and cook on high for 3 minutes. Once done, release pressure using quick release. Remove lid. Serve and enjoy.
Nutrition Info: Calories 303 Fat 11 g Carbohydrates 17.6 g Sugar 17.3 g Protein 34.6 g Cholesterol 78 mg

516. Sage Salmon Fillet

Servings: 1   Cooking Time: 25 Minutes
Ingredients:

4 oz salmon fillet	1 teaspoon sesame oil
½ teaspoon salt	½ teaspoon sage

Directions:
Rub the fillet with salt and sage. Place the fish in the tray and sprinkle it with sesame oil. Cook the fish for 25 minutes at 365F. Flip the fish carefully onto another side after 12 minutes of cooking.
Nutrition Info: Per Serving:calories 191, fat 11.6, fiber 0.1, carbs 0.2, protein 22

517. Seafood Stew Cioppino

Servings: 6   Cooking Time: 40 Minutes
Ingredients:

¼ cup Italian parsley, chopped	½ onion, chopped
¼ tsp dried basil	1 lb. mahi mahi, cut into ½-inch cubes
¼ tsp dried thyme	
½ cup dry white wine like pinot grigio	1 lb. raw shrimp
½ lb. King crab legs, cut at each joint	1 tbsp olive oil
	2 bay leaves
½ tsp red pepper flakes (adjust to desired spiciness)	2 cups clam juice
	50 live clams, washed
	6 cloves garlic, minced
1 28-oz can crushed tomatoes	Pepper and salt to taste

Directions:
On medium fire, place a stockpot and heat oil. Add onion and for 4 minutes sauté until soft. Add bay leaves, thyme, basil, red pepper flakes and garlic. Cook for a minute while stirring a bit. Add clam juice and tomatoes. Once simmering, place fire to medium low and cook for 20 minutes uncovered. Add white wine and clams. Cover and cook for 5 minutes or until clams have slightly opened. Stir pot then add fish pieces, crab legs and shrimps. Do not stir soup to maintain the fish's shape. Cook while covered for 4 minutes or until clams are fully opened; fish and shrimps are

opaque and cooked.   Season with pepper and salt to taste.   Transfer Cioppino to serving bowls and garnish with parsley before serving.
Nutrition Info: Calories per Serving: 371; Carbs: 15.5 g; Protein: 62 g; Fat: 6.8 g

518.   Shrimp And Lemon Sauce

Servings: 4   Cooking Time: 15 Minutes
Ingredients:

1 pound shrimp, peeled and deveined	Salt and black pepper to the taste
1/3 cup lemon juice	1 cup black olives, pitted and halved
4 egg yolks	
2 tablespoons olive oil	1 tablespoon thyme, chopped
1 cup chicken stock	

Directions:
In a bowl, mix the lemon juice with the egg yolks and whisk well.   Heat up a pan with the oil over medium heat, add the shrimp and cook for 2 minutes on each side and transfer to a plate. Heat up a pan with the stock over medium heat, add some of this over the egg yolks and lemon juice mix and whisk well.   Add this over the rest of the stock, also add salt and pepper, whisk well and simmer for 2 minutes.   Add the shrimp and the rest of the ingredients, toss and serve right away.
Nutrition Info:calories 237, fat 15.3, fiber 4.6, carbs 15.4, protein 7.6

519.   Feta Tomato Sea Bass

Servings: 4   Cooking Time: 8 Minutes
Ingredients:

4 sea bass fillets	1/2 cup feta cheese, crumbled
1 1/2 cups water	
1 tbsp olive oil	1 cup can tomatoes, diced
1 tsp garlic, minced	
1 tsp basil, chopped	Pepper
1 tsp parsley, chopped	Salt

Directions:
Season fish fillets with pepper and salt.   Pour 2 cups of water into the instant pot then place steamer rack in the pot.   Place fish fillets on steamer rack in the pot.   Seal pot with lid and cook on high for 5 minutes.   Once done, release pressure using quick release.   Remove lid. Remove fish fillets from the pot and clean the pot. Add oil into the inner pot of instant pot and set the pot on sauté mode.   Add garlic and sauté for 1 minute.   Add tomatoes, parsley, and basil and stir well and cook for 1 minute.   Add fish fillets and top with crumbled cheese and cook for a minute.   Serve and enjoy.
Nutrition Info: Calories 219 Fat 10.1 g Carbohydrates 4 g Sugar 2.8 g Protein 27.1 g Cholesterol 70 mg

520.   Salmon And Broccoli

Servings: 4   Cooking Time: 20 Minutes
Ingredients:

2 tablespoons balsamic vinegar	1 big red onion, roughly chopped
1 broccoli head, florets separated	1 tablespoon olive oil
4 pieces salmon fillets, skinless	Sea salt and black pepper to the taste

Directions:

In a baking dish, combine the salmon with the broccoli and the rest of the ingredients, introduce in the oven and bake at 390 degrees F for 20 minutes.   Divide the mix between plates and serve.
Nutrition Info:calories 302, fat 15.5, fiber 8.5, carbs 18.9, protein 19.8

521.   Halibut And Quinoa Mix

Servings: 4   Cooking Time: 12 Minutes
Ingredients:

4 halibut fillets, boneless	2 teaspoons oregano, dried
2 tablespoons olive oil	A pinch of salt and black pepper
1 teaspoon rosemary, dried	1 cup cherry tomatoes, halved
2 teaspoons cumin, ground	1 avocado, peeled, pitted and sliced
1 tablespoons coriander, ground	1 cucumber, cubed
2 teaspoons cinnamon powder	½ cup black olives, pitted and sliced
2 cups quinoa, cooked	Juice of 1 lemon

Directions:
In a bowl, combine the fish with the rosemary, cumin, coriander, cinnamon, oregano, salt and pepper and toss.   Heat up a pan with the oil over medium heat, add the fish, and sear for 2 minutes on each side.   Introduce the pan in the oven and bake the fish at 425 degrees F for 7 minutes. Meanwhile, in a bowl, mix the quinoa with the remaining ingredients, toss and divide between plates.   Add the fish next to the quinoa mix and serve right away.
Nutrition Info:calories 364, fat 15.4, fiber 11.2, carbs 56.4, protein 24.5

522.   Crab Stew

Servings: 2   Cooking Time: 13 Minutes
Ingredients:

1/2 lb lump crab meat	2 cups fish stock
2 tbsp heavy cream	1/2 tsp garlic, chopped
1 tbsp olive oil	
1/2 lb shrimp, shelled and chopped	1/4 onion, chopped
	Pepper
1 celery stalk, chopped	Salt

Directions:
Add oil into the inner pot of instant pot and set the pot on sauté mode.   Add onion and sauté for 3 minutes.   Add garlic and sauté for 30 seconds. Add remaining ingredients except for heavy cream and stir well.   Seal pot with lid and cook on high for 10 minutes.   Once done, release pressure using quick release. Remove lid.   Stir in heavy cream and serve.
Nutrition Info: Calories 376 Fat 25.5 g Carbohydrates 5.8 g Sugar 0.7 g Protein 48.1 g Cholesterol 326 mg

523.   Crazy Saganaki Shrimp

Servings: 4   Cooking Time: 10 Minutes
Ingredients:

¼ tsp salt	½ cup Chardonnay
½ cup crumbled Greek feta cheese	12 jumbo shrimps,

1 medium bulb. fennel, cored and finely chopped
1 small Chile pepper, seeded and minced
1 tbsp extra virgin olive oil

peeled and deveined with tails left on
2 tbsp lemon juice, divided
5 scallions sliced thinly
Pepper to taste

Directions:
In medium bowl, mix salt, lemon juice and shrimp. On medium fire, place a saganaki pan (or large nonstick saucepan) and heat oil. Sauté Chile pepper, scallions, and fennel for 4 minutes or until starting to brown and is already soft. Add wine and sauté for another minute. Place shrimps on top of fennel, cover and cook for 4 minutes or until shrimps are pink. Remove just the shrimp and transfer to a plate. Add pepper, feta and 1 tbsp lemon juice to pan and cook for a minute or until cheese begins to melt. To serve, place cheese and fennel mixture on a serving plate and top with shrimps.

Nutrition Info: Calories per serving: 310; Protein: 49.7g; Fat: 6.8g; Carbs: 8.4g

524. Grilled Tuna

Servings: 3   Cooking Time: 6 Minutes
Ingredients:
3 tuna fillets
3 teaspoons teriyaki sauce

½ teaspoon minced garlic
1 teaspoon olive oil

Directions:
Whisk together teriyaki sauce, minced garlic, and olive oil. Bruhs every tuna fillet with teriyaki mixture. Preheat grill to 390F. Grill the fish for 3 minutes from each side.

Nutrition Info: Per Serving:calories 382, fat 32.6, fiber 0, carbs 1.1, protein 21.4

525. Rosemary Salmon

Servings: 5   Cooking Time: 10 Minutes
Ingredients:
2-pound salmon fillet
2 tablespoons avocado oil
2 teaspoons fresh rosemary, chopped
½ teaspoon minced garlic

½ teaspoon dried cilantro
½ teaspoon salt
1 teaspoon butter
½ teaspoon white pepper

Directions:
Whisk together avocado oil, fresh rosemary, minced garlic, dried cilantro, salt, and white pepper. Rub the salmon fillet with the rosemary mixture generously and leave fish in the fridge for 20 minutes to marinate. After this, put butter in the saucepan or big skillet and melt it. Then put heat on maximum and place a salmon fillet in the hot butter. Roast it for 1 minute from each side. After this, preheat grill to 385F and grill the fillet for 8 minutes (for 4 minutes from each side). Cut the cooked salmon on the servings.

Nutrition Info: Per Serving:calories 257, fat 12.8, fiber 0.5, carbs 0.9, protein 35.3

526. Easy Seafood French Stew

Servings: 12   Cooking Time: 45 Minutes
Ingredients:
Pepper and Salt
1/2 lb. littleneck

3 cups tomatoes, peeled, seeded, and

clams
1/2 lb. mussels
1 lb. shrimp, peeled and deveined
1 large lobster
2 lbs. assorted small whole fresh fish, scaled and cleaned
2 tbsp parsley, finely chopped
2 tbsp garlic, chopped
1 cup fennel, julienned
Juice and zest of one orange

chopped
1 cup leeks, julienned
Pinch of Saffron
1 cup white wine
Water
1 lb. fish bones
2 sprigs thyme
8 peppercorns
1 bay leaf
3 cloves garlic
Salt and pepper
1/2 cup chopped celery
1/2 cup chopped onion
2 tbsp olive oil

Directions:
Do the stew: Heat oil in a large saucepan. Sauté the celery and onions for 3 minutes. Season with pepper and salt. Stir in the garlic and cook for about a minute. Add the thyme, peppercorns, and bay leaves. Stir in the wine, water and fish bones. Let it boil then before reducing to a simmer. Take the pan off the fire and strain broth into another container. For the Bouillabaisse: Bring the strained broth to a simmer and stir in the parsley, leeks, orange juice, orange zest, garlic, fennel, tomatoes and saffron. Sprinkle with pepper and salt. Stir in the lobsters and fish. Let it simmer for eight minutes before stirring in the clams, mussels and shrimps. For six minutes, allow to cook while covered before seasoning again with pepper and salt. Assemble in a shallow dish all the seafood and pour the broth over it.

Nutrition Info: Calories per serving: 348; Carbs: 20.0g; Protein: 31.8g; Fat: 15.2g

527. Lime Squid And Capers Mix

Servings: 6   Cooking Time: 20 Minutes
Ingredients:
1 pound baby squid, cleaned, body and tentacles chopped
½ teaspoon lime zest, grated
1 tablespoon lime juice
½ teaspoon orange zest, grated
3 tablespoons olive oil
1 teaspoon red pepper flakes, crushed

1 tablespoon parsley, chopped
4 garlic cloves, minced
1 shallot, chopped
2 tablespoons capers, drained
1 cup chicken stock
2 tablespoons red wine vinegar
Salt and black pepper to the taste

Directions:
Heat up a pan with the oil over medium-high heat, add the lime zest, lime juice, orange zest and the rest of the ingredients except the squid and the parsley, stir, bring to a simmer and cook over medium heat for 10 minutes. Add the remaining ingredients, stir, cook everything for 10 minutes more, divide into bowls and serve.

Nutrition Info:calories 302, fat 8.5, fiber 9.8, carbs 21.8, protein 11.3

528. Salmon And Pineapple Sauce

Servings: 4   Cooking Time: 15 Minutes
Ingredients:

1 cup pineapple, chopped
14 oz salmon fillet
¾ teaspoon ground turmeric
¼ teaspoon cayenne pepper

½ teaspoon salt
1 teaspoon butter
1 teaspoon olive oil
1 tablespoon water
¼ teaspoon ground thyme
¼ cup of water

Directions:
Rub the salmon fillet with salt and ground turmeric. Brush the fish with oil and grill in the grill for 3 minutes from each side at 385F. Meanwhile, make the pineapple dip: blend the pineapple until smooth and transfer in the skillet. Add water, butter, ground thyme, and cayenne pepper. Brin the pineapple dip to boil and cook it without lid for 5 minutes over the high heat. Cut the salmon fillet on 4 servings and arrange them in the serving plates. Then top every salmon piece with pineapple dip.
Nutrition Info: Per Serving: calories 172, fat 8.4, fiber 0.7, carbs 5.8, protein 19.5

529. Wrapped Scallops

Servings: 12   Cooking Time: 6 Minutes
Ingredients:
12 medium scallops
12 thin bacon slices
2 teaspoons lemon juice
A pinch of chili powder

2 teaspoons olive oil
A pinch of cloves, ground
Salt and black pepper to the taste

Directions:
Wrap each scallop in a bacon slice and secure with toothpicks. Heat up a pan with the oil over medium-high heat, add the scallops and the rest of the ingredients, cook for 3 minutes on each side, divide between plates and serve.
Nutrition Info: calories 297, fat 24.3, fiber 9.6, carbs 22.4, protein 17.6

530. Walnut Salmon Mix

Servings: 4   Cooking Time: 25 Minutes
Ingredients:
12 oz salmon fillet
1/3 cup walnuts
1 tablespoon panko breadcrumbs
1 tablespoon dried oregano

1 tablespoon sunflower oil
½ teaspoon salt
½ teaspoon ground black pepper
1 tablespoon mustard

Directions:
Put the walnuts, panko bread crumbs, dried oregano, sunflower oil, salt, and ground black pepper in the blender. Blend the ingredients until you get smooth and sticky mass. After this, line the baking tray with baking paper. Brush the salmon fillet with mustard from all sides and coat in the blended walnut mixture generously. Bake the salmon for 25 minutes at 365F. Flip the salmon fillet on another side after 15 minutes of cooking.
Nutrition Info: Per Serving: calories 233, fat 15.9, fiber 1.9, carbs 4.7, protein 20.1

531. Pan Fried Tuna With Herbs And Nut

Servings: 4   Cooking Time: 5 Minutes

Ingredients:
¼ cup almonds, chopped finely
¼ cup fresh tangerine juice
½ tsp fennel seeds, chopped finely
½ tsp ground pepper, divided
1 tbsp olive oil

½ tsp sea salt, divided
2 tbsp. fresh mint, chopped finely
2 tbsp. red onion, chopped finely
4 pieces of 6-oz Tuna steak cut in half

Directions:
Mix fennel seeds, olive oil, mint, onion, tangerine juice and almonds in small bowl. Season with ¼ each of pepper and salt. Season fish with the remaining pepper and salt. On medium high fire, place a large nonstick fry pan and grease with cooking spray. Pan fry tuna until desired doneness is reached or for one minute per side. Transfer cooked tuna in serving plate, drizzle with dressing and serve.
Nutrition Info: Calories per Serving: 272; Fat: 9.7 g; Protein: 42 g; Carbohydrates: 4.2 g

532. Tarragon Cod Fillets

Servings: 4   Cooking Time: 12 Minutes
Ingredients:
4 cod fillets, boneless
1 tablespoon tarragon, chopped
Sea salt and black pepper to the taste
2 tablespoons olive oil

¼ cup capers, drained
2 tablespoons parsley, chopped
1 tablespoon olive oil
1 tablespoon lemon juice

Directions:
Heat up a pan with the oil over medium-high heat, add the fish and cook for 3 minutes on each side. Add the rest of the ingredients, cook everything for 7 minutes more, divide between plates and serve.
Nutrition Info: calories 162, fat 9.6, fiber 4.3, carbs 12.4, protein 16.5

533. Cayenne Cod And Tomatoes

Servings: 4   Cooking Time: 25 Minutes
Ingredients:
Salt and black pepper to the taste
1 teaspoon sweet paprika
1 teaspoon cayenne pepper
2 tablespoons olive oil
1 yellow onion, chopped

1 teaspoon lime juice
2 garlic cloves, minced
4 cod fillets, boneless
A pinch of cloves, ground
½ cup chicken stock
½ pound cherry tomatoes, cubed

Directions:
Heat up a pan with the oil over medium-high heat add the cod, salt, pepper and the cayenne, cook for 4 minutes on each side and divide between plates. Heat up the same pan over medium-high heat, add the onion and garlic and sauté for 5 minutes. Add the rest of the ingredients, stir, bring to a simmer and cook for 10 minutes more. Divide the mix next to the fish and serve.
Nutrition Info: calories 232, fat 16.5, fiber 11.1, carbs 24.8, protein 16.5

534. Cod And Mustard Sauce

Servings: 4   Cooking Time: 45 Minutes

Ingredients:

1-pound cod fillet	1 tablespoon olive oil
1 carrot, peeled	1 teaspoon coriander
1 bell pepper, chopped	seeds
1 white onion, chopped	1 teaspoon salt
1 eggplant, peeled, chopped	1 teaspoon dried dill
2 tablespoons butter	1 teaspoon honey
	1 tablespoon Mustard

Directions:

Chop the cod fillet roughly. Line the baking tray with baking paper and arrange the fish in it. After this, mix up together mustard, honey, dried dill, salt, coriander seeds, olive oil, and butter. Chop the carrot roughly. Put all vegetables in the baking tray and sprinkle with honey mixture. Preheat the oven to 365F. Bake the sheet-pan fish for 45 minutes. When all the vegetables and fish are soft, the meal is cooked.

Nutrition Info: Per Serving:calories 257, fat 11.6, fiber 6, carbs 15.9, protein 25.1

535. Garlic Scallops And Peas Mix

Servings: 6   Cooking Time: 20 Minutes

Ingredients:

12 ounces scallops	1 cup snow peas, sliced
2 tablespoons olive oil	½ tablespoon balsamic vinegar
4 garlic cloves, minced	1 cup scallions, sliced
A pinch of salt and black pepper	1 tablespoon basil, chopped
½ cup chicken stock	

Directions:

Heat up a pan with half of the oil over medium-high heat, add the scallops, cook for 5 minutes on each side and transfer to a bowl. Heat up the pan again with the rest of the oil over medium heat, add the scallions and the garlic and sauté for 2 minutes. Add the rest of the ingredients, stir, bring to a simmer and cook for 5 minutes more. Add the scallops to the pan, cook everything for 3 minutes, divide into bowls and serve.

Nutrition Info:calories 296, fat 11.8, fiber 9.8, carbs 26.5, protein 20.5

536. Shrimp And Beans Salad

Servings: 4   Cooking Time: 4 Minutes

Ingredients:

1 pound shrimp, peeled and deveined	30 ounces canned cannellini beans, drained and rinsed
2 tablespoons olive oil	A pinch of salt and black pepper
1 cup cherry tomatoes, halved	For the dressing:
1 teaspoon lemon zest, grated	3 tablespoons red wine vinegar
½ cup red onion, chopped	2 garlic cloves, minced
4 handfuls baby arugula	½ cup olive oil

Directions:

Heat up a pan with 2 tablespoons oil over medium-high heat, add the shrimp and cook for 2 minutes on each side. In a salad bowl, combine the shrimp with the beans and the rest of the ingredients except the ones for the dressing and

toss. In a separate bowl, combine the vinegar with ½ cup oil and the garlic and whisk well. Pour over the salad, toss and serve right away.

Nutrition Info:calories 207, fat 12.3, fiber 6.6, carbs 15.4, protein 8.7

537. Lemoney Prawns

Servings: 2   Cooking Time: 3 Minutes

Ingredients:

1/2 lb prawns	1/2 cup fish stock
1 tbsp fresh lemon juice	1 tbsp olive oil
1 tbsp lemon zest, grated	1 tbsp garlic, minced
	Pepper
	Salt

Directions:

Add all ingredients into the inner pot of instant pot and stir well. Seal pot with lid and cook on high for 3 minutes. Once done, release pressure using quick release. Remove lid. Drain prawns and serve.

Nutrition Info: Calories 215 Fat 9.5 g Carbohydrates 3.9 g Sugar 0.4 g Protein 27.6 g Cholesterol 239 mg

538. Pesto And Lemon Halibut

Servings: 4   Cooking Time: 10 Minutes

Ingredients:

1 tbsp fresh lemon juice	2 tbsp olive oil
1 tbsp lemon rind, grated	2/3 cups firmly packed basil leaves
2 garlic cloves, peeled	1/8 tsp freshly ground black pepper
¼ cup Parmesan Cheese, freshly grated	¼ tsp salt, divided
	4 pcs 6-oz halibut fillets

Directions:

Preheat grill to medium fire and grease grate with cooking spray. Season fillets with pepper and 1/8 tsp salt. Place on grill and cook until halibut is flaky around 4 minutes per side. Meanwhile, make your lemon pesto by combining lemon juice, lemon rind, garlic, olive oil, Parmesan cheese, basil leaves and remaining salt in a blender. Pulse mixture until finely minced but not pureed. Once fish is done cooking, transfer to a serving platter, pour over the lemon pesto sauce, serve and enjoy.

Nutrition Info: Calories per Serving: 277.4; Fat: 13g; Protein: 38.7g; Carbs: 1.4g

539. Stuffed Branzino

Servings: 7   Cooking Time: 40 Minutes

Ingredients:

6 oz fennel bulb, trimmed	1 teaspoon salt
1 teaspoon ground coriander	1 teaspoon dried cilantro
½ teaspoon ground black pepper	1 tablespoon butter, unsalted
1 tablespoon lemon juice	1.5-pound whole branzino, trimmed, peeled
1 teaspoon dried oregano	1 tablespoon sunflower oil

Directions:

Slice fennel bulb. Rub the branzino with ground coriander, black pepper, salt, oregano, and cilantro. Then sprinkle it with lemon juice and sunflower oil. After this, fill the branzino with butter and sliced

fennel and wrap the fish in the foil. Bake the fish for 40 minutes at 365F. Then discard the foil from the fish and cut it on the servings.
Nutrition Info: Per Serving:calories 245, fat 8.4, fiber 0.9, carbs 2.1, protein 39.2

540. Tomato Olive Fish Fillets

Servings: 4   Cooking Time: 8 Minutes
Ingredients:

2 lbs halibut fish fillets	1 cup olives, pitted
2 oregano sprigs	28 oz can tomatoes, diced
2 rosemary sprigs	1 tbsp garlic, minced
2 tbsp fresh lime juice	1 onion, chopped
	2 tbsp olive oil

Directions:
Add oil into the inner pot of instant pot and set the pot on sauté mode. Add onion and sauté for 3 minutes. Add garlic and sauté for a minute. Add lime juice, olives, herb sprigs, and tomatoes and stir well. Seal pot with lid and cook on high for 3 minutes. Once done, release pressure using quick release. Remove lid. Add fish fillets and seal pot again with lid and cook on high for 2 minutes. Once done, release pressure using quick release. Remove lid. Serve and enjoy.
Nutrition Info: Calories 333 Fat 19.1 g Carbohydrates 31.8 g Sugar 8.4 g Protein 13.4 g Cholesterol 5 mg

541. Steamed Mussels Thai Style

Servings: 4   Cooking Time: 15 Minutes
Ingredients:

¼ cup minced shallots	1 tbsp chopped fresh mint
½ tsp Madras curry	2 lbs. mussel, cleaned and debearded
1 cup dry white wine	2 tbsp butter
1 small bay leaf	4 medium garlic cloves, minced
1 tbsp chopped fresh basil	
1 tbsp chopped fresh cilantro	

Directions:
In a large heavy bottomed pot, on medium high fire add to pot the curry powder, bay leaf, wine plus the minced garlic and shallots. Bring to a boil and simmer for 3 minutes. Add the cleaned mussels, stir, cover, and cook for 3 minutes. Stir mussels again, cover, and cook for another 2 or 3 minutes. Cooking is done when majority of shells have opened. With a slotted spoon, transfer cooked mussels in a large bowl. Discard any unopened mussels. Continue heating pot with sauce. Add butter and the chopped herbs. Season with pepper and salt to taste. Once good, pour over mussels, serve and enjoy.
Nutrition Info: Calories per Serving: 407.2; Protein: 43.4g; Fat: 21.2g; Carbs: 10.8g

542. Oregano Citrus Salmon

Servings: 2   Cooking Time: 15 Minutes
Ingredients:

2 salmon fillets (5 oz each fish fillet)	¾ teaspoon ground coriander
½ teaspoon garlic powder	1 tablespoon butter
¾ teaspoon chili flakes	½ teaspoon dried oregano
½ teaspoon salt	1 orange, peeled

Directions:
In the shallow bowl make the spice mix from garlic powder, chili flakes, ground coriander, salt, and dried oregano. Then coat the salmon fillets in the spice mix. Slice the orange and place it in the skillet. Add butter and roast the sliced orange until the butter is melted. Then remove the sliced orange from the skillet. Add salmon fillets and roast them for 4 minutes from each side over the medium heat. After this, top the salmon with roasted sliced orange and close the lid. Cook the fish for 5 minutes more over the low heat.
Nutrition Info: Per Serving:calories 285, fat 14.7, fiber 2.5, carbs 11.6, protein 28.6

543. Nutmeg Sea Bass

Servings: 4   Cooking Time: 10 Minutes
Ingredients:

1 teaspoon fresh ginger, minced	1 teaspoon minced garlic
10 oz seabass fillet (4 fillets)	¼ teaspoon ground nutmeg
1 tablespoon butter	½ teaspoon salt

Directions:
Toss butter in the skillet and melt it. Add minced garlic, ground nutmeg, salt, and fresh ginger. Roast the mixture for 1 minute. Then add seabass fillet. Fryt the fish for 3 minutes from each side.
Nutrition Info: Per Serving:calories 205, fat 13.5, fiber 0.8, carbs 0.6, protein 19.7

544. Shrimp Kebabs

Servings: 2   Cooking Time: 5 Minutes
Ingredients:

4 King prawns, peeled	½ teaspoon salt
1 tablespoon lemon juice	1 tablespoon tomato sauce
¾ teaspoon ground coriander	1 tablespoon olive oil

Directions:
Skew the shrimps on the skewers and sprinkle them with lemon juice, ground coriander, salt, and tomato sauce. Then drizzle the shrimps with olive oil. Preheat grill to 385F. Grill the shrimp kebabs for 2 minutes from each side.
Nutrition Info: Per Serving:calories 106, fat 7.5, fiber 0.4, carbs 0.6, protein 9.1

545. Easy Broiled Lobster Tails

Servings: 2   Cooking Time: 10 Minutes
Ingredients:

1 6-oz frozen lobster tails	1 tsp lemon pepper seasoning
1 tbsp olive oil	

Directions:
Preheat oven broiler. With kitchen scissors, cut thawed lobster tails in half lengthwise. Brush with oil the exposed lobster meat. Season with lemon pepper. Place lobster tails in baking sheet with exposed meat facing up. Place on top broiler rack and broil for 10 minutes until lobster meat is lightly browned on the sides and center meat is opaque. Serve and enjoy.
Nutrition Info: Calories per Serving: 175.6; Protein: 3g; Fat: 10g; Carbs: 18.4g

546. Cajun Garlic Shrimp Noodle Bowl

Servings: 2   Cooking Time: 15 Minutes

Ingredients:

½ teaspoon salt
1 onion, sliced
1 red pepper, sliced
1 tablespoon butter
1 teaspoon garlic granules
1 teaspoon onion powder
2 large zucchinis, cut into noodle strips

1 teaspoon paprika
20 jumbo shrimps, shells removed and deveined
3 cloves garlic, minced
3 tablespoon ghee
A dash of cayenne pepper
A dash of red pepper flakes

Directions:

Prepare the Cajun seasoning by mixing the onion powder, garlic granules, pepper flakes, cayenne pepper, paprika and salt. Toss in the shrimp to coat in the seasoning.   In a skillet, heat the ghee and sauté the garlic. Add in the red pepper and onions and continue sautéing for 4 minutes.   Add the Cajun shrimp and cook until opaque. Set aside. In another pan, heat the butter and sauté the zucchini noodles for three minutes.   Assemble by the placing the Cajun shrimps on top of the zucchini noodles.

Nutrition Info: Calories per Serving: 712; Fat: 30.0g; Protein: 97.8g; Carbs: 20.2g

547. Red Peppers & Pineapple Topped Mahi-mahi

Servings: 4   Cooking Time: 30 Minutes

Ingredients:

¼ tsp black pepper
1 cup whole wheat couscous
1 red bell pepper, diced
2 1/3 cups low sodium chicken broth
2 cups chopped fresh pineapple

¼ tsp salt
2 tbsp. chopped fresh chives
2 tsp. olive oil
4 pieces of skinless, boneless mahi mahi (dolphin fish) fillets (around 4-oz each)

Directions:

On high fire, add 1 1/3 cups broth to a small saucepan and heat until boiling. Once boiling, add couscous. Turn off fire, cover and set aside to allow liquid to be fully absorbed around 5 minutes.   On medium high fire, place a large nonstick saucepan and heat oil.   Season fish on both sides with pepper and salt. Add mahi mahi to hot pan and pan fry until golden around one minute each side. Once cooked, transfer to plate.   On same pan, sauté bell pepper and pineapples until soft, around 2 minutes on medium high fire.   Add couscous to pan along with chives, and remaining broth.   On top of the mixture in pan, place fish. With foil, cover pan and continue cooking until fish is steaming and tender underneath the foil, around 3-5 minutes.

Nutrition Info: Calories per serving: 302; Protein: 43.1g; Fat: 4.8g; Carbs: 22.0g

548. Kale, Beets And Cod Mix

Servings: 4   Cooking Time: 20 Minutes

Ingredients:

2 tablespoons apple cider vinegar

Salt and black pepper to the taste

½ cup chicken stock
1 red onion, sliced
4 golden beets, trimmed, peeled and cubed
2 tablespoons olive oil

4 cups kale, torn
2 tablespoons walnuts, chopped
1 pound cod fillets, boneless, skinless and cubed

Directions:

Heat up a pan with the oil over medium-high heat, add the onion and the beets and cook for 3-4 minutes.   Add the rest of the ingredients except the fish and the walnuts, stir, bring to a simmer and cook for 5 minutes more.   Add the fish, cook for 10 minutes, divide between plates and serve.

Nutrition Info:calories 285, fat 7.6, fiber 6.5, carbs 16.7, protein 12.5

549. Shrimp Scampi

Servings: 6   Cooking Time: 8 Minutes

Ingredients:

1 lb whole wheat penne pasta
1 lb frozen shrimp
2 tbsp garlic, minced
1/2 tbsp Italian seasoning

1/4 tsp cayenne
1/4 cup olive oil
3 1/2 cups fish stock
Pepper
Salt

Directions:

Add all ingredients into the inner pot of instant pot and stir well.   Seal pot with lid and cook on high for 6 minutes.   Once done, release pressure using quick release. Remove lid.   Stir well and serve.

Nutrition Info: Calories 435 Fat 12.6 g Carbohydrates 54.9 g Sugar 0.1 g Protein 30.6 g Cholesterol 116 mg

550. Orange Rosemary Seared Salmon

Servings: 4   Cooking Time: 10 Minutes

Ingredients:

1 cup fresh orange juice
1 tablespoon coconut oil
1 tablespoon tapioca starch
2 garlic cloves, minced
2 tablespoon fresh lemon juice

½ cup chicken stock
2 teaspoon fresh rosemary, minced
2 teaspoon orange zest
4 salmon fillets, skins removed
Salt and pepper to taste

Directions:

Season the salmon fillet on both sides.   In a skillet, heat coconut oil over medium high heat. Cook the salmon fillets for 5 minutes on each side. Set aside.   In a mixing bowl, combine the orange juice, chicken stock, lemon juice and orange zest. In the skillet, sauté the garlic and rosemary for 2 minutes and pour the orange juice mixture. Bring to a boil. Lower the heat to medium low and simmer. Season with salt and pepper to taste. Pour the sauce all over the salmon fillet then serve.

Nutrition Info: Calories per Serving: 493; Fat: 17.9g; Protein: 66.7g; Carbs: 12.8g

551. Dill Halibut

Servings: 3   Cooking Time: 10 Minutes

Ingredients:

13 oz halibut fillet
1/3 cup cream
¼ cup dill, chopped

¼ teaspoon turmeric
¼ teaspoon ground

½ teaspoon garlic powder
paprika
1 teaspoon salt
1 teaspoon olive oil

Directions:
Chop the fish fillet on the big cubes and sprinkle them with garlic powder, turmeric, ground paprika, and salt.   Pour olive oil in the skillet and preheat it well.   Then place fish in the hot oil and roast it for 2 minutes from each side over the medium heat. Add cream and stir gently with the help of the spatula.   Bring the mixture to boil and add dill. Close the lid and cook the fish on the medium heat for 5 minutes. Till the fish and creamy sauce are cooked.   Serve the halibut cubes with creamy sauce.
Nutrition Info: Per Serving:calories 170, fat 5.9, fiber 0.7, carbs 3.6, protein 25.1

552. Salmon And Mango Mix

Servings: 2   Cooking Time: 25 Minutes
Ingredients:
2 salmon fillets, skinless and boneless
Salt and pepper to the taste
2 tablespoons olive oil
2 garlic cloves, minced
2 mangos, peeled and cubed
1 red chili, chopped
1 small piece ginger, grated
Juice of 1 lime
1 tablespoon cilantro, chopped

Directions:
In a roasting pan, combine the salmon with the oil, garlic and the rest of the ingredients except the cilantro, toss, introduce in the oven at 350 degrees F and bake for 25 minutes.   Divide everything between plates and serve with the cilantro sprinkled on top.
Nutrition Info:calories 251, fat 15.9, fiber 5.9, carbs 26.4, protein 12.4

553. Delicious Shrimp Alfredo

Servings: 4   Cooking Time: 3 Minutes
Ingredients:
12 shrimp, remove shells
1/4 cup parmesan cheese
2 cups whole wheat rotini noodles
1 tbsp garlic, minced
1 cup fish broth
15 oz alfredo sauce
1 onion, chopped
Salt

Directions:
Add all ingredients except parmesan cheese into the instant pot and stir well.   Seal pot with lid and cook on high for 3 minutes.   Once done, release pressure using quick release. Remove lid. Stir in cheese and serve.
Nutrition Info: Calories 669 Fat 23.1 g Carbohydrates 76 g Sugar 2.4 g Protein 37.8 g Cholesterol 190 mg

554. Cod And Mushrooms Mix

Servings: 4   Cooking Time: 25 Minutes
Ingredients:
2 cod fillets, boneless
4 tablespoons olive oil
4 ounces mushrooms, sliced
Sea salt and black pepper to the taste
12 cherry tomatoes,
1 avocado, pitted, peeled and cubed
1 red chili pepper, chopped
1 tablespoon cilantro, chopped
2 tablespoons balsamic vinegar

halved
8 ounces lettuce leaves, torn
1 ounce feta cheese, crumbled

Directions:
Put the fish in a roasting pan, brush it with 2 tablespoons oil, sprinkle salt and pepper all over and broil under medium-high heat for 15 minutes. Meanwhile, heat up a pan with the rest of the oil over medium heat, add the mushrooms, stir and sauté for 5 minutes.   Add the rest of the ingredients, toss, cook for 5 minutes more and divide between plates.   Top with the fish and serve right away.
Nutrition Info:calories 257, fat 10, fiber 3.1, carbs 24.3, protein 19.4

555. Baked Shrimp Mix

Servings: 4   Cooking Time: 32 Minutes
Ingredients:
4 gold potatoes, peeled and sliced
2 fennel bulbs, trimmed and cut into wedges
2 garlic cloves, minced
3 tablespoons olive oil
½ cup kalamata olives, pitted and halved
2 shallots, chopped
2 pounds shrimp, peeled and deveined
1 teaspoon lemon zest, grated
2 teaspoons oregano, dried
4 ounces feta cheese, crumbled
2 tablespoons parsley, chopped

Directions:
In a roasting pan, combine the potatoes with 2 tablespoons oil, garlic and the rest of the ingredients except the shrimp, toss, introduce in the oven and bake at 450 degrees F for 25 minutes. Add the shrimp, toss, bake for 7 minutes more, divide between plates and serve.
Nutrition Info:calories 341, fat 19, fiber 9, carbs 34, protein 10

556. Lemon And Dates Barramundi

Servings: 2   Cooking Time: 12 Minutes
Ingredients:
2 barramundi fillets, boneless
1 shallot, sliced
4 lemon slices
Juice of ½ lemon
Zest of 1 lemon, grated
2 tablespoons olive oil
6 ounces baby spinach
¼ cup almonds, chopped
4 dates, pitted and chopped
¼ cup parsley, chopped
Salt and black pepper to the taste

Directions:
Season the fish with salt and pepper and arrange on 2 parchment paper pieces.   Top the fish with the lemon slices, drizzle the lemon juice, and then top with the other ingredients except the oil. Drizzle 1 tablespoon oil over each fish mix, wrap the parchment paper around the fish shaping to packets and arrange them on a baking sheet. Bake at 400 degrees F for 12 minutes, cool the mix a bit, unfold, divide everything between plates and serve.
Nutrition Info:calories 232, fat 16.5, fiber 11.1, carbs 24.8, protein 6.5

557. Cheesy Crab And Lime Spread

Servings: 8   Cooking Time: 25 Minutes

Ingredients:

1 pound crab meat, flaked

4 ounces cream cheese, soft

1 teaspoon lime juice

1 tablespoon chives, chopped

1 teaspoon lime zest, grated

Directions:

In a baking dish greased with cooking spray, combine the crab with the rest of the ingredients and toss.   Introduce in the oven at 350 degrees F, bake for 25 minutes, divide into bowls and serve.

Nutrition Info:calories 284, fat 14.6, fiber 5.8, carbs 16.5, protein 15.4

558. Honey Lobster

Servings: 2   Cooking Time: 10 Minutes

Ingredients:

2 lobster tails

2 teaspoons butter, melted

¼ teaspoon ground paprika

1 teaspoon honey

1 teaspoon lemon juice

¼ teaspoon dried dill

Directions:

Cut the top of the lobster tail shell to the tip of the tail with the help of the scissors. It will look like "lobster meat in a blanket".   Mix up together melted butter, honey, ground paprika, lemon juice, and dried dill.   Brush the lobster tails with butter mixture carefully from the top and down. Preheat the oven to 365F.   Line the baking tray with parchment and arrange the lobster tails in it. Bake the lobster tails for 10 minutes.

Nutrition Info: Per Serving:calories 91, fat 3.9, fiber 0.1 carbs 3.1, protein 0.1

559. Fried Salmon

Servings: 2   Cooking Time: 8 Minutes

Ingredients:

5 oz salmon fillet

¼ teaspoon salt

½ teaspoon ground black pepper

1 tablespoon sunflower oil

¼ teaspoon lime juice

Directions:

Cut the salmon fillet on 2 lengthwise pieces. Sprinkle every fish piece with salt, ground black pepper, and lime juice.   Pour sunflower oil in the skillet and preheat it until shimmering.   Then place fish fillets in the hot oil and cook them for 3 minutes from each side.

Nutrition Info: Per Serving:calories 157, fat 11.4, fiber 0.1, carbs 0.3, protein 13.8

560. Smoked Salmon And Veggies Mix

Servings: 4   Cooking Time: 20 Minutes

Ingredients:

3 red onions, cut into wedges

¾ cup green olives, pitted and halved

3 red bell peppers, roughly chopped

½ teaspoon smoked paprika

Salt and black pepper to the taste

3 tablespoons olive oil

4 salmon fillets, skinless and boneless

2 tablespoons chives, chopped

Directions:

In a roasting pan, combine the salmon with the onions and the rest of the ingredients, introduce in the oven and bake at 390 degrees F for 20 minutes. Divide the mix between plates and serve.

Nutrition Info:calories 301, fat 5.9, fiber 11.9, carbs 26.4, protein 22.4

561. Berries And Grilled Calamari

Servings: 4   Cooking Time: 5 Minutes

Ingredients:

¼ cup dried cranberries

¼ cup extra virgin olive oil

¼ cup olive oil

¼ cup sliced almonds

½ lemon, juiced

¾ cup blueberries

1 ½ pounds calamari tube, cleaned

1 granny smith apple, sliced thinly

1 tablespoon fresh lemon juice

2 tablespoons apple cider vinegar

6 cups fresh spinach

Freshly grated pepper to taste

Sea salt to taste

Directions:

In a small bowl, make the vinaigrette by mixing well the tablespoon of lemon juice, apple cider vinegar, and extra virgin olive oil. Season with pepper and salt to taste. Set aside.   Turn on the grill to medium fire and let the grates heat up for a minute or two.   In a large bowl, add olive oil and the calamari tube. Season calamari generously with pepper and salt.   Place seasoned and oiled calamari onto heated grate and grill until cooked or opaque. This is around two minutes per side.   As you wait for the calamari to cook, you can combine almonds, cranberries, blueberries, spinach, and the thinly sliced apple in a large salad bowl. Toss to mix. Remove cooked calamari from grill and transfer on a chopping board. Cut into ¼-inch thick rings and throw into the salad bowl.   Drizzle with vinaigrette and toss well to coat salad.   Serve and enjoy!

Nutrition Info: Calories per Serving: 567; Fat: 24.5g; Protein: 54.8g; Carbs: 30.6g

562. Salmon And Zucchini Rolls

Servings: 8   Cooking Time: 0 Minutes

Ingredients:

8 slices smoked salmon, boneless

1 cup ricotta cheese, soft

2 teaspoons lemon zest, grated

1 tablespoon dill, chopped

2 zucchinis, sliced lengthwise in 8 pieces

1 small red onion, sliced

Salt and pepper to the taste

Directions:

In a bowl, mix the ricotta cheese with the rest of the ingredients except the salmon and the zucchini and whisk well.   Arrange the zucchini slices on a working surface, and divide the salmon on top. Spread the cheese mix all over, roll and secure with toothpicks and serve right away.

Nutrition Info:calories 297, fat 24.3, fiber 11.6, carbs 15.4, protein 11.6

563. Scallions And Salmon Tartar

Servings: 4   Cooking Time: 0 Minutes

Ingredients:

4 tablespoons scallions, chopped

2 teaspoons lemon

1 pound salmon, skinless, boneless and minced

juice
1 tablespoon chives, minced
1 tablespoon olive oil
Salt and black pepper to the taste
1 tablespoon parsley, chopped

Directions:
In a bowl, combine the scallions with the salmon and the rest of the ingredients, stir well, divide into small moulds between plates and serve.
Nutrition Info:calories 224, fat 14.5, fiber 5.2, carbs 12.7, protein 5.3

564.	Flavors Cioppino

Servings: 6   Cooking Time: 5 Minutes
Ingredients:
1 lb codfish, cut into chunks
1 1/2 lbs shrimp
28 oz can tomatoes, diced
1 cup dry white wine
1 bay leaf
1 tsp cayenne
1 tsp oregano
1 shallot, chopped
1 tsp garlic, minced
1 tbsp olive oil
1/2 tsp salt

Directions:
Add oil into the inner pot of instant pot and set the pot on sauté mode.   Add shallot and garlic and sauté for 2 minutes.   Add wine, bay leaf, cayenne, oregano, and salt and cook for 3 minutes.   Add remaining ingredients and stir well.   Seal pot with a lid and select manual and cook on low for 0 minutes.   Once done, release pressure using quick release. Remove lid.   Serve and enjoy.
Nutrition Info: Calories 281 Fat 5 g Carbohydrates 10.5 g Sugar 4.9 g Protein 40.7 g Cholesterol 266 mg

565.	Warm Caper Tapenade On Cod

Servings: 4   Cooking Time: 30 Minutes
Ingredients:
¼ cup chopped cured olives
¼ tsp freshly ground pepper
1 ½ tsp chopped fresh oregano
1 cup halved cherry tomatoes
1 lb. cod fillet
1 tbsp capers, rinsed and chopped
1 tbsp minced shallot
1 tsp balsamic vinegar
3 tsp extra virgin olive oil, divided

Directions:
Grease baking sheet with cooking spray and preheat oven to 450oF.   Place cod on prepared baking sheet. Rub with 2 tsp oil and season with pepper.   Roast in oven for 15 to 20 minutes or until cod is flaky.   While waiting for cod to cook, on medium fire, place a small fry pan and heat 1 tsp oil.   Sauté shallots for a minute.   Add tomatoes and cook for two minutes or until soft.   Add capers and olives. Sauté for another minute.   Add vinegar and oregano. Turn off fire and stir to mix well.   Evenly divide cod into 4 servings and place on a plate.   To serve, top cod with Caper-Olive-Tomato Tapenade and enjoy.
Nutrition Info: Calories per Serving: 107; Fat: 2.9g; Protein: 17.6g; Carbs: 2.0g

566.	Spicy Tomato Crab Mix

Servings: 4   Cooking Time: 12 Minutes
Ingredients:
1 lb crab meat
1 cup grape tomatoes, cut into half
1 tsp paprika
1 tbsp olive oil
Pepper

2 tbsp green onion, chopped
Salt

Directions:
Add oil into the inner pot of instant pot and set the pot on sauté mode.   Add paprika and onion and sauté for 2 minutes.   Add the rest of the ingredients and stir well.   Seal pot with lid and cook on high for 10 minutes.   Once done, release pressure using quick release. Remove lid.   Serve and enjoy.
Nutrition Info: Calories 142 Fat 5.7 g Carbohydrates 4.3 g Sugar 1.3 g Protein 14.7 g Cholesterol 61 mg

567.	Salmon Bake

Servings: 6   Cooking Time: 25 Minutes
Ingredients:
1 teaspoon baking powder
½ cup skim milk
1 ½ cup wheat flour, whole grain
½ teaspoon salt
1 egg, beaten
2 oz Cheddar cheese, shredded
8 oz salmon, canned
1 teaspoon olive oil
1 teaspoon butter
½ teaspoon paprika
½ teaspoon ground black pepper
1 tablespoon sour cream

Directions:
Make the pie dough: pour skim milk in the saucepan and reheat it until it is warm but not hot. Then add baking powder, flour, salt, and egg. Knead the non-sticky dough. Add more flour if needed.   Make the bun from the dough and cover it with a towel. Let it rest for at least 10 minutes in a warm place.   Meanwhile, make the filling for the pie: chop the salmon and combine it with cheese, paprika, sour cream, and ground black pepper. Stir well.   Cut the dough on the two pieces.   Roll up one piece of dough and arrange it in the non-sticky round springform.   Put the filling over the dough.   Roll up the second part of the dough and cover the filing.   Secure the edges of the pie with the help of the fork or fingertip. Bake the pie for 25 minutes at 360F.   When the pie is cooked, chill it to the room temperature and cut on 6 servings.
Nutrition Info: Per Serving:calories 238, fat 8.4, fiber 1, carbs 25.7, protein 14.6

568.	Baked Trout And Fennel

Servings: 4   Cooking Time: 22 Minutes
Ingredients:
2 tablespoons olive oil
1 yellow onion, sliced
3 teaspoons Italian seasoning
4 rainbow trout fillets, boneless
1 fennel bulb, sliced
¼ cup panko breadcrumbs
½ cup kalamata olives, pitted and halved
Juice of 1 lemon

Directions:
Spread the fennel the onion and the rest of the ingredients except the trout and the breadcrumbs on a baking sheet lined with parchment paper, toss them and cook at 400 degrees F for 10 minutes. Add the fish dredged in breadcrumbs and seasoned with salt and pepper and cook it at 400 degrees F for 6 minutes on each side.   Divide the mix between plates and serve.

Nutrition Info:calories 306, fat 8.9, fiber 11.1, carbs 23.8, protein 14.5

569. Salmon And Corn Salad

Servings: 4   Cooking Time: 0 Minutes
Ingredients:

½ cup pecans, chopped	2 tablespoons olive oil
2 cups baby arugula	2 tablespoon lemon juice
1 cup corn	
¼ pound smoked salmon, skinless, boneless and cut into small chunks	Sea salt and black pepper to the taste

Directions:
In a salad bowl, combine the salmon with the corn and the rest of the ingredients, toss and serve right away.
Nutrition Info:calories 284, fat 18.4, fiber 5.4, carbs 22.6, protein 17.4

570. Minty Sardines Salad

Servings: 4   Cooking Time: 0 Minutes
Ingredients:

4 ounces canned sardines in olive oil, skinless, boneless and flaked	A pinch of salt and black pepper
2 teaspoons avocado oil	1 avocado, peeled, pitted and cubed
2 tablespoons mint, chopped	1 cucumber, cubed
	2 tomatoes, cubed
	2 spring onions, chopped

Directions:
In a bowl, combine the sardines with the oil and the rest of the ingredients, toss, divide into small cups and keep in the fridge for 10 minutes before serving.
Nutrition Info:calories 261, fat 7.6, fiber 2.2, carbs 22.8, protein 12.5

571. Smoked Salmon And Watercress Salad

Servings: 4   Cooking Time: 0 Minutes
Ingredients:

2 bunches watercress	Salt and black pepper to the taste
1 pound smoked salmon, skinless, boneless and flaked	1 big cucumber, sliced
2 teaspoons mustard	2 tablespoons chives, chopped
¼ cup lemon juice	
½ cup Greek yogurt	

Directions:
In a salad bowl, combine the salmon with the watercress and the rest of the ingredients toss and serve right away.
Nutrition Info:calories 244, fat 16.7, fiber 4.5, carbs 22.5, protein 15.6

572. Easy Salmon Stew

Servings: 6   Cooking Time: 8 Minutes
Ingredients:

2 lbs salmon fillet, cubed	1 tbsp olive oil
1 onion, chopped	Pepper
2 cups fish broth	salt

Directions:
Add oil into the inner pot of instant pot and set the pot on sauté mode.   Add onion and sauté for 2 minutes.   Add remaining ingredients and stir well.   Seal pot with lid and cook on high for 6 minutes.   Once done, release pressure using quick release. Remove lid.   Stir and serve.
Nutrition Info: Calories 243 Fat 12.6 g Carbohydrates 0.8 g Sugar 0.3 g Protein 31 g Cholesterol 78 mg

573. Oregano Swordfish Mix

Servings: 4   Cooking Time: 20 Minutes
Ingredients:

4 swordfish fillets (oz each fillet)	4 teaspoons capers
4 sprig fresh rosemary	½ teaspoon salt
½ teaspoon dried oregano	1 teaspoon butter
1 tablespoon olive oil	1 tablespoon lemon juice
	¼ teaspoon lemon zest, grated

Directions:
Toss butter in the skillet and bring it to boil.   Add rosemary sprigs, lemon zest, and dried oregano. Boil the ingredients for 20 seconds.   Then add swordfish fillets.   Roast the fish for 2 minutes from each side over the high heat.   Then reduce the heat to medium.   Sprinkle the fish with olive oil, salt, lemon juice, and capers.   Close the lid and cook the swordfish for 15 minutes over the low heat.
Nutrition Info: Per Serving:calories 206, fat 10, fiber 0.3, carbs 0.5, protein 27.1

574. Cheddar Tuna Bake

Servings: 4   Cooking Time: 35 Minutes
Ingredients:

½ cup Cheddar cheese, shredded	2 tomatoes, chopped
7 oz tuna filet, chopped	½ teaspoon salt
1 teaspoon ground coriander	1 teaspoon olive oil
	½ teaspoon dried oregano

Directions:
Brush the casserole mold with olive oil.   Mix up together chopped tuna fillet with dried oregano and ground coriander.   Place the fish in the mold and flatten well to get the layer.   Then add chopped tomatoes and shredded cheese.   Cover the casserole with foil and secure the edges.   Bake the meal for 35 minutes at 355F.
Nutrition Info: Per Serving:calories 260, fat 21.5, fiber 0.8, carbs 2.7, protein 14.6

575. Tarragon Trout And Beets

Servings: 4   Cooking Time: 35 Minutes
Ingredients:

1 pound medium beets, peeled and cubed	1 tablespoon chives, chopped
3 tablespoons olive oil	1 tablespoon tarragon, chopped
4 trout fillets, boneless	3 tablespoon spring onions, chopped
Salt and black pepper to the taste	2 tablespoons lemon juice
½ cup chicken stock	

Directions:
Spread the beets on a baking sheet lined with parchment paper, add salt, pepper and 1 tablespoon oil, toss and bake at 450 degrees F for 20 minutes.   Heat up a pan with the rest of the

oil over medium-high heat, add the trout and the remaining ingredients, and cook for 4 minutes on each side. Add the baked beets, cook the mix for 5 minutes more, divide everything between plates and serve.

Nutrition Info:calories 232, fat 5.5, fiber 7.5, carbs 20.9, protein 16.8

576.	Cod And Brussels Sprouts

Servings: 4   Cooking Time: 20 Minutes

Ingredients:

1 teaspoon garlic powder
1 teaspoon smoked paprika
2 tablespoons olive oil
4 cod fillets, boneless

2 pounds Brussels sprouts, trimmed and halved
½ cup tomato sauce
1 teaspoon Italian seasoning
1 tablespoon chives, chopped

Directions:

In a roasting pan, combine the sprouts with the garlic powder and the other ingredients except the cod and toss. Put the cod on top, cover the pan with tin foil and bake at 450 degrees F for 20 minutes. Divide the mix between plates and serve.

Nutrition Info:calories 188, fat 12.8, fiber 9.2, carbs 22.2, protein 16.8

577.	Salmon Tortillas

Servings: 2   Cooking Time: 10 Minutes

Ingredients:

2 corn tortillas
8 oz wild salmon fillet
1 teaspoon balsamic vinegar
¾ teaspoon cayenne pepper
¾ teaspoon salt

1 teaspoon Italian herbs
1 teaspoon olive oil
¼ cup green olives, pitted
1 tablespoon fresh cilantro, chopped

Directions:

Sprinkle salmon fillet with balsamic vinegar, cayenne pepper, salt, Italian herbs, and olive oil. Massage the salmon fillet well with the help of the fingertips. Then preheat skillet well and place salmon fillet inside. Roast the fish for 10 minutes totally. Meanwhile, slice green olives and mix them up with fresh cilantro. Chill the cooked salmon gently and chop it. Arrange the fish on the corn tortillas and sprinkle with cilantro mixture. Fold up the tortillas in the shape of tacos.

Nutrition Info: Per Serving:calories 233, fat 9.6, fiber 2.9, carbs 14.1, protein 20.6

578.	Tasty Tuna Scaloppine

Servings: 4   Cooking Time: 10 Minutes

Ingredients:

¼ cup chopped almonds
¼ cup fresh tangerine juice
½ tsp fennel seeds
½ tsp ground black pepper, divided
½ tsp salt
1 tbsp extra virgin olive oil

2 tbsp chopped fresh mint
2 tbsp chopped red onion
4 6-oz sushi-grade Yellowfin tuna steaks, each split in half horizontally
Cooking spray

Directions:

In a small bowl mix fennel seeds, olive oil, mint, onion, tangerine juice, almonds, ¼ tsp pepper and ¼ tsp salt. Combine thoroughly. Season fish with remaining salt and pepper. On medium high fire, place a large nonstick pan and grease with cooking spray. Pan fry fish in two batches cooking each side for a minute. Fish is best served with a side of salad greens or a half cup of cooked brown rice.

Nutrition Info: Calories per serving: 405; Protein: 27.5g; Fat: 11.9g; Carbs: 27.5

579.	Tuna And Tomato Salad

Servings: 6   Cooking Time: 10 Minutes

Ingredients:

½ cup white beans, canned, drained
4 oz tuna fillet
1 teaspoon fresh basil, chopped
1 scallion, chopped
½ cup cherry tomatoes, halved
4 Kalamata olives
¼ teaspoon ground black pepper

½ red onion, peeled, sliced
1 tablespoon sesame oil
½ tablespoon lemon juice
¼ tablespoon Dijon Mustard
½ teaspoon butter
½ teaspoon salt

Directions:

Rub the tuna fillet with ground black pepper and sprinkle with lemon juice. Place butter in the skillet and melt it. Add tuna and cook it for 8 minutes (for 4 minutes from each side) over the medium heat. After this, chill the cooked tuna well and chop. In the salad bowl, combine together white beans, chopped basil, scallion, halved cherry tomatoes, sliced red onion, and salt. Slice Kalamata olives and add in the salad bowl. Churn together Dijon mustard and sesame oil. The salad dressing is cooked. Shake the salad well and sprinkle with oil dressing. Mix up the cooked salad directly before serving.

Nutrition Info: Per Serving:calories 150, fat 5.1, fiber 3.2, carbs 12.1, protein 15

580.	Leftover Salmon Salad Power Bowls

Servings: 1   Cooking Time: 10 Minutes

Ingredients:

½ cup raspberries
½ cup zucchini, sliced
1 lemon, juice squeezed
1 tablespoon balsamic glaze
2 sprigs of thyme, chopped

2 tablespoon olive oil
4 cups seasonal greens
4 ounces leftover grilled salmon
Salt and pepper to taste

Directions:

Heat oil in a skillet over medium flame and sauté the zucchini. Season with salt and pepper to taste. In a mixing bowl, mix all ingredients together. Toss to combine everything. Sprinkle with nut cheese.

Nutrition Info: Calories per Serving: 450.3; Fat: 35.5 g; Protein: 23.4g; Carbs: 9.3 g

581. Roasted Pollock Fillet With Bacon And Leeks

Servings: 2   Cooking Time: 30 Minutes

Ingredients:

¼ cup olive oil
½ cup white wine
1 ½ lbs. Pollock fillets
1 sprig fresh thyme
1 tbsp chopped fresh thyme
2 tbsp. olive oil
4 leeks, sliced

Directions:

Grease a 9x13 baking dish and preheat oven to 4000F.   In baking pan add olive oil and leeks. Toss to combine.   Pop into the oven and roast for 10 minutes.   Remove from oven; add white wine and 1 tbsp chopped thyme. Return to oven and roast for another 10 minutes.   Remove pan from oven and add fish on top. With a spoon, spoon olive oil mixture onto fish until coated fully. Return to oven and roast for another ten minutes.   Remove from oven, garnish with a sprig of thyme and serve.

Nutrition Info: Calories per Serving: 442; Carbs: 13.6 g; Protein: 42.9 g; Fat: 24 g

582. Coriander Shrimps

Servings: 6   Cooking Time: 5 Minutes

Ingredients:

1 hot chili pepper
¼ cup fresh coriander leaves
½ teaspoon ground cumin
2 garlic cloves, peeled
½ teaspoon salt
1 tablespoon lemon juice
2 tablespoons olive oil
2-pounds shrimps, peeled

Directions:

Place in the blender: hot chili pepper, fresh coriander leaves, ground cumin, garlic cloves, salt, lemon juice, and olive oil. Blend the spices until you get the smooth texture of the mixture.   After this, place peeled shrimps in the big bowl.   Pour the blended spice mass over the shrimps. Mix up well.   Then preheat skillet well.   Place the shrimps and all spicy mixture in the skillet. Roast the seafood for 5 minutes over the medium heat. Stir the shrimps with the help of the wooden spatula from time to time.   Then remove the shrimps from the heat and let them rest for 10 minutes before serving.

Nutrition Info: Per Serving:calories 223, fat 7.3, fiber 0.1, carbs 2.8, protein 34.6

583. Lemon Rainbow Trout

Servings: 2   Cooking Time: 15 Minutes

Ingredients:

2 rainbow trout
Juice of 1 lemon
3 tablespoons olive oil
4 garlic cloves, minced
A pinch of salt and black pepper

Directions:

Line a baking sheet with parchment paper, add the fish and the rest of the ingredients and rub.   Bake at 400 degrees F for 15 minutes, divide between plates and serve with a side salad.

Nutrition Info: calories 521, fat 29, fiber 5, carbs 14, protein 52

584. Salmon With Pesto

Servings: 1 Fillet   Cooking Time: 10 Minutes

Ingredients:

2 cups fresh basil
2 cloves garlic
4 TB. fresh lemon juice
1 tsp. salt
1 tsp. ground black pepper
3 TB. grated Parmesan cheese
3 TB. toasted pine nuts
1/4 cup plus 2 TB. extra-virgin olive oil
2 (6-oz.) salmon fillets
1/2 medium lemon

Directions:

In a food processor fitted with a chopping blade, pulse basil, garlic, 2 tablespoons lemon juice, 1/2 teaspoon salt, and 1/2 teaspoon black pepper 15 times.   Add Parmesan cheese, pine nuts, and 1/4 cup extra-virgin olive oil, and pulse 15 more times. Set aside.   Set salmon fillets on a plate. Drizzle both sides with remaining 2 tablespoons lemon juice, and season with remaining 1/2 teaspoon salt and remaining 1/2 teaspoon black pepper.   In a large, nonstick skillet over medium heat, heat remaining 2 tablespoons extra-virgin olive oil. Add salmon, and cook for 5 minutes per side.   Place salmon on a serving plate, spoon 2 tablespoons pesto over each piece, and serve warm.

585. Baked Sea Bass

Servings: 4   Cooking Time: 12 Minutes

Ingredients:

4 sea bass fillets, boneless
Sal and black pepper to the taste
2 cups potato chips, crushed
1 tablespoon mayonnaise

Directions:

Season the fish fillets with salt and pepper, brush with the mayonnaise and dredge each in the potato chips.   Arrange the fillets on a baking sheet lined with parchment paper and bake at 400 degrees F for 12 minutes.   Divide the fish between plates and serve with a side salad.

Nutrition Info: calories 228, fat 8.6, fiber 0.6, carbs 9.3, protein 25

586. Italian Tuna Pasta

Servings: 6   Cooking Time: 5 Minutes

Ingredients:

15 oz whole wheat pasta
2 tbsp capers
2 cups can tomatoes, crushed
3 oz tuna
2 anchovies
1 tsp garlic, minced
1 tbsp olive oil
Salt

Directions:

Add oil into the inner pot of instant pot and set the pot on sauté mode.   Add anchovies and garlic and sauté for 1 minute.   Add remaining ingredients and stir well. Pour enough water into the pot to cover the pasta.   Seal pot with a lid and select manual and cook on low for 4 minutes. Once done, release pressure using quick release. Remove lid.   Stir and serve.

Nutrition Info: Calories 339 Fat 6 g Carbohydrates 56.5 g Sugar 5.2 g Protein 15.2 g Cholesterol 10 mg

587. Mustard Cod

Servings: 2   Cooking Time: 20 Minutes

Ingredients:

1 tablespoon Dijon mustard
2 teaspoons
¾ cup black olives, chopped

sunflower oil
1 white onion, diced
1/3 teaspoon minced garlic
2 tomatoes, chopped

1 teaspoon capers, drained
1 tablespoon fresh parsley
10 oz cod fillets (5 oz each fish fillet)

Directions:
Preheat sunflower oil in the skillet over the medium heat.   Then place the fish fillets in the hot oil and roast them for 2 minutes from each side. Transfer the fish in the plate.   After this, add diced onion in the skillet.   Then add minced garlic, tomatoes, and capers. Mix up well and close the lid.   Cook the vegetables for 5 minutes over the medium heat.   Then ad roasted cod fillets and stir puttanesca well.   Close the lid and cook the meal for 10 minutes over the medium-low heat. Transfer the cooked cod in the serving plates and top with the cooked vegetables.
Nutrition Info: Per Serving:calories 285, fat 12.2, fiber 4.7, carbs 13.9, protein 32.6

588.   Ginger Scallion Sauce Over Seared Ahi

Servings: 4   Cooking Time: 6 Minutes
Ingredients:
1 bunch scallions, bottoms removed, finely chopped
1 tbsp rice wine vinegar
1 tbsp. Bragg's liquid amino

16-oz ahi tuna steaks
2 tbsp. fresh ginger, peeled and grated
3 tbsp. coconut oil, melted
Pepper and salt to taste

Directions:
In a small bowl mix together vinegar, 2 tbsp. oil, soy sauce, ginger and scallions. Put aside.   On medium fire, place a large saucepan and heat remaining oil. Once oil is hot and starts to smoke, sear tuna until deeply browned or for two minutes per side.   Place seared tuna on a serving platter and let it stand for 5 minutes before slicing into 1-inch thick strips.   Drizzle ginger-scallion mixture over seared tuna, serve and enjoy.
Nutrition Info: Calories per Serving: 247; Protein: 29g; Fat: 1g; Carbs: 8g

589.   Creamy Scallops

Servings: 4   Cooking Time: 7 Minutes
Ingredients:
1 teaspoon fresh rosemary
½ teaspoon dried cumin
½ teaspoon garlic, diced

½ cup heavy cream
8 oz bay scallops
1 teaspoon olive oil
½ teaspoon salt
¼ teaspoon chili flakes

Directions:
Preheat olive oil in the skillet until hot.   Then sprinkle scallops with salt, chili flakes, and dried cumin and place in the hot oil.   Add fresh rosemary and diced garlic.   Roast the scallops for 2 minutes from each side.   After this, add heavy cream and bring the mixture to boil. Boil it for 1 minute.
Nutrition Info: Per Serving:calories 114, fat 7.3, fiber 0.2, carbs 2.2, protein 9.9

590.   Fish And Rice (sayadieh)

Servings: 1 Cup   Cooking Time: 1½hours
Ingredients:
1 lb. whitefish fillets (cod, tilapia, or haddock)
2 tsp. salt
2 tsp. ground black pepper
1/4 cup plus 2 TB. extra-virgin olive oil
2 large yellow onions, sliced

5 cups water
1 tsp. turmeric
1 tsp. ground coriander
1/2 tsp. ground cumin
1/4 tsp. ground cinnamon
2 cups basmati rice
1/2 cup sliced almonds

Directions:
Season both sides of whitefish with 1 teaspoon salt and 1 teaspoon black pepper.   In a skillet over medium heat, heat 1/4 cup extra-virgin olive oil. Add fish, and cook for 3 minutes per side. Remove fish from the pan.   Add yellow onions to the skillet, reduce heat to medium-low, and cook for 15 minutes or until golden brown and caramelized. In a 3-quart pot over medium heat, add 1/2 of cooked onions, water, turmeric, coriander, cumin, cinnamon, remaining 1 teaspoon salt, and remaining 1 teaspoon black pepper. Simmer for 20 minutes.   Add basmati rice, cover, and cook for 30 minutes.   Cut fish into 1/2-inch pieces, fluff rice, and gently fold fish into rice. Cover and cook for 10 more minutes.   Remove from heat, and let sit for 10 minutes before serving.   Meanwhile, in a small saucepan over low heat, heat remaining 2 tablespoons extra-virgin olive oil. Add almonds, and toast for 3 minutes.   Spoon fish and rice onto a serving plate, top with remaining onions and toasted almonds, and serve.

591.   Creamy Bacon-fish Chowder

Servings: 8   Cooking Time: 30 Minutes
Ingredients:
1 1/2 lbs. cod
1 1/2 tsp dried thyme
1 large onion, chopped
1 medium carrot, coarsely chopped
1 tbsp butter, cut into small pieces
3 1/2 cups baking potato, peeled and cubed

1 tsp salt, divided
3 slices uncooked bacon
3/4 tsp freshly ground black pepper, divided
4 1/2 cups water
4 bay leaves
4 cups 2% reduced-fat milk

Directions:
In a large skillet, add the water and bay leaves and let it simmer. Add the fish. Cover and let it simmer some more until the flesh flakes easily with fork. Remove the fish from the skillet and cut into large pieces. Set aside the cooking liquid.   Place Dutch oven in medium heat and cook the bacon until crisp. Remove the bacon and reserve the bacon drippings. Crush the bacon and set aside.   Stir potato, onion and carrot in the pan with the bacon drippings, cook over medium heat for 10 minutes. Add the cooking liquid, bay leaves, 1/2 tsp salt, 1/4 tsp pepper and thyme, let it boil. Lower the heat and let simmer for 10 minutes. Add the milk and butter, simmer until the potatoes becomes tender, but do not boil. Add the fish, 1/2 tsp salt, 1/2 tsp pepper.

Remove the bay leaves.   Serve sprinkled with the crushed bacon.

Nutrition Info: Calories per serving: 400; Carbs: 34.5g; Protein: 20.8g; Fat: 19.7g

592.   Healthy Poached Trout

Servings: 2   Cooking Time: 10 Minutes

Ingredients:

1 8-oz boneless, skin on trout fillet	2 leeks, halved
2 cups chicken broth or water	6-8 slices lemon
	salt and pepper to taste

Directions:

On medium fire, place a large nonstick skillet and arrange leeks and lemons on pan in a layer. Cover with soup stock or water and bring to a simmer. Meanwhile, season trout on both sides with pepper and salt. Place trout on simmering pan of water. Cover and cook until trout is flaky, around 8 minutes.   In a serving platter, spoon leek and lemons on bottom of plate, top with trout and spoon sauce into plate. Serve and enjoy.

Nutrition Info: Calories per serving: 360.2; Protein: 13.8g; Fat: 7.5g; Carbs: 51.5g

593.   Creamy Curry Salmon

Servings: 2   Cooking Time: 20 Minutes

Ingredients:

2 salmon fillets, boneless and cubed	1 cup Greek yogurt
1 tablespoon olive oil	2 teaspoons curry powder
1 tablespoon basil, chopped	1 garlic clove, minced
Sea salt and black pepper to the taste	½ teaspoon mint, chopped

Directions:

Heat up a pan with the oil over medium-high heat, add the salmon and cook for 3 minutes.   Add the rest of the ingredients, toss, cook for 15 minutes more, divide between plates and serve.

Nutrition Info:calories 284, fat 14.1, fiber 8.5, carbs 26.7, protein 31.4

594.   Cod And Cabbage

Servings: 4   Cooking Time: 15 Minutes

Ingredients:

3 cups green cabbage, shredded	1 sweet onion, sliced
A pinch of salt and black pepper	4 teaspoons olive oil
½ cup feta cheese, crumbled	4 cod fillets, boneless
	¼ cup green olives, pitted and chopped

Directions:

Grease a roasting pan with the oil, add the fish, the cabbage and the rest of the ingredients, introduce in the pan and cook at 450 degrees F for 15 minutes. Divide the mix between plates and serve.

Nutrition Info:calories 270, fat 10, fiber 3, carbs 12, protein 31

595.   Pecan Salmon Fillets

Servings: 6   Cooking Time: 15 Minutes

Ingredients:

3 tablespoons olive oil	1 tablespoon lemon juice
3 tablespoons mustard	3 teaspoons parsley, chopped
5 teaspoons honey	Salt and pepper to the taste
1 cup pecans,	

chopped
6 salmon fillets, boneless

Directions:

In a bowl, mix the oil with the mustard and honey and whisk well.   Put the pecans and the parsley in another bowl.   Season the salmon fillets with salt and pepper, arrange them on a baking sheet lined with parchment paper, brush with the honey and mustard mix and top with the pecans mix. Introduce in the oven at 400 degrees F, bake for 15 minutes, divide between plates, drizzle the lemon juice on top and serve.

Nutrition Info:calories 282, fat 15.5, fiber 8.5, carbs 20.9, protein 16.8

596.   Shrimp And Mushrooms Mix

Servings: 4   Cooking Time: 12 Minutes

Ingredients:

1 pound shrimp, peeled and deveined	2 teaspoons ginger, minced
2 green onions, sliced	2 teaspoons garlic, minced
½ pound white mushrooms, sliced	3 tablespoons olive oil
2 tablespoons balsamic vinegar	2 tablespoons dill, chopped
2 tablespoons sesame seeds, toasted	

Directions:

Heat up a pan with the oil over medium-high heat, add the green onions and the garlic and sauté for 2 minutes.   Add the rest of the ingredients except the shrimp and cook for 6 minutes more.   Add the shrimp, cook for 4 minutes, divide everything between plates and serve.

Nutrition Info:calories 245, fat 8.5, fiber 45.8, carbs 11.8, protein 17.7

597.   Leeks And Calamari Mix

Servings: 6   Cooking Time: 15 Minutes

Ingredients:

2 tablespoon avocado oil	1 red onion, chopped
2 leeks, chopped	1 tablespoon parsley, chopped
Salt and black to the taste	1 tablespoon chives, chopped
1 pound calamari rings	2 tablespoons tomato paste

Directions:

Heat up a pan with the avocado oil over medium heat, add the leeks and the onion, stir and sauté for 5 minutes.   Add the rest of the ingredients, toss, simmer over medium heat for 10 minutes, divide into bowls and serve.

Nutrition Info:calories 238, fat 9, fiber 5.6, carbs 14.4, protein 8.4

598.   Cod With Lentils

Servings: 4   Cooking Time: 30 Minutes

Ingredients:

1 red pepper, chopped	1 teaspoon salt
1 yellow onion, diced	1 tablespoon tomato paste
1 teaspoon ground black pepper	1 teaspoon chili pepper
1 teaspoon butter	3 tablespoons fresh cilantro, chopped
1 jalapeno pepper, chopped	8 oz cod, chopped
½ cup lentils	

3 cups chicken stock

Directions:
Place butter, red pepper, onion, and ground black pepper in the saucepan. Roast the vegetables for 5 minutes over the medium heat. Then add chopped jalapeno pepper, lentils, and chili pepper. Mix up the mixture well and add chicken stock and tomato paste. Stir until homogenous. Add cod. Close the lid and cook chili for 20 minutes over the medium heat.

Nutrition Info: Per Serving:calories 187, fat 2.3, fiber 8.8, carbs 21.3, protein 20.6

---

599.   Honey Garlic Shrimp

Servings: 4   Cooking Time: 5 Minutes

Ingredients:

1 lb shrimp, peeled and deveined	1 tbsp olive oil
1/4 cup honey	1/4 cup fish stock
1 tbsp garlic, minced	Pepper
1 tbsp ginger, minced	Salt

Directions:
Add shrimp into the large bowl. Add remaining ingredients over shrimp and toss well. Transfer shrimp into the instant pot and stir well. Seal pot with lid and cook on high for 5 minutes. Once done, release pressure using quick release. Remove lid. Serve and enjoy.

Nutrition Info: Calories 240 Fat 5.6 g Carbohydrates 20.9 g Sugar 17.5 g Protein 26.5 g Cholesterol 239 mg

---

600.   Pepper Salmon Skewers

Servings: 5   Cooking Time: 15 Minutes

Ingredients:

1.5-pound salmon fillet	1 teaspoon dried cilantro
½ cup Plain yogurt	1 teaspoon sunflower oil
1 teaspoon paprika	½ teaspoon ground nutmeg
1 teaspoon turmeric	
1 teaspoon red pepper	
1 teaspoon salt	

Directions:
For the marinade: mix up together Plain yogurt, paprika, turmeric red pepper, salt, and ground nutmeg. Chop the salmon fillet roughly and put it in the yogurt mixture. Mix up well and marinate for 25 minutes. Then skew the fish on the skewers. Sprinkle the skewers with sunflower oil and place in the tray. Bake the salmon skewers for 15 minutes at 375F.

Nutrition Info: Per Serving:calories 217, fat 9.9, fiber 0.6, carbs 4.2, protein 28.1

Beans & Grains Recipes

601. Curried Chicken, Chickpeas And Raita Salad

Servings: 8   Cooking Time: 15 Minutes

Ingredients:

1 cup red grapes, halved
3-4 cups rotisserie chicken, meat coarsely shredded
2 tbsp cilantro
1 cup plain yogurt
2 medium tomatoes, chopped
1 tsp ground cumin
1 tbsp curry powder
2 tbsp olive oil
1 tbsp minced peeled ginger
1 medium onion, chopped
1 tbsp minced garlic
¼ tsp cayenne
½ tsp turmeric
1 tsp ground cumin
1 19-oz can chickpeas, rinsed, drained and patted dry
1 tbsp olive oil
½ cup sliced and toasted almonds
2 tbsp chopped mint
2 cups cucumber, peeled, cored and chopped
1 cup plain yogurt

Directions:

To make the chicken salad, on medium low fire, place a medium nonstick saucepan and heat oil. Sauté ginger, garlic and onion for 5 minutes or until softened while stirring occasionally. Add 1 ½ tsp salt, cumin and curry. Sauté for two minutes. Increase fire to medium high and add tomatoes. Stirring frequently, cook for 5 minutes. Pour sauce into a bowl, mix in chicken, cilantro and yogurt. Stir to combine and let it stand to cool to room temperature. To make the chickpeas, on a nonstick fry pan, heat oil for 3 minutes. Add chickpeas and cook for a minute while stirring frequently. Add ¼ tsp salt, cayenne, turmeric and cumin. Stir to mix well and cook for two minutes or until sauce is dried. Transfer to a bowl and let it cool to room temperature. To make the raita, mix ½ tsp salt, mint, cucumber and yogurt. Stir thoroughly to combine and dissolve salt. To assemble, in four 16-oz lidded jars or bowls layer the following: curried chicken, raita, chickpeas and garnish with almonds. You can make this recipe one day ahead and refrigerate for 6 hours before serving.

Nutrition Info: Calories per serving: 381; Protein: 36.1g; Carbs: 27.4g; Fat: 15.5g

602. Bulgur Tomato Pilaf

Servings: 1 Cup   Cooking Time: 27 Minutes

Ingredients:

1 lb. ground beef
3 TB. extra-virgin olive oil
1 large yellow onion, finely chopped
2 medium tomatoes, diced
11/2 tsp. salt
1 tsp. ground black pepper
2 cups plain tomato sauce
2 cups water
2 cups bulgur wheat, grind #2

Directions:

In a large, 3-quart pot over medium heat, brown beef for 5 minutes, breaking up chunks with a wooden spoon. Add extra-virgin olive oil and yellow onion, and cook for 5 minutes. Stir in tomatoes, salt, and black pepper, and cook for 5 minutes. Add tomato sauce and water, and simmer for 10 minutes. Add bulgur wheat, and cook for 2 minutes. Remove from heat, cover, and let sit for 5 minutes. Uncover, fluff bulgur with a fork, cover, and let sit for 5 more minutes. Serve warm.

603. Garbanzo And Kidney Bean Salad

Servings: 4   Cooking Time: 0 Minutes

Ingredients:

1 (15 ounce) can kidney beans, drained
1 lemon, zested and juiced
1 medium tomato, chopped
1 teaspoon capers, rinsed and drained
1/2 cup chopped fresh parsley
1 (15.5 ounce) can garbanzo beans, drained
1/2 teaspoon salt, or to taste
1/4 cup chopped red onion
3 tablespoons extra virgin olive oil

Directions:

In a salad bowl, whisk well lemon juice, olive oil and salt until dissolved. Stir in garbanzo, kidney beans, tomato, red onion, parsley, and capers. Toss well to coat. Allow flavors to mix for 30 minutes by setting in the fridge. Mix again before serving.

Nutrition Info: Calories per serving: 329; Protein: 12.1g; Carbs: 46.6g; Fat: 12.0g

604. Rice & Currant Salad Mediterranean Style

Servings: 4   Cooking Time: 50 Minutes

Ingredients:

1 cup basmati rice
salt
2 1/2 Tablespoons lemon juice
1 teaspoon grated orange zest
2 Tablespoons fresh orange juice
1/4 cup olive oil
1/2 teaspoon cinnamon
Salt and pepper to taste
4 chopped green onions
1/2 cup dried currants
3/4 cup shelled pistachios or almonds
1/4 cup chopped fresh parsley

Directions:

Place a nonstick pot on medium high fire and add rice. Toast rice until opaque and starts to smell, around 10 minutes. Add 4 quarts of boiling water to pot and 2 tsp salt. Boil until tender, around 8 minutes uncovered. Drain the rice and spread out on a lined cookie sheet to cool completely. In a large salad bowl, whisk well the oil, juices and spices. Add salt and pepper to taste. Add half of the green onions, half of parsley, currants, and nuts. Toss with the cooled rice and let stand for at least 20 minutes. If needed adjust seasoning with pepper and salt. Garnish with remaining parsley and green onions.

Nutrition Info: Calories per serving: 450; Carbs: 50.0g; Protein: 9.0g; Fat: 24.0g

605. Stuffed Tomatoes With Green Chili

Servings: 6   Cooking Time: 55 Minutes

Ingredients:

4 oz Colby-Jack shredded cheese	1 tbsp fresh lime juice
¼ cup water	1 tbsp olive oil
1 cup uncooked quinoa	1 tbsp chopped fresh oregano
6 large ripe tomatoes	1 cup chopped onion
¼ tsp freshly ground black pepper	2 cups fresh corn kernels
¾ tsp ground cumin	2 poblano chilies
1 tsp salt, divided	

Directions:

Preheat broiler to high.   Slice lengthwise the chilies and press on a baking sheet lined with foil. Broil for 8 minutes. Remove from oven and let cool for 10 minutes. Peel the chilies and chop coarsely and place in medium sized bowl.   Place onion and corn in baking sheet and broil for ten minutes. Stir two times while broiling. Remove from oven and mix in with chopped chilies.   Add black pepper, cumin, ¼ tsp salt, lime juice, oil and oregano. Mix well.   Cut off the tops of tomatoes and set aside. Leave the tomato shell intact as you scoop out the tomato pulp.   Drain tomato pulp as you press down with a spoon. Reserve 1 ¼ cups of tomato pulp liquid and discard the rest. Invert the tomato shells on a wire rack for 30 mins and then wipe the insides dry with a paper towel.   Season with ½ tsp salt the tomato pulp.   On a sieve over a bowl, place quinoa. Add water until it covers quinoa. Rub quinoa grains for 30 seconds together with hands; rinse and drain. Repeat this procedure two times and drain well at the end.   In medium saucepan bring to a boil remaining salt, ¼ cup water, quinoa and tomato liquid.   Once boiling, reduce heat and simmer for 15 minutes or until liquid is fully absorbed. Remove from heat and fluff quinoa with fork. Transfer and mix well the quinoa with the corn mixture.   Spoon ¾ cup of the quinoa-corn mixture into the tomato shells, top with cheese and cover with the tomato top. Bake in a preheated 350oF oven for 15 minutes and then broil high for another 1.5 minutes.

Nutrition Info: Calories per serving: 276; Carbs: 46.3g; Protein: 13.4g; Fat: 4.1g

606. Red Wine Risotto

Servings: 8   Cooking Time: 25 Minutes

Ingredients:

Pepper to taste	2 cloves garlic, minced
1 cup finely shredded Parmigian-Reggiano cheese, divided	1 medium onion, freshly chopped
2 tsp tomato paste	2 tbsp extra-virgin olive oil
1 ¾ cups dry red wine	4 ½ cups reduced sodium beef broth
¼ tsp salt	
1 ½ cups Italian 'risotto' rice	

Directions:

On medium high fire, bring to a simmer broth in a medium fry pan. Lower fire so broth is steaming but not simmering.   On medium low heat, place a Dutch oven and heat oil.   Sauté onions for 5 minutes. Add garlic and cook for 2 minutes.   Add rice, mix well, and season with salt.   Into rice, add a generous splash of wine and ½ cup of broth. Lower fire to a gentle simmer, cook until liquid is fully absorbed while stirring rice every once in a while.   Add another splash of wine and ½ cup of broth. Stirring once in a while.   Add tomato paste and stir to mix well.   Continue cooking and adding wine and broth until broth is used up. Once done cooking, turn off fire and stir in pepper and ¾ cup cheese.   To serve, sprinkle with remaining cheese and enjoy.

Nutrition Info: Calories per Serving: 231; Carbs: 33.9g; Protein: 7.9g; Fat: 5.7g

607. Chicken Pasta Parmesan

Servings: 1   Cooking Time: 20 Minutes

Ingredients:

¼ cup prepared marinara sauce	½ cup cooked whole wheat spaghetti
1 oz reduced fat mozzarella cheese, grated	2 tbsp seasoned dry breadcrumbs
1 tbsp olive oil	4 oz skinless chicken breast

Directions:

On medium high fire, place an ovenproof skillet and heat oil.   Pan fry chicken for 3 to 5 minutes per side or until cooked through.   Pour marinara sauce, stir and continue cooking for 3 minutes. Turn off fire, add mozzarella and breadcrumbs on top.   Pop into a preheated broiler on high and broil for 10 minutes or until breadcrumbs are browned and mozzarella is melted.   Remove from broiler, serve and enjoy.

Nutrition Info: Calories per Serving: 529; Carbs: 34.4g; Protein: 38g; Fat: 26.6g

608. Orange, Dates And Asparagus On Quinoa Salad

Servings: 8   Cooking Time: 25 Minutes

Ingredients:

¼ cup chopped pecans, toasted	2 cups water
½ cup white onion, finely chopped	5 dates, pitted and chopped
½ jalapeno pepper, diced	¼ tsp freshly ground black pepper
½ lb. asparagus, sliced into 2-inch lengths, steamed and chilled	¼ tsp salt
	1 garlic clove, minced
½ tsp salt	1 tbsp extra virgin olive oil
1 cup fresh orange sections	2 tbsp chopped fresh mint
1 cup uncooked quinoa	2 tbsp fresh lemon juice
1 tsp olive oil	Mint sprigs – optional
2 tbsp minced red onion	

Directions:

On medium high fire, place a large nonstick pan and heat 1 tsp oil.   Add white onion and sauté for two minutes.   Add quinoa and for 5 minutes sauté it.   Add salt and water. Bring to a boil, once boiling, slow fire to a simmer and cook for 15 minutes while covered.   Turn off fire and leave for 15 minutes, to let quinoa absorb the remaining water.   Transfer quinoa to a large salad bowl. Add jalapeno pepper, asparagus, dates, red onion,

pecans and oranges. Toss to combine. Make the dressing by mixing garlic, pepper, salt, olive oil and lemon juice in a small bowl. Pour dressing into quinoa salad along with chopped mint, mix well. If desired, garnish with mint sprigs before serving.
Nutrition Info: Calories per Serving: 265.2; Carbs: 28.3g; Protein: 14.6g; Fat: 10.4g

609. Tasty Lasagna Rolls

Servings: 6   Cooking Time: 20 Minutes
Ingredients:

¼ tsp crushed red pepper	¼ tsp salt
½ cup shredded mozzarella cheese	1 tbsp extra virgin olive oil
½ cups parmesan cheese, shredded	12 whole wheat lasagna noodles
1 14-oz package tofu, cubed	2 tbsp Kalamata olives, chopped
1 25-oz can of low-sodium marinara sauce	3 cloves minced garlic
	3 cups spinach, chopped

Directions:
Put enough water on a large pot and cook the lasagna noodles according to package instructions. Drain, rinse and set aside until ready to use. In a large skillet, sauté garlic over medium heat for 20 seconds. Add the tofu and spinach and cook until the spinach wilts. Transfer this mixture in a bowl and add parmesan olives, salt, red pepper and 2/3 cup of the marinara sauce. In a pan, spread a cup of marinara sauce on the bottom. To make the rolls, place noodle on a surface and spread ¼ cup of the tofu filling. Roll up and place it on the pan with the marinara sauce. Do this procedure until all lasagna noodles are rolled. Place the pan over high heat and bring to a simmer. Reduce the heat to medium and let it cook for three more minutes. Sprinkle mozzarella cheese and let the cheese melt for two minutes. Serve hot.
Nutrition Info: Calories per Serving: 304; Carbs: 39.2g; Protein: 23g; Fat: 19.2g

610. Raisins, Nuts And Beef On Hashweh Rice

Servings: 8   Cooking Time: 50 Minutes
Ingredients:

½ cup dark raisins, soaked in 2 cups water for an hour	½ cup fresh parsley leaves, roughly chopped
1/3 cup slivered almonds, toasted and soaked in 2 cups water overnight	¾ tsp cloves, divided
1/3 cup pine nuts, toasted and soaked in 2 cups water overnight	1 tsp garlic powder
Pepper and salt to taste	1 ¾ tsp allspice, divided
¾ tsp ground cinnamon, divided	1 lb. lean ground beef or lean ground lamb
	1 small red onion, finely chopped
	Olive oil
	1 ½ cups medium grain rice

Directions:
For 15 to 20 minutes, soak rice in cold water. You will know that soaking is enough when you can snap a grain of rice easily between your thumb and index finger. Once soaking is done, drain rice well. Meanwhile, drain pine nuts, almonds and raisins

for at least a minute and transfer to one bowl. Set aside. On a heavy cooking pot on medium high fire, heat 1 tbsp olive oil. Once oil is hot, add red onions. Sauté for a minute before adding ground meat and sauté for another minute. Season ground meat with pepper, salt, ½ tsp ground cinnamon, ½ tsp ground cloves, 1 tsp garlic powder, and 1 ¼ tsp allspice. Sauté ground meat for 10 minutes or until browned and cooked fully. Drain fat. In same pot with cooked ground meat, add rice on top of meat. Season with a bit of pepper and salt. Add remaining cinnamon, ground cloves, and allspice. Do not mix. Add 1 tbsp olive oil and 2 ½ cups of water. Bring to a boil and once boiling, lower fire to a simmer. Cook while covered until liquid is fully absorbed, around 20 to 25 minutes. Turn of fire. To serve, place a large serving platter that fully covers the mouth of the pot. Place platter upside down on mouth of pot, and invert pot. The inside of the pot should now rest on the platter with the rice on bottom of plate and ground meat on top of it. Garnish the top of the meat with raisins, almonds, pine nuts, and parsley. Serve and enjoy.
Nutrition Info: Calories per serving: 357; Carbs: 39.0g; Protein: 16.7g; Fat: 15.9g

611. Yangchow Chinese Style Fried Rice

Servings: 4   Cooking Time: 20 Minutes
Ingredients:

4 cups cold cooked rice	1/2 cup peas
1 medium yellow onion, diced	5 tbsp olive oil
	6 oz roast pork
4 oz frozen medium shrimp, thawed, shelled, deveined and chopped finely	3 large eggs
	Salt and freshly ground black pepper
	1/2 tsp cornstarch

Directions:
Combine the salt and ground black pepper and 1/2 tsp cornstarch, coat the shrimp with it. Chop the roasted pork. Beat the eggs and set aside. Stir-fry the shrimp in a wok on high fire with 1 tbsp heated oil until pink, around 3 minutes. Set the shrimp aside and stir fry the roasted pork briefly. Remove both from the pan. In the same pan, stir-fry the onion until soft, Stir the peas and cook until bright green. Remove both from pan. Add 2 tbsp oil in the same pan, add the cooked rice. Stir and separate the individual grains. Add the beaten eggs, toss the rice. Add the roasted pork, shrimp, vegetables and onion. Toss everything together. Season with salt and pepper to taste.
Nutrition Info: Calories per serving: 556; Carbs: 60.2g; Protein: 20.2g; Fat: 25.2g

612. Cinnamon Quinoa Bars

Servings: 4   Cooking Time: 30 Minutes
Ingredients:

2 ½ cups cooked quinoa	4 large eggs
1/3 cup unsweetened almond milk	Seeds from ½ whole vanilla bean pod or 1 tbsp vanilla extract
1/3 cup pure maple syrup	1 ½ tbsp cinnamon
	1/4 tsp salt

Directions:

Preheat oven to 3750F.   Combine all ingredients into large bowl and mix well.   In an 8 x 8 Baking pan, cover with parchment paper.   Pour batter evenly into baking dish.   Bake for 25-30 minutes or until it has set. It should not wiggle when you lightly shake the pan because the eggs are fully cooked.   Remove as quickly as possible from pan and parchment paper onto cooling rack.   Cut into 4 pieces.   Enjoy on its own, with a small spread of almond or nut butter or wait until it cools to enjoy the next morning.
Nutrition Info: Calories per serving: 285; Carbs: 46.2g; Protein: 8.5g; Fat: 7.4g

613.   Cucumber Olive Rice

Servings: 8   Cooking Time: 10 Minutes
Ingredients:

2 cups rice, rinsed	2 tbsp olive oil
1/2 cup olives, pitted	2 cups vegetable broth
1 cup cucumber, chopped	1/2 tsp dried oregano
1 tbsp red wine vinegar	1 red bell pepper, chopped
1 tsp lemon zest, grated	1/2 cup onion, chopped
1 tbsp fresh lemon juice	1 tbsp olive oil
	Pepper
	Salt

Directions:
Add oil into the inner pot of instant pot and set the pot on sauté mode.   Add onion and sauté for 3 minutes.   Add bell pepper and oregano and sauté for 1 minute.   Add rice and broth and stir well. Seal pot with lid and cook on high for 6 minutes. Once done, allow to release pressure naturally for 10 minutes then release remaining using quick release. Remove lid.   Add remaining ingredients and stir everything well to mix.   Serve immediately and enjoy it.
Nutrition Info: Calories 229 Fat 5.1 g Carbohydrates 40.2 g Sugar 1.6 g Protein 4.9 g Cholesterol 0 mg

614.   Chorizo-kidney Beans Quinoa Pilaf

Servings: 4   Cooking Time: 35 Minutes
Ingredients:

¼ pound dried Spanish chorizo diced (about 2/3 cup)	1 large clove garlic minced
¼ teaspoon red pepper flakes	1 small red bell pepper finely diced
¼ teaspoon smoked paprika	1 small red onion finely diced
½ teaspoon cumin	1 tablespoon tomato paste
½ teaspoon sea salt	1 15-ounce can kidney beans rinsed and drained
1 3/4 cups water	
1 cup quinoa	

Directions:
Place a nonstick pot on medium high fire and heat for 2 minutes. Add chorizo and sauté for 5 minutes until lightly browned.   Stir in peppers and onion. Sauté for 5 minutes.   Add tomato paste, red pepper flakes, salt, paprika, cumin, and garlic. Sauté for 2 minutes.   Stir in quinoa and mix well. Sauté for 2 minutes.   Add water and beans. Mix well. Cover and simmer for 20 minutes or until liquid is fully absorbed.   Turn off fire and fluff

quinoa. Let it sit for 5 minutes more while uncovered.   Serve and enjoy.
Nutrition Info: Calories per serving: 260; Protein: 9.6g; Carbs: 40.9g; Fat: 6.8g

615.   Belly-filling Cajun Rice & Chicken

Servings: 6   Cooking Time: 20 Minutes
Ingredients:

1 tablespoon oil	1 tablespoon tomato paste
1 onion, diced	
3 cloves of garlic, minced	2 cups chicken broth
1-pound chicken breasts, sliced	1 ½ cups white rice, rinsed
1 tablespoon Cajun seasoning	1 bell pepper, chopped

Directions:
Press the Sauté on the Instant Pot and pour the oil. Sauté the onion and garlic until fragrant.   Stir in the chicken breasts and season with Cajun seasoning.   Continue cooking for 3 minutes. Add the tomato paste and chicken broth. Dissolve the tomato paste before adding the rice and bell pepper.   Close the lid and press the rice button. Once done cooking, do a natural release for 10 minutes.   Then, do a quick release.   Once cooled, evenly divide into serving size, keep in your preferred container, and refrigerate until ready to eat.
Nutrition Info: Calories per serving: 337; Carbohydrates: 44.3g; Protein: 26.1g; Fat: 5.0g

616.   Chicken And White Bean

Servings: 8   Cooking Time: 70 Minutes
Ingredients:

2 tbsp fresh cilantro, chopped	1 cup corn kernels
2 cups grated Monterey Jack cheese	2 15-oz cans shite beans, drained and rinsed
3 cups water	2 garlic cloves
1/8 tsp cayenne pepper	1 medium onion, diced
2 tsp pure chile powder	2 tbsp extra virgin olive oil
2 tsp ground cumin	1 lb. chicken breasts, boneless and skinless
1 4-oz can chopped green chiles	

Directions:
Slice chicken breasts into ½-inch cubes and with pepper and salt, season it.   On high fire, place a large nonstick fry pan and heat oil.   Sauté chicken pieces for three to four minutes or until lightly browned.   Reduce fire to medium and add garlic and onion.   Cook for 5 to 6 minutes or until onions are translucent.   Add water, spices, chilies, corn and beans. Bring to a boil.   Once boiling, slow fire to a simmer and continue simmering for an hour, uncovered.   To serve, garnish with a sprinkling of cilantro and a tablespoon of cheese.
Nutrition Info: Calories per serving: 433; Protein: 30.6g; Carbs: 29.5g; Fat: 21.8g

617.Quinoa & Black Bean Stuffed Sweet Potatoes

Servings: 8   Cooking Time: 60 Minutes
Ingredients:

4 sweet potatoes	1 tbsp chili powder
½ onion, diced	

1 garlic glove, crushed and diced
½ large bell pepper diced (about 2/3 cups)
Handful of diced cilantro
½ cup cooked quinoa
½ cup black beans
1 tbsp olive oil

½ tbsp cumin
½ tbsp paprika
½ tbsp oregano
2 tbsp lime juice
2 tbsp honey
Sprinkle salt
1 cup shredded cheddar cheese
Chopped spring onions, for garnish (optional)

Directions:
Preheat oven to 400oF.   Wash and scrub outside of potatoes. Poke with fork a few times and then place on parchment paper on cookie sheet. Bake for 40-45 minutes or until it is cooked.   While potatoes are baking, sauté onions, garlic, olive oil and spices in a pan on the stove until onions are translucent and soft.   In the last 10 minutes while the potatoes are cooking, in a large bowl combine the onion mixture with the beans, quinoa, honey, lime juice, cilantro and ½ cup cheese. Mix well. When potatoes are cooked, remove from oven and let cool slightly. When cool to touch, cut in half (hot dog style) and scoop out most of the insides. Leave a thin ring of potato so that it will hold its shape. You can save the sweet potato guts for another recipe, such as my veggie burgers (recipe posted below).   Fill with bean and quinoa mixture. Top with remaining cheddar cheese.   (If making this a freezer meal, stop here. Individually wrap potato skins in plastic wrap and place on flat surface to freeze. Once frozen, place all potatoes in large zip lock container or Tupperware.)   Return to oven for an additional 10 minutes or until cheese is melted.
Nutrition Info: Calories per serving: 243; Carbs: 37.6g; Protein: 8.5g; Fat: 7.3g

618.   Feta, Eggplant And Sausage Penne

Servings: 6   Cooking Time: 30 Minutes
Ingredients:
¼ cup chopped fresh parsley
½ cup crumbled feta cheese
6 cups hot cooked penne
1 14.5oz can diced tomatoes
1 tsp dried oregano

¼ tsp ground black pepper
2 tbsp tomato paste
4 garlic cloves, minced
½ lb. bulk pork breakfast sausage
4 ½ cups cubed peeled eggplant

Directions:
On medium high fire, place a nonstick, big fry pan and cook for seven minutes garlic, sausage and eggplant or until eggplants are soft and sausage are lightly browned.   Stir in diced tomatoes, black pepper, oregano and tomato paste. Cover and simmer for five minutes while occasionally stirring. Remove pan from fire, stir in pasta and mix well. Transfer to a serving dish, garnish with parsley and cheese before serving.
Nutrition Info: Calories per Serving: 376; Carbs: 50.8g; Protein: 17.8g; Fat: 11.6g

619.   Bell Peppers 'n Tomato-chickpea Rice

Servings: 4   Cooking Time: 35 Minutes
Ingredients:
2 tablespoons olive oil
1/2 chopped red bell pepper
1/2 chopped green bell pepper
1/2 chopped yellow pepper
1/2 chopped red pepper
1 medium onion, chopped

1 clove garlic, minced
2 cups cooked jasmine rice
1 teaspoon tomato paste
1 cup chickpeas
salt to taste
1/2 teaspoon paprika
1 small tomato, chopped
Parsley for garnish

Directions:
In a large mixing bowl, whisk well olive oil, garlic, tomato paste, and paprika. Season with salt generously.   Mix in rice and toss well to coat in the dressing.   Add remaining ingredients and toss well to mix.   Let salad rest to allow flavors to mix for 15 minutes.   Toss one more time and adjust salt to taste if needed.   Garnish with parsley and serve.
Nutrition Info: Calories per serving: 490; Carbs: 93.0g; Protein: 10.0g; Fat: 8.0g

620.   Lipsmacking Chicken Tetrazzini

Servings: 8   Cooking Time: 3 Hours
Ingredients:
Toasted French bread slices
¾ cup thinly sliced green onion
2/3 cup grated parmesan cheese
10 oz dried spaghetti or linguine, cooked and drained
¼ tsp ground nutmeg
¼ tsp ground black pepper

2 tbsp dry sherry
¼ cup chicken broth or water
1 16oz jar of Alfredo pasta sauce
2 4.5oz jars of sliced mushrooms, drained
2.5 lbs. skinless chicken breasts cut into ½ inch slices

Directions:
In a slow cooker, mix mushrooms and chicken. In a bowl, mix well nutmeg, pepper, sherry, broth and alfredo sauce before pouring over chicken and mushrooms.   Set on high heat, cover and cook for two to three hours.   Once chicken is cooked, pour over pasta, garnish with green onion and serve with French bread on the side.
Nutrition Info: Calories per Serving: 505; Carbs: 24.7g; Protein: 35.1g; Fat: 30.2g

621.   Spaghetti In Lemon Avocado White Sauce

Servings: 6   Cooking Time: 30 Minutes
Ingredients:
Freshly ground black pepper
Zest and juice of 1 lemon
1 avocado, pitted and peeled
1-pound spaghetti

Salt
1 tbsp Olive oil
8 oz small shrimp, shelled and deveined
¼ cup dry white wine
1 large onion, finely sliced

Directions:

Let a big pot of water boil. Once boiling add the spaghetti or pasta and cook following manufacturer's instructions until al dente. Drain and set aside. In a large fry pan, over medium fire sauté wine and onions for ten minutes or until onions are translucent and soft. Add the shrimps into the fry pan and increase fire to high while constantly sautéing until shrimps are cooked around five minutes. Turn the fire off. Season with salt and add the oil right away. Then quickly toss in the cooked pasta, mix well. In a blender, until smooth, puree the lemon juice and avocado. Pour into the fry pan of pasta, combine well. Garnish with pepper and lemon zest then serve.

Nutrition Info: Calories per Serving: 206; Carbs: 26.3g; Protein: 10.2g; Fat: 8.0g

622.   Kidney Beans And Beet Salad

Servings: 4   Cooking Time: 15 Minutes

Ingredients:

1 14.5-ounce can kidney beans, drained and rinsed	4 beets, scrubbed and stems removed
1 tablespoon pomegranate syrup or juice	4 green onions, chopped
2 tablespoons olive oil	Juice of 1 lemon
	Salt and pepper to taste

Directions:

Bring a pot of water to boil and add beets. Simmer for 10 minutes or until tender. Drain beets and place in ice bath for 5 minutes. Peel bets and slice in halves. Toss to mix the pomegranate syrup, olive oil, lemon juice, green onions, and kidney beans in a salad bowl. Stir in beets. Season with pepper and salt to taste. Serve and enjoy.

Nutrition Info: Calories per serving: 175; Protein: 6.0g; Carbs: 22.0g; Fat: 7.0g

623.   Filling Macaroni Soup

Servings: 6   Cooking Time: 45 Minutes

Ingredients:

1 cup of minced beef or chicken or a combination of both	2 cups broth (chicken, vegetable or beef)
1 cup carrots, diced	½ tbsp olive oil
1 cup milk	1 cup uncooked whole wheat pasta like macaroni, shells, even angel hair broken to pieces
½ medium onion, sliced thinly	
3 garlic cloves, minced	
Salt and pepper to taste	1 cup water

Directions:

In a heavy bottomed pot on medium high fire heat oil. Add garlic and sauté for a minute or two until fragrant but not browned. Add onions and sauté for 3 minutes or until soft and translucent. Add a cup of minced meat. You can also use whatever leftover frozen meat you have. Sauté the meat well until cooked around 8 minutes. While sautéing, season meat with pepper and salt. Add water and broth and bring to a boil. Once boiling, add pasta. I use any leftover pasta that I have in the pantry. If all you have left is spaghetti, lasagna, angel hair or fettuccine, just break them into pieces—around 1-inch in length before adding

to the pot. Slow fire to a simmer and cook while covered until pasta is soft. Halfway through cooking the pasta, around 8 minutes I add the carrots. Once the pasta is soft, turn off fire and add milk. Mix well and season to taste again if needed. Serve and enjoy.

Nutrition Info: Calories per Serving: 125; Carbs: 11.4g; Protein: 10.1g; Fat: 4.3g

624.   Simple Penne Anti-pasto

Servings: 4   Cooking Time: 15 Minutes

Ingredients:

¼ cup pine nuts, toasted	½ cup grated Parmigiano-Reggiano cheese, divided
8oz penne pasta, cooked and drained	3 oz chopped prosciutto
1 6oz jar drained, sliced, marinated and quartered artichoke hearts	1/3 cup pesto
	½ cup pitted and chopped Kalamata olives
1 7 oz jar drained and chopped sun-dried tomato halves packed in oil	1 medium red bell pepper

Directions:

Slice bell pepper, discard membranes, seeds and stem. On a foiled lined baking sheet, place bell pepper halves, press down by hand and broil in oven for eight minutes. Remove from oven, put in a sealed bag for 5 minutes before peeling and chopping. Place chopped bell pepper in a bowl and mix in artichokes, tomatoes, prosciutto, pesto and olives. Toss in ¼ cup cheese and pasta. Transfer to a serving dish and garnish with ¼ cup cheese and pine nuts. Serve and enjoy!

Nutrition Info: Calories per Serving: 606; Carbs: 70.3g; Protein: 27.2g; Fat: 27.6g

625.   Squash And Eggplant Casserole

Servings: 2   Cooking Time: 45 Minutes

Ingredients:

½ cup dry white wine	Salt and pepper to taste
1 eggplant, halved and cut to 1-inch slices	¼ cup parmesan cheese, grated
1 large onion, cut into wedges	1 cup instant polenta
1 red bell pepper, seeded and cut to julienned strips	2 tbsp fresh oregano, chopped
1 small butternut squash, cut into 1-inch slices	1 garlic clove, chopped
1 tbsp olive oil	2 tbsp slivered almonds
12 baby corn	5 tbsp parsley, chopped
2 cups low sodium vegetable broth	Grated zest of 1 lemon

Directions:

Preheat the oven to 350 degrees Fahrenheit. In a casserole, heat the oil and add the onion wedges and baby corn. Sauté over medium high heat for five minutes. Stir occasionally to prevent the onions and baby corn from sticking at the bottom of the pan. Add the butternut squash to the casserole and toss the vegetables. Add the eggplants and the red pepper. Cover the vegetables and cook over low to medium heat. Cook for about ten minutes before adding the wine. Let the wine sizzle before stirring in the broth. Bring to a boil and cook in the oven for 30 minutes. While the casserole is cooking inside the oven, make the topping by spreading the slivered almonds on a baking tray and toasting under the grill until they are lightly browned. Place the toasted almonds in a small bowl and mix the remaining ingredients for the toppings. Prepare the polenta. In a large saucepan, bring 3 cups of water to boil over high heat. Add the polenta and continue whisking until it absorbs all the water. Reduce the heat to medium until the polenta is thick. Add the parmesan cheese and oregano. Serve the polenta on plates and add the casserole on top. Sprinkle the toppings on top.

Nutrition Info: Calories per Serving: 579.3; Carbs: 79.2g; Protein: 22.2g; Fat: 19.3g

626. Blue Cheese And Grains Salad

Servings: 4   Cooking Time: 40 Minutes

Ingredients:

¼ cup thinly sliced scallions
½ cup millet, rinsed
½ cup quinoa, rinsed
1 ½ tsp olive oil
1 Bartlett pear, cored and diced
1/8 tsp ground black pepper
2 cloves garlic, minced
2 oz blue cheese
2 tbsp fresh lemon juice
2 tsp dried rosemary
4 4-oz boneless, skinless chicken breasts
6 oz baby spinach
olive oil cooking spray
¼ cup fresh raspberries
1 tbsp pure maple syrup
1 tsp fresh thyme leaf
2 tbsp grainy mustard
6 tbsp balsamic vinegar

Directions:

Bring millet, quinoa, and 2 ¼ cups water on a small saucepan to a boil. Once boiling, slow fire to a simmer and stir once. Cover and cook until water is fully absorbed and grains are soft around 15 minutes. Turn off fire, fluff grains with a fork and set aside to cool a bit. Arrange one oven rack to highest position and preheat broiler. Line a baking sheet with foil, and grease with cooking spray. Whisk well pepper, oil, rosemary, lemon juice and garlic. Rub onto chicken. Place chicken on prepared pan, pop into the broiler and broil until juices run clear and no longer pin inside around 12 minutes. Meanwhile, make the dressing by combining all ingredients in a blender. Blend until smooth. Remove chicken from oven, cool slightly before cutting into strips, against the grain. To assemble, place grains in a large salad bowl. Add in dressing and spinach, toss to mix well. Add scallions and pear, mix gently and evenly divide into four plates. Top each salad with cheese and chicken. Serve and enjoy.

Nutrition Info: Calories per Serving: 530.4; Carbs: 77g; Protein: 21.4g; Fat: 15.2g

627. Creamy Artichoke Lasagna

Servings: 8   Cooking Time: 70 Minutes

Ingredients:

1 cup shredded mozzarella cheese
2 cups light cream
¼ cup all-purpose flour
1 egg
4 cloves garlic, minced
½ cup pine nuts
3 tbsp olive oil
1 cup vegetable broth
¾ tsp salt
1 cup snipped fresh basil
1 cup finely shredded Parmesan cheese
1 15-oz carton ricotta cheese
9 dried lasagna noodles, cooked, rinsed in cold water and drained
15 fresh baby artichokes
¼ cup lemon juice
3 cups water

Directions:

Prepare in a medium bowl lemon juice and water. Put aside. Slice off artichoke base and remove yellowed outer leaves and cut into quarters. Immediately soak sliced artichokes in prepared liquid and drain after a minute. Over medium fire, place a big saucepan with 2 tbsp oil and fry half of garlic, pine nuts and artichokes. Stir frequently and cook until artichokes are soft around ten minutes. Turn off fire and transfer mixture to a big bowl and quickly stir in salt, egg, ½ cup of basil, ½ cup of parmesan cheese and ricotta cheese. Mix thoroughly. In a small bowl mix flour and broth. In same pan, add 1 tbsp oil and fry remaining garlic for half a minute. Add light cream and flour mixture. Stir constantly and cook until thickened. Remove from fire and stir in ½ cup of basil. In a separate bowl mix ½ cup parmesan and mozzarella cheese. Assemble the lasagna by layering the following in a greased rectangular glass dish: lasagna, 1/3 of artichoke mixture, 1/3 of sauce, sprinkle with the dried cheeses and repeat layering procedure until all ingredients are used up. For forty minutes, bake lasagna in a pre-heated oven of 350oF. Remove lasagna from oven and before serving, let it stand for fifteen minutes.

Nutrition Info: Calories per Serving: 425; Carbs: 41.4g; Protein: 21.3g; Fat: 19.8g

628. Brown Rice Pilaf With Butternut Squash

Servings: 8   Cooking Time: 50 Minutes

Ingredients:

Pepper to taste
A pinch of cinnamon
1 tsp salt
2 tbsp chopped fresh oregano
½ cup chopped fennel fronds
1 ¾ cups water + 2 tbsp, divided
1 cup instant or parboiled brown rice
½ cup white wine
1 tbsp tomato paste
1 garlic clove, minced
1 large onion, finely chopped
3 tbsp extra virgin olive oil
2 lbs. butternut squash, peeled, halved and seeded

Directions:

In a large hole grater, grate squash. On medium low fire, place a large nonstick skillet and heat oil for 2 minutes. Add garlic and onions. Sauté for 8 minutes or until lightly colored and soft. Add 2 tbsp water and tomato paste. Stir well to combine and cook for 3 minutes. Add rice, mix well to coat in mixture and cook for 5 minutes while stirring frequently. If needed, add squash in batches until it has wilted so that you can cover pan. Add remaining water and increase fire to medium high. Add wine, cover and boil. Once boiling, lower fire to a simmer and cook for 20 to 25 minutes or until liquid is fully absorbed. Stir in pepper, cinnamon, salt, oregano, and fennel fronds.

Turn off fire, cover and let it stand for 5 minutes before serving.
Nutrition Info: Calories per Serving: 147; Carbs: 22.1g; Protein: 2.3g; Fat: 5.5g

629. Cranberry And Roasted Squash Delight

Servings: 8   Cooking Time: 60 Minutes
Ingredients:

¼ cup chopped walnuts
¼ tsp thyme
½ tbsp chopped Italian parsley
1 cup diced onion
1 cup fresh cranberries
1 small orange, peeled and segmented
2 tsp canola oil, divided
4 cups cooked wild rice
4 cups diced winter squash, peeled and cut into ½-inch cubes
Pepper to taste

Directions:
Grease roasting pan with cooking spray and preheat oven to 400oF.   In prepped roasting pan place squash cubes, add a teaspoon of oil and toss to coat. Place in oven and roast until lightly browned, around 40 minutes.   On medium high fire, place a nonstick fry pan and heat remaining oil. Once hot, add onions and sauté until lightly browned and tender, around 5 minutes.   Add cranberries and continue stir frying for a minute. Add remaining ingredients into pan and cook until heated through around four to five minutes.   Best served warm.
Nutrition Info: Calories per Serving: 166.2; Protein: 4.8g; Carbs: 29.1g; Fat: 3.4g

630. Spanish Rice Casserole With Cheesy Beef

Servings: 2   Cooking Time: 32 Minutes
Ingredients:

2 tablespoons chopped green bell pepper
1/4 teaspoon Worcestershire sauce
1/4 teaspoon ground cumin
1/4 cup shredded Cheddar cheese
1/4 cup finely chopped onion
1/4 cup chile sauce
1/3 cup uncooked long grain rice
1/2-pound lean ground beef
1/2 teaspoon salt
1/2 teaspoon brown sugar
1/2 pinch ground black pepper
1/2 cup water
1/2 (14.5 ounce) can canned tomatoes
1 tablespoon chopped fresh cilantro

Directions:
Place a nonstick saucepan on medium fire and brown beef for 10 minutes while crumbling beef. Discard fat.   Stir in pepper, Worcestershire sauce, cumin, brown sugar, salt, chile sauce, rice, water, tomatoes, green bell pepper, and onion. Mix well and cook for 10 minutes until blended and a bit tender.   Transfer to an ovenproof casserole and press down firmly. Sprinkle cheese on top and cook for 7 minutes at 400oF preheated oven. Broil for 3 minutes until top is lightly browned.   Serve and enjoy with chopped cilantro.
Nutrition Info: Calories per serving: 460; Carbohydrates: 35.8g; Protein: 37.8g; Fat: 17.9g

631. Kidney Bean And Parsley-lemon Salad

Servings: 6   Cooking Time: 0 Minutes
Ingredients:

¼ cup lemon juice (about 1 ½ lemons)
¼ cup olive oil
¾ cup chopped fresh parsley
¾ teaspoon salt
1 can (15 ounces) chickpeas, rinsed and drained, or 1 ½ cups cooked chickpeas
1 medium cucumber, peeled, seeded and diced
1 small red onion, diced
2 cans (15 ounces each) red kidney beans, rinsed and drained, or 3 cups cooked kidney beans
2 stalks celery, sliced in half or thirds lengthwise and chopped
2 tablespoons chopped fresh dill or mint
3 cloves garlic, pressed or minced
Small pinch red pepper flakes

Directions:
Whisk well in a small bowl the pepper flakes, salt, garlic, and lemon juice until emulsified.   In a serving bowl, combine the prepared kidney beans, chickpeas, onion, celery, cucumber, parsley and dill (or mint).   Drizzle salad with the dressing and toss well to coat.   Serve and enjoy.
Nutrition Info: Calories per serving: 228; Protein: 8.5g; Carbs: 26.2g; Fat: 11.0g

632. Italian White Bean Soup

Servings: 4   Cooking Time: 50 Minutes
Ingredients:

1 (14 ounce) can chicken broth
1 bunch fresh spinach, rinsed and thinly sliced
1 clove garlic, minced
1 stalk celery, chopped
1 tablespoon lemon juice
1 tablespoon vegetable oil
1 onion, chopped
1/4 teaspoon ground black pepper
1/8 teaspoon dried thyme
2 (16 ounce) cans white kidney beans, rinsed and drained
2 cups water

Directions:
Place a pot on medium high fire and heat pot for a minute. Add oil and heat for another minute. Stir in celery and onion. Sauté for 7 minutes.   Stir in garlic and cook for another minute.   Add water, thyme, pepper, chicken broth, and beans. Cover and simmer for 15 minutes.   Remove 2 cups of the bean and celery mixture with a slotted spoon and set aside.   With an immersion blender, puree remaining soup in pot until smooth and creamy. Return the 2 cups of bean mixture. Stir in spinach and lemon juice. Cook for 2 minutes until heated through and spinach is wilted.   Serve and enjoy.
Nutrition Info: Calories per serving: 245; Protein: 12.0g; Carbs: 38.1g; Fat: 4.9g

633. Mexican Quinoa Bake

Servings: 4   Cooking Time: 40 Minutes
Ingredients:

3 cups sweet potato, peeled, diced very small (about 1 large sweet potato)
2 cups cooked quinoa
1 red bell pepper, diced
1 large carrot, diced
3 Tbs canned green chiles

1 cup shredded sharp cheddar cheese
2 Tbs chili powder
T Tbs paprika
1 1/4 cup salsa of your choice

1 small onion, diced
3 garlic cloves, minced
2 cups cooked black beans

Directions:
Preheat oven to 4000F.   Dice, chop, measure and prep all ingredients.   Combine all ingredients in one big bowl and toss ingredients well.   Spray a 9 X 13-inch pan with cooking spray and pour all ingredients in.   Bake for 35-40 minutes or until sweet potato pieces are slightly mushy, cheese is melted and items are heated all the way through. Let sit for about 5 minutes, scoop into bowls and enjoy!
Nutrition Info: Calories per serving: 414; Carbs: 56.6g; Protein: 22.0g; Fat: 13.0g

634.   Citrus Quinoa & Chickpea Salad

Servings: 4   Cooking Time: 0 Minutes
Ingredients:
2 cups cooked quinoa
1 can chickpeas, drained & rinsed
1 ripe avocado, diced
1 red bell pepper, diced
1/2 red onion, diced
1/4 cup lime juice

1/2 tbsp garlic powder
1/2 tbsp paprika
1/4-1/2 cup chopped cilantro
1 tbsp chopped jalapenos
Sea salt to taste

Directions:
Add all ingredients in a large bowl and mix well. Enjoy right away or refrigerate for later.
Nutrition Info: Calories per serving: 300; Carbs: 43.5g; Protein: 10.3g; Fat: 10.9g

635.   Chickpea Salad Moroccan Style

Servings: 6   Cooking Time: 0 Minutes
Ingredients:
1/3 cup crumbled low-fat feta cheese
¼ cup fresh mint, chopped
¼ cup fresh cilantro, chopped
1 red bell pepper, diced
2 plum tomatoes, diced
3 cups BPA free canned chickpeas or garbanzo beans

3 green onions, sliced thinly
1 large carrot, peeled and julienned
Pinch of cayenne pepper
¼ tsp salt
¼ tsp pepper
2 tsp ground cumin
3 tbsp fresh lemon juice
3 tbsp olive oil

Directions:
Make the dressing by whisking cayenne, black pepper, salt, cumin, lemon juice and oil in a small bowl and set aside.   Mix together feta, mint, cilantro, red pepper, tomatoes, onions, carrots and chickpeas in a large salad bowl.   Pour dressing over salad and toss to coat well.   Serve and enjoy.
Nutrition Info: Calories per serving: 300; Protein: 13.2g; Carbs: 35.4g; Fat: 12.8g

636.   Garlicky Peas And Clams On Veggie Spiral

Servings: 4   Cooking Time: 15 Minutes
Ingredients:

2 tbsp chopped fresh basil
½ cup pre-shredded Parmesan cheese
1 cup frozen green peas
¼ tsp crushed red pepper
1 cup organic vegetable broth

¼ cup dry white wine
3 cans chopped clams, clams and juice separated
1 ½ tsp bottled minced garlic
2 tbsp olive oil
6 cups zucchini, spiral

Directions:
Bring a pot of water to a rolling boil and blanch zucchini for 4 minutes on high fire. Drain and let stand for a couple of minutes to continue cooking. On medium high fire, add a large nonstick saucepan and heat oil. Add and sauté for a minute the garlic. Pour in wine, broth and clam juice. Once liquid is boiling, low fire to a simmer and add pepper.   Continue cooking and stirring for 5 minutes.   Add peas and clams, cook until heated through or around two minutes.   Toss in zucchini, mix well. Cook until heated through.   Add basil and cheese, toss to mix well then remove from fire. Transfer equally to four serving bowls and enjoy.
Nutrition Info: Calories per Serving: 210; Carbs: 24.0g; Protein: 8.5g; Fat: 9.2g

637.   Leek, Bacon And Pea Risotto

Servings: 4   Cooking Time: 60 Minutes
Ingredients:
Salt and pepper to taste
2 tbsp fresh lemon juice
½ cup grated parmesan cheese
¾ cup frozen peas
1 cup dry white wine

2 ½ cups Arborio rice
4 slices bacon (cut into strips)
12 cups low sodium chicken broth
2 leeks cut lengthwise

Directions:
In a saucepan, bring the broth to a simmer over medium flame.   On another skillet, cook bacon and stir continuously to avoid the bacon from burning. Cook more for five minutes and add the leeks and cook for two more minutes.   Increase the heat to medium high and add the rice until the grains become translucent.   Add the wine and stir until it evaporates.   Add 1 cup of broth to the mixture and reduce the heat to medium low. Stir constantly for two minutes.   Gradually add the remaining broth until the rice becomes al dente and it becomes creamy.   Add the peas and the rest of the broth.   Remove the skillet or turn off the heat and add the Parmesan cheese.   Cover the skillet and let the cheese melt. Season the risotto with lemon juice, salt and pepper.   Serve the risotto with more parmesan cheese.
Nutrition Info: Calories per Serving: 742; Carbs: 57.6g; Protein: 38.67g; Fat: 39.6g

638.   Chickpea Fried Eggplant Salad

Servings: 4   Cooking Time: 10 Minutes
Ingredients:
1 cup chopped dill
1 cup chopped parsley
1 cup cooked or canned chickpeas,

3 tbsp Za'atar spice, divided
oil for frying, preferably extra

drained
1 large eggplant, thinly sliced (no more than 1/4 inch in thickness)
1 small red onion, sliced in 1/2 moons
1/2 English cucumber, diced
3 Roma tomatoes, diced
virgin olive oil
Salt
1 large lime, juice of
1/3 cup extra virgin olive oil
1–2 garlic cloves, minced
Salt & Pepper to taste

Directions:
On a baking sheet, spread out sliced eggplant and season with salt generously. Let it sit for 30 minutes. Then pat dry with paper towel. Place a small pot on medium high fire and fill halfway with oil. Heat oil for 5 minutes. Fry eggplant in batches until golden brown, around 3 minutes per side. Place cooked eggplants on a paper towel lined plate. Once eggplants have cooled, assemble the eggplant on a serving dish. Sprinkle with 1 tbsp of Za'atar. Mix dill, parsley, red onions, chickpeas, cucumbers, and tomatoes in a large salad bowl. Sprinkle remaining Za'atar and gently toss to mix. Whisk well the vinaigrette ingredients in a small bowl. Drizzle 2 tbsp of the dressing over the fried eggplant. Add remaining dressing over the chickpea salad and mix. Add the chickpea salad to the serving dish with the fried eggplant. Serve and enjoy.
Nutrition Info: Calories per serving: 642; Protein: 16.6g; Carbs: 25.9g; Fat: 44.0g

| 639. | Turkey And Quinoa Stuffed Peppers |

Servings: 6   Cooking Time: 55 Minutes
Ingredients:
3 large red bell peppers
2 tsp chopped fresh rosemary
2 tbsp chopped fresh parsley
3 tbsp chopped pecans, toasted
1/2 cup chicken stock
¼ cup extra virgin olive oil
½ lb. fully cooked smoked turkey sausage, diced
½ tsp salt
2 cups water
1 cup uncooked quinoa

Directions:
On high fire, place a large saucepan and add salt, water and quinoa. Bring to a boil. Once boiling, reduce fire to a simmer, cover and cook until all water is absorbed around 15 minutes. Uncover quinoa, turn off fire and let it stand for another 5 minutes. Add rosemary, parsley, pecans, olive oil, chicken stock and turkey sausage into pan of quinoa. Mix well. Slice peppers lengthwise in half and discard membranes and seeds. In another boiling pot of water, add peppers, boil for 5 minutes, drain and discard water. Grease a 13 x 9 baking dish and preheat oven to 350oF. Place boiled bell pepper onto prepared baking dish, evenly fill with the quinoa mixture and pop into oven. Bake for 15 minutes.
Nutrition Info: Calories per Serving: 255.6; Carbs: 21.6g; Protein: 14.4g; Fat: 12.4g

| 640. | Pastitsio An Italian Dish |

Servings: 8   Cooking Time: 30 Minutes

Ingredients:
2 tbsp chopped fresh flat leaf parsley
¾ cup shredded mozzarella cheese
1 3oz package of fat free cream cheese
½ cup 1/3 less fat cream cheese
1 can 14.5-oz of diced tomatoes, drained
2 cups fat free milk
1 tbsp all-purpose flour
¾ tsp kosher salt
5 garlic cloves, minced
1 ½ cups chopped onion
1 tbsp olive oil
1 lb. ground sirloin
Cooking spray
8 oz penne, cooked and drained

Directions:
On medium high fire, place a big nonstick saucepan and for five minutes sauté beef. Keep on stirring to break up the pieces of ground meat. Once cooked, remove from pan and drain fat. Using same pan, heat oil and fry onions until soft around four minutes while occasionally stirring. Add garlic and continue cooking for another minute while constantly stirring. Stir in beef and flour, cook for another minute. Mix constantly. Add the fat free cream cheese, less fat cream cheese, tomatoes and milk. Cook until mixture is smooth and heated. Toss in pasta and mix well. Transfer pasta into a greased rectangular glass dish and top with mozzarella. Cook in a preheated broiler for four minutes. Remove from broiler and garnish with parsley before serving.
Nutrition Info: Calories per Serving: 263; Carbs: 17.8g; Protein: 24.1g; Fat: 10.6g

| 641. | Rice And Chickpea Stew |

Servings: 6   Cooking Time: 60 Minutes
Ingredients:
½ cup chopped fresh cilantro
¼ tsp freshly ground pepper
¼ tsp salt
2/3 cup brown basmati rice
3 cups peeled and diced sweet potato
2 15-oz cans chickpeas, rinsed
4 cups reduced-sodium chicken broth
1 cup orange juice
2 tsp ground coriander
2 tsp ground cumin
3 medium onions, halved and thinly sliced
1 tbsp extra virgin olive oil

Directions:
On medium fire, place a large nonstick fry pan and heat oil. Sauté onions for 8 minutes or until soft and translucent. Add coriander and cumin, sauté for half a minute. Add broth and orange juice. Add salt, rice, sweet potato, and chickpeas. Bring to a boil, once boiling lower fire to a simmer, cover and cook. Stir occasionally, cook for 45 minutes or until potatoes and rice are tender. Season with pepper. Stew will be thick, if you want a less thick soup, just add water and adjust salt and pepper to taste. To serve, garnish with cilantro.
Nutrition Info: Calories per serving: 332; Protein: 13.01g; Carbs: 55.5g; Fat: 7.5g

| 642. | Mediterranean Diet Pasta With Mussels |

Servings: 4   Cooking Time: 20 Minutes
Ingredients:
1 tbsp finely grated   Big pinch of saffron

lemon zest
¼ cup chopped fresh parsley
Freshly ground pepper to taste
¼ tsp salt
Big pinch of crushed red pepper
¾ cup dry white wine
2 lbs. mussels, cleaned

threads soaked in 2 tbsp of water
1 can of 15 oz crushed tomatoes with basil
2 large cloves garlic, chopped
¼ cup extra virgin olive oil
8 oz whole wheat linguine or spaghetti

Directions:
Cook your pasta following the package label, drain and set aside while covering it to keep it warm. On medium heat, place a large pan and heat oil. Sauté for two to three minutes the garlic and add the saffron plus liquid and the crushed tomatoes. Let it simmer for five minutes. On high heat and in a different pot, boil the wine and mussels for four to six minutes or until it opens. Then transfer the mussels into a clean bowl while disposing of the unopened ones. Then, with a sieve strain the mussel soup into the tomato sauce, add the red pepper and continue for a minute to simmer the sauce. Lastly, season with pepper and salt. Then transfer half of the sauce into the pasta bowl and toss to mix. Then ladle the pasta into 4 medium sized serving bowls, top with mussels, remaining sauce, lemon zest and parsley in that order before serving.
Nutrition Info: Calories per Serving: 402; Carbs: 26.0g; Protein: 35.0g; Fat: 17.5g

643.	**Brussels Sprouts 'n White Bean Medley**

Servings: 4   Cooking Time: 15 Minutes
Ingredients:
1 tsp salt
2 tbsp olive oil
3 cans white beans, drained and rinsed
3 medium onions, peeled and sliced
3 tbsp lemon juice

4 ½ cups Brussels sprouts, cleaned and sliced in half
6 garlic cloves, smashed, peeled, and minced
Pepper to taste

Directions:
Place a saucepan on medium high fire and heat for 2 minutes. Add oil and heat for a minute. Sauté garlic and onions for 3 minutes. Stir in Brussels Sprouts and sauté for 5 minutes. Stir in white beans and sauté for 5 minutes. Season with pepper and salt.
Nutrition Info: Calories per serving: 371; Protein: 21.4g; Carbs: 57.8g; Fat: 8.1g

644.	**Sun-dried Tomatoes And Chickpeas**

Servings: 6   Cooking Time: 22 Minutes
Ingredients:
1 red bell pepper
1/2 cup parsley, chopped
1/4 cup red wine vinegar
2 14.5-ounce cans chickpeas, drained and rinsed

2 cloves garlic, chopped
2 cups water
2 tablespoons extra-virgin olive oil
4 sun-dried tomatoes
Salt to taste

Directions:
Lengthwise, slice bell pepper in half. Place on baking sheet with skin side up. Broil on top rack for 5 minutes until skin is blistered. In a brown paper bag, place the charred bell pepper halves. Fold bag and leave in there for 10 minutes. Remove pepper and peel off skin. Slice into thin strips. Meanwhile, microwave 2 cups of water to boiling. Add the sun-dried tomatoes and leave in to reconstitute for 10 minutes. Drain and slice into thin strips. Whisk well olive oil, garlic, and red wine vinegar. Mix in parsley, sun-dried tomato, bell pepper, and chickpeas. Season with salt to taste and serve.
Nutrition Info: Calories per serving: 195; Protein: 8.0g; Carbs: 26.0g; Fat: 7.0g

645.	**Puttanesca Style Bucatini**

Servings: 4   Cooking Time: 40 Minutes
Ingredients:
1 tbsp capers, rinsed
1 tsp coarsely chopped fresh oregano
1 tsp finely chopped garlic
2 cups coarsely chopped canned no-salt-added whole peeled tomatoes with their juice

1/8 tsp salt
12-oz bucatini pasta
3 tbsp extra virgin olive oil, divided
4 anchovy fillets, chopped
8 black Kalamata olives, pitted and sliced into slivers

Directions:
Cook bucatini pasta according to package directions. Drain, keep warm, and set aside. On medium fire, place a large nonstick saucepan and heat 2 tbsp oil. Sauté anchovies until it starts to disintegrate. Add garlic and sauté for 15 seconds. Add tomatoes, sauté for 15 to 20 minutes or until no longer watery. Season with 1/8 tsp salt. Add oregano, capers, and olives. Add pasta, sautéing until heated through. To serve, drizzle pasta with remaining olive oil and enjoy.
Nutrition Info: Calories per Serving: 207.4; Carbs: 31g; Protein: 5.1g; Fat: 7g

646.	**Garlic Avocado-pesto And Zucchini Pasta**

Servings: 2   Cooking Time: 0 Minutes
Ingredients:
salt and pepper to taste
1 tbsp pine nuts
1 tbsp cashew nuts
1 lemon juice
4 cloves garlic, minced
1 small ripe avocado

2 cups zucchini, spiral
2 tbsp olive oil
2 tbsp grated Pecorino Cheese
½ cup packed fresh basil leaves

Directions:
In a food processor grind pine nuts and cashew nuts to a fine powder. Add basil leaves, cheese, olive oil, ripe avocado, garlic, lemon juice, salt and pepper to taste and process until you have a smooth mixture. Arrange zucchini pasta on two plates and top evenly with the Avocado pesto mixture. Serve and enjoy.
Nutrition Info: Calories per Serving: 353; Carbs: 17.0g; Protein: 5.5g; Fat: 31.9g

647.	**Mushroom Chickpea Marsala**

Servings: 4   Cooking Time: 20 Minutes

Ingredients:

2 tbsp olive oil	1 tsp rubbed sage
8 oz. baby portobello mushrooms, sliced	1/2 tsp black pepper
	1/4 tsp salt
2 garlic cloves, minced	2 tbsp chopped fresh parsley
1 cup dry Marsala wine	1-14 oz. can or 1 3/4 cups cooked
2 tbsp lemon juice, or to taste	chickpeas, rinsed and drained

Directions:
On medium fire, place a large saucepan and heat oil. Add mushrooms, cover and cook for 5 minutes. Stir in garlic and cook for 2 minutes. Add wine, lemon juice, sage, salt and pepper. Deglaze pot. Simmer for 10 minutes while covered. Add chickpeas and mix well. Cook for 3 minutes. Remove pot from fire and stir in parsley. Serve and enjoy.

Nutrition Info: Calories per serving: 159; Protein: 6.1g; Carbs: 16.8g; Fat: 8.5g

---

648. Creamy Alfredo Fettuccine

Servings: 4   Cooking Time: 25 Minutes

Ingredients:

Grated parmesan cheese	½ tsp salt
½ cup freshly grated parmesan cheese	1 cup whipping cream
	2 tbsp butter
1/8 tsp freshly ground black pepper	8 oz dried fettuccine, cooked and drained

Directions:
On medium high fire, place a big fry pan and heat butter. Add pepper, salt and cream and gently boil for three to five minutes. Once thickened, turn off fire and quickly stir in ½ cup of parmesan cheese. Toss in pasta, mix well. Top with another batch of parmesan cheese and serve.

Nutrition Info: Calories per Serving: 202; Carbs: 21.1g; Protein: 7.9g; Fat: 10.2g

---

649. Chickpea-crouton Kale Caesar Salad

Servings: 4   Cooking Time: 35 Minutes

Ingredients:

1 large bunch Tuscan kale, stem removed & thinly sliced	2 tablespoons olive oil
	1 lemon, zested and juiced
½ cup toasted pepitas	1 clove garlic
1 cup chickpeas, rinsed and drained	2 teaspoons capers, drained
1 tbsp Dijon mustard	2 tablespoons nutritional yeast
1 tbsp nutritional yeast	1 teaspoon Dijon mustard
2 tbsp olive oil	salt and pepper, to taste
salt and pepper, to taste	
½ cup silken tofu	

Directions:
Heat oven to 3500F. Toss the chickpeas in the garlic, Dijon, nutritional yeast, olive oil, and salt and pepper. Roast for 30-35 minutes, until browned and crispy. In a blender, add all dressing ingredients. Puree until smooth and creamy. In a large salad bowl, toss the kale with dressing to taste, massaging lightly to tenderize the kale. Top with the chickpea croutons, pepitas, and enjoy!

Nutrition Info: Calories per serving: 327; Protein: 11.9g; Carbs: 20.3g; Fat: 23.8g

---

650. Lemon Asparagus Risotto

Servings: 5   Cooking Time: 6 Minutes

Ingredients:

1 tablespoons olive oil	2 teaspoon thyme leaves
1 shallot, chopped	
1 clove of garlic, minced	Salt and pepper to taste
1 ½ cup Arborio rice	1 bunch asparagus spears, trimmed
1/3 cup white wine	
3 cups vegetable broth	1 tablespoons butter
	2 tablespoons parmesan cheese, grated
1 teaspoon lemon zest	

Directions:
Heat olive oil in a pot for 2 minutes. Sauté the shallot and garlic until fragrant, around 2 minutes. Add the Arborio rice and stir for 2 minutes before adding the white wine. Pour in the vegetable broth. Season with salt and pepper to taste. Stir in the lemon zest and thyme leaves. Cover and cook on medium fire for 15 minutes. Stir in the asparagus spears and allow to simmer for 3 minutes. Add the butter and sprinkle with parmesan cheese. Turn off fire and let it sit covered for 10 minutes.

Nutrition Info: Calories per serving: 179; Carbohydrates: 21.4g; Protein:5.7g; Fat: 12.9g

---

651. Seafood Paella With Couscous

Servings: 4   Cooking Time: 15 Minutes

Ingredients:

½ cup whole wheat couscous	¼ tsp freshly ground pepper
4 oz small shrimp, peeled and deveined	
	¼ tsp salt
4 oz bay scallops, tough muscle removed	½ tsp fennel seed
	½ tsp dried thyme
¼ cup vegetable broth	1 clove garlic, minced
1 cup freshly diced tomatoes and juice	1 medium onion, chopped
Pinch of crumbled saffron threads	2 tsp extra virgin olive oil

Directions:
Put on medium fire a large saucepan and add oil. Stir in the onion and sauté for three minutes before adding: saffron, pepper, salt, fennel seed, thyme, and garlic. Continue to sauté for another minute. Then add the broth and tomatoes and let boil. Once boiling, reduce the fire, cover and continue to cook for another 2 minutes. Add the scallops and increase fire to medium and stir occasionally and cook for two minutes. Add the shrimp and wait for two minutes more before adding the couscous. Then remove from fire, cover and set aside for five minutes before carefully mixing.

Nutrition Info: Calories per Serving: 117; Carbs: 11.7g; Protein: 11.5g; Fat: 3.1g

---

652. Greek Farro Salad

Servings: 4   Cooking Time: 15 Minutes

Ingredients:

½ teaspoon fine-grain sea salt	2 cups cooked chickpeas (or one 14-ounce can, rinsed
1 cup farro, rinsed	

1 tablespoon olive oil
2 garlic cloves, pressed or minced
½ small red onion, chopped and then rinsed under water to mellow the flavor
1 avocado, sliced into strips
1 cucumber, sliced into thin rounds
15 pitted Kalamata olives, sliced into rounds
1-pint cherry tomatoes, sliced into rounds
and drained)
5 ounces mixed greens
Lemon wedges
⅛ teaspoon salt
1 ¼ cups plain Greek yogurt
1 ½ tablespoon lightly packed fresh dill, roughly chopped
1 ½ tablespoon lightly packed fresh mint, torn into pieces
1 tablespoon lemon juice (about ½ lemon)
1 tablespoon olive oil

Directions:
In a blender, blend and puree all herbed yogurt ingredients and set aside. Then cook the farro by placing in a pot filled halfway with water. Bring to a boil, reduce fire to a simmer and cook for 15 minutes or until farro is tender. Drain well. Mix in salt, garlic, and olive oil and fluff to coat. Evenly divide the cooled farro into 4 bowls. Evenly divide the salad ingredients on the 4 farro bowl. Top with ¼ of the yogurt dressing. Serve and enjoy.
Nutrition Info: Calories per serving: 428; Protein: 17.7g; Carbs: 47.6g; Fat: 24.5g

653. Exotic Chickpea Tagine

Servings: 4   Cooking Time: 45 Minutes
Ingredients:
4 tsp sliced toasted almonds
1 cup whole wheat couscous, cooked according to manufacturer's instructions
Freshly squeezed juice of ½ lemon, plus additional to taste
1 19-oz can chickpeas, drained and rinsed
½ cup water
¼ cup packed dried apricots, sliced
1 medium zucchini, quartered and cut into ½-inch chunks
4 plum tomatoes, cored and chopped
¼ tsp turmeric
1 whole cinnamon stick
1 tsp ground cumin
2 tsp honey, plus additional to taste
½ tsp harissa paste plus additional to taste
3 quarter-sized pieces of peeled fresh ginger
2 garlic cloves, roughly chopped
2 small carrots, sliced lengthwise, then cut into ½-inch thick slices
1 ½ cups cubed, peeled butternut squash
½ tsp salt plus additional to taste
1 red onion, quartered and thickly sliced
1 ½ tbsp extra virgin olive oil

Directions:
On medium low fire, place a heavy and large pot. Heat oil and sauté onions and salt until onions are soft and translucent. Add carrots and sauté for another 5 minutes. Add ginger, garlic and butternut squash. Sauté for 5 minutes and lower fire to medium. Add turmeric, cinnamon stick, cumin,

honey and harissa. Sauté for a minute or until fragrant. Stir in apricots, zucchini and tomatoes. Add water and bring to a boil. Once boiling, lower fire to a simmer, cover and cook for 20 minutes or until vegetables are tender. Stir in lemon juice and chickpeas. Increase fire to medium and continue cooking dish uncovered for 5 to 10 minutes or until sauce has thickened. Season dish to taste. Adjust seasoning like lemon, honey and harissa if needed. Serve tagine over couscous and garnished with sliced almonds.
Nutrition Info: Calories per serving: 345; Protein: 13.2g; Carbs: 54.1g; Fat: 10.0g

654. Amazingly Good Parsley Tabbouleh

Servings: 4   Cooking Time: 15 Minutes
Ingredients:
¼ cup chopped fresh mint
¼ cup lemon juice
¼ tsp salt
½ cup bulgur
½ tsp minced garlic
1 small cucumber, peeled, seeded and diced
1 cup water
2 cups finely chopped flat-leaf parsley
2 tbsp extra virgin olive oil
2 tomatoes, diced
4 scallions, thinly sliced
Pepper to taste

Directions:
Cook bulgur according to package instructions. Drain and set aside to cool for at least 15 minutes. In a small bowl, mix pepper, salt, garlic, oil, and lemon juice. Transfer bulgur into a large salad bowl and mix in scallions, cucumber, tomatoes, mint, and parsley. Pour in dressing and toss well to coat. Place bowl in ref until chilled before serving.
Nutrition Info: Calories per Serving: 134.8; Carbs: 13g; Protein: 7.2g; Fat: 6g

655. Zucchini And Brown Rice

Servings: 1 Cup   Cooking Time: 50 Minutes
Ingredients:
2 TB. extra-virgin olive oil
2 large zucchini, diced
1 (16-oz.) can artichoke hearts, rinsed and drained
1 TB. fresh dill
1 tsp. ground black pepper
1 tsp. salt
4 cups chicken or vegetable broth
2 cups basmati brown rice

Directions:
In a large, 3-quart pot over medium heat, heat extra-virgin olive oil. Add zucchini, and cook for 3 minutes. Add artichoke hearts, and cook for 2 minutes. Add dill, black pepper, salt, and chicken broth, and bring to a simmer. Stir in basmati brown rice, cover, reduce heat to low, and cook for 40 minutes. Remove from heat, uncover, fluff with a fork, cover, and let sit for another 15 minutes. Serve with Greek yogurt.

656. Perfect Herb Rice

Servings: 4   Cooking Time: 4 Minutes
Ingredients:
1 cup brown rice, rinsed
1 tbsp olive oil
1 1/2 cups water
1/2 cup fresh mix herbs, chopped
1 tsp salt
Directions:

Add all ingredients into the inner pot of instant pot and stir well. Seal pot with lid and cook on high for 4 minutes. Once done, allow to release pressure naturally for 10 minutes then release remaining using quick release. Remove lid. Stir well and serve.

Nutrition Info: Calories 264 Fat 9.9 g Carbohydrates 36.7 g Sugar 0.4 g Protein 7.3 g Cholesterol 0 mg

---

657. Fiber Packed Chicken Rice

Servings: 6   Cooking Time: 16 Minutes

Ingredients:

1 lb chicken breast, skinless, boneless, and cut into chunks	2 cups wild rice
	1 small onion, chopped
14.5 oz can cannellini beans	1 tbsp garlic, chopped
4 cups chicken broth	1 tbsp olive oil
1 tbsp Italian seasoning	Pepper
	Salt

Directions:

Add oil into the inner pot of instant pot and set the pot on sauté mode. Add garlic and onion and sauté for 2 minutes. Add chicken and cook for 2 minutes. Add remaining ingredients and stir well. Seal pot with lid and cook on high for 12 minutes. Once done, release pressure using quick release. Remove lid. Stir well and serve.

Nutrition Info: Calories 399 Fat 6.4 g Carbohydrates 53.4 g Sugar 3 g Protein 31.6 g Cholesterol 50 mg

---

658. Baked Parmesan And Eggplant Pasta

Servings: 8   Cooking Time: 50 Minutes

Ingredients:

½ cup grated Parmesan cheese, divided	½ tsp dried basil
	2 cups Italian seasoned breadcrumbs
8-oz mozzarella cheese, shredded and divided	½ lb. ground beef
6 cups spaghetti sauce	6 cups eggplant, spiralized
	1 tbsp olive oil

Directions:

Grease a 9x13 baking dish and preheat oven to 3500F. On medium high fire, place a nonstick large saucepan and heat oil. Sauté ground beef until cooked around 8 minutes. Pour in spaghetti sauce and cook until heated through. Scoop out two cups of spaghetti meat sauce and set aside. Add eggplant spirals in saucepan and mix well. Scoop out half of eggplant spaghetti into baking dish, top with half of mozzarella cheese and cover with breadcrumbs. Top again with the remaining spaghetti, mozzarella and Parmesan cheese. Pop into oven and bake until tops are golden brown around 35 minutes. Remove from oven and evenly slice into 8 pieces. Serve and enjoy while warm.

Nutrition Info: Calories per Serving: 297; Carbs: 26.6g; Protein: 22.9g; Fat: 11.1g

---

659. Greek Couscous Salad And Herbed Lamb Chops

Servings: 4   Cooking Time: 30 Minutes

Ingredients:

¼ tsp salt	2 ½ lbs. lamb loin chops, trimmed of fat
½ cup crumbled feta	
½ cup whole wheat couscous	2 medium tomatoes, chopped
1 cup water	2 tbsp finely chopped fresh dill
1 medium cucumber, peeled and chopped	
1 tbsp finely chopped fresh parsley	2 tsp extra virgin olive oil
1 tbsp minced garlic	3 tbsp lemon juice

Directions:

On medium saucepan, add water and bring to a boil. Ibn a small bowl, mix salt, parsley, and garlic. Rub onto lamb chops. On medium high fire, place a large nonstick saucepan and heat oil. Pan fry lamb chops for 5 minutes per side or to desired doneness. Once done, turn off fire and keep warm. On saucepan of boiling water, add couscous. Once boiling, lower fire to a simmer, cover and cook for two minutes. After two minutes, turn off fire, cover and let it stand for 5 minutes. Fluff couscous with a fork and place into a medium bowl. Add dill, lemon juice, feta, cucumber, and tomatoes in bowl of couscous and toss well to combine. Serve lamb chops with a side of couscous and enjoy.

Nutrition Info: Calories per Serving: 524.1; Carbs: 12.3g; Protein: 61.8g; Fat: 25.3g

---

660. Fresh Herbs And Clams Linguine

Servings: 4   Cooking Time: 10 Minutes

Ingredients:

½ tsp freshly ground black pepper	2 cups vertically sliced red onion
¾ tsp salt	2 tbsp olive oil
2 tbsp butter	2 tsp grated lemon zest
1.5 lbs. littleneck clams	
½ cup white wine	1 tbsp chopped fresh oregano
4 garlic cloves, sliced	1/3 cup parsley leaves
¼ tsp crushed red pepper	8-oz linguine, cooked and drained

Directions:

Chop finely lemon rind, oregano and parsley. Set aside. On medium high fire, place a nonstick fry pan with olive oil and fry for four minutes garlic, red pepper and onion. Add clams and wine and cook until shells have opened, around five minutes. Throw any unopened clam. Transfer mixture into a large serving bowl. Add pepper, salt, butter and pasta. Toss to mix well. Serve with parsley garnish.

Nutrition Info: Calories per Serving: 507; Carbs: 53.9g; Protein: 34.2g; Fat: 16.8g

---

661. Garbanzo And Lentil Soup

Servings: 8   Cooking Time: 90 Minutes

Ingredients:

1 14.5-oz can petite diced tomatoes, undrained	1 cup lentils
	½ tsp ground cumin
2 15-oz cans Garbanzo beans, rinsed and drained	1 tsp turmeric
	1 tsp garam masala
	1 tsp minced garlic
6 cups vegetable broth	2 tsp grated fresh ginger
¼ tsp ground	1 cup diced carrots

cayenne pepper
1 cup chopped celery
2 onions, chopped

Directions:
On medium high fire, place a heavy bottomed large pot and grease with cooking spray. Add onions and sauté until tender, around three to four minutes. Add celery and carrots. Cook for another five minutes. Add cayenne pepper, cumin, turmeric, ginger, garam masala and garlic, cook for half a minute. Add diced tomatoes, garbanzo beans, lentils and vegetable broth. Bring to a boil. Once boiling, slow fire to a simmer and cook while covered for 90 minutes. Occasionally stir soup. If you want a thicker and creamier soup, you can puree ½ of the pot's content and mix in. Once lentils are soft, turn off fire and serve.
Nutrition Info: Calories per serving: 196; Protein: 10.1g; Carbs: 33.3g; Fat: 3.6g

662. Pasta And Tuna Salad

Servings: 4   Cooking Time: 12 Minutes
Ingredients:
¼ cup mayonnaise
½ cup chopped zucchini
2 cups whole wheat macaroni, uncooked
¼ cup sliced carrots
1/3 cup diced onion
2 5-oz cans low-sodium tuna, water pack

Directions:
In a pot of boiling water, cook macaroni according to manufacturer's instructions. Drain macaroni, run under cold tap water until cool and set aside. Drain and discard tuna liquid. Place tuna in a salad bowl. Add zucchini, carrots, drained macaroni and onion. Toss to mix. Add mayonnaise and mix well. Serve and enjoy.
Nutrition Info: Calories per Serving: 168.2; Carbs: 24.6g; Protein: 5.3g; Fat: 5.4g

663. Quinoa Buffalo Bites

Servings: 4   Cooking Time: 15 Minutes
Ingredients:
2 cups cooked quinoa
1 cup shredded mozzarella
1/2 cup buffalo sauce
1/4 cup +1 Tbsp flour
1 egg
1/4 cup chopped cilantro
1 small onion, diced

Directions:
Preheat oven to 350oF. Mix all ingredients in large bowl. Press mixture into greased mini muffin tins. Bake for approximately 15 minutes or until bites are golden. Enjoy on its own or with blue cheese or ranch dip.
Nutrition Info: Calories per serving: 212; Carbs: 30.6g; Protein: 15.9g; Fat: 3.0g

664. Feta On Tomato-black Bean

Servings: 8   Cooking Time: 0 Minutes
Ingredients:
1/2 red onion, sliced
1/4 cup crumbled feta cheese
1/4 cup fresh dill, chopped
2 14.5-ounce cans black beans, drained and rinsed
2 tablespoons extra-virgin olive oil
4 Roma or plum tomatoes, diced
Juice of 1 lemon
Salt to taste

Directions:

Except for feta, mix well all ingredients in a salad bowl. Sprinkle with feta. Serve and enjoy.
Nutrition Info: Calories per serving: 121; Protein: 6.0g; Carbs: 15.0g; Fat: 5.0g

665. Black Beans And Quinoa

Servings: 6   Cooking Time: 30 Minutes
Ingredients:
½ cup chopped cilantro
2 15-oz cans black beans, rinsed and drained
1 cup frozen corn kernels
Pepper and salt to taste
¼ tsp cayenne pepper
1 tsp ground cumin
1 ½ cups vegetable broth
¾ cup quinoa
3 cloves garlic, chopped
1 onion, chopped
1 tsp vegetable oil

Directions:
On medium fire, place a saucepan and heat oil. Add garlic and onions. Sauté for 5 minutes or until onions are soft. Add quinoa. Pour vegetable broth and bring to a boil while increasing fire. As you wait for broth to boil, season quinoa mixture with pepper, salt, cayenne pepper, and cumin. Once boiling, reduce fire to a simmer, cover and simmer around 20 minutes or until liquid is fully absorbed. Once liquid is fully absorbed, stir in black beans and frozen corn. Continue cooking until heated through, around 5 minutes. To serve, add cilantro, toss well to mix, and enjoy.
Nutrition Info: Calories per serving: 262; Carbs: 47.1g; Protein: 13.0g; Fat: 2.9g

666. Veggie Pasta With Shrimp, Basil And Lemon

Servings: 4   Cooking Time: 5 Minutes
Ingredients:
2 cups baby spinach
½ tsp salt
2 tbsp fresh lemon juice
2 tbsp extra virgin olive oil
3 tbsp drained capers
¼ cup chopped fresh basil
1 lb. peeled and deveined large shrimp
4 cups zucchini, spirals

Directions:
Bring a pot of water to a rolling boil and blanch zucchini and shrimp for 3 minutes or until desired softness is achieved. Remove from fire, drain and let stand for a minute while draining. Meanwhile, in a large salad bowl, mix salt, lemon juice, olive oil, capers and basil. Toss in zucchini and shrimps. Toss to mix well. Evenly divide into 4 serving plates, top with ¼ cup of spinach, serve and enjoy.
Nutrition Info: Calories per Serving: 51; Carbs: 4.4g; Protein: 1.8g; Fat: 3.4g

667. Nutty And Fruity Amaranth Porridge

Servings: 2   Cooking Time: 30 Minutes
Ingredients:
¼ cup pumpkin seeds
½ cup blueberries
1 medium pear, chopped
1 tsp cinnamon
2 cups filtered water
2/3 cups whole-grain amaranth

141

1 tbsp raw honey

Directions:

In a nonstick pan with cover, boil water and amaranth. Slow fire to a simmer and continue cooking until liquid is absorbed completely, around 25-30 minutes. Turn off fire. Mix in cinnamon, honey and pumpkin seeds. Mix well. Pour equally into two bowls. Garnish with pear and blueberries. Serve and enjoy.

Nutrition Info: Calories per Serving: 393.4; Carbs: 68.5g; Protein: 10.5g; Fat: 8.6g

---

668. Kasha With Onions And Mushrooms

Servings: 4   Cooking Time: 40 Minutes

Ingredients:

½ tsp pepper	12oz shiitake
½ tsp rubbed sage	mushrooms
¾ cup carrot juice	2 large onions, thinly
1 cup water	sliced
1 cup whole grain	2 tsp sugar
kasha	Salt to taste
1 tbsp olive oil	

Directions:

In a large skillet, heat oil over medium high heat and add onions and sugar. Cook until the onions are brown. Add the sage, mushrooms and pepper stir constantly until the mushrooms are tender. Set aside. In the same skillet, place kasha and cook over medium heat. Stir constantly until lightly toasted. Combine carrot juice, water and salt in a saucepan and bring to a boil over medium heat. Add kasha and cook until tender. Fluff with fork and transfer the contents to the skillet with the onion and sugar mixture. Toss until well combined. Serve and enjoy.

Nutrition Info: Calories per Serving: 254.5; Carbs: 46.8 g; Protein: 6.7g; Fat: 4.5g

---

669. Chickpea Alfredo Sauce

Servings: 4   Cooking Time: 0 Minutes

Ingredients:

¼ teaspoon ground nutmeg	1 tablespoon white miso paste
¼ teaspoon sea salt or to taste	1-½ cups water
1 clove garlic minced	2 tablespoons lemon juice
2 cups chickpeas, rinsed and drained	3 tablespoons nutritional yeast

Directions:

Add all ingredients in a blender. Puree until smooth and creamy.

Nutrition Info: Calories per serving: 123; Protein: 6.2g; Carbs: 20.2g; Fat: 2.4g

---

670. Lime-cilantro Rice Chipotle Style

Servings: 10   Cooking Time: 17 Minutes

Ingredients:

1 can vegetable broth	2 cups long grain
¾ cup water	white rice, rinsed
2 tablespoons canola oil	Zest of 1 lime
3 tablespoons juice of lime juice	½ cup cilantro, chopped
	½ teaspoon salt

Directions:

Place everything in the pot and give a good stir. Give a good stir and close the lid. Seal off the vent. Press the Rice button and adjust the cooking time to 17 minutes. Do natural pressure release. Fluff the rice before serving. Once cooled, evenly divide into serving size, keep in your preferred container, and refrigerate until ready to eat.

Nutrition Info: Calories per serving: 166; Carbohydrates: 31.2g; Protein:2.7g; Fat: 3.1g

---

671.Lentils And Rice (mujaddara With Rice)

Servings: 1 Cup   Cooking Time: 1 Hour 10 Minutes

Ingredients:

1/4 cup extra-virgin olive oil	1 large yellow onion, finely chopped
2 tsp. salt	6 cups water
2 cups green or brown lentils, picked over and rinsed	1 cup long-grain rice or brown rice
	1 TB. cumin

Directions:

In a large, 3-quart pot over medium-low heat, heat extra-virgin olive oil. Add yellow onion and 1 teaspoon salt, and cook, stirring intermittently, for 10 minutes. Add green lentils and water, and cook, stirring intermittently, for 20 minutes. Stir in long-grain rice, remaining 1 teaspoon salt, and cumin. Cover and cook, stirring intermittently, for 40 minutes. Serve warm or at room temperature with tzatziki sauce or a Mediterranean salad.

---

672. Gorgonzola And Chicken Pasta

Servings: 8   Cooking Time: 40 Minutes

Ingredients:

12 oz pastas, cooked and drained	8 oz stemmed fresh cremini or shiitake
¼ cup snipped fresh Italian parsley	mushrooms
2/3 cup Parmesan cheese	3 tbsp olive oil
1 cup crumbled	½ tsp ground pepper
Gorgonzola cheese	½ tsp salt
2 cups whipping cream	1 ½ lbs. skinless chicken breast, cut into ½-inch slices

Directions:

Season chicken breasts with ¼ tsp pepper and ¼ tsp salt. On medium high fire, place a nonstick pan with 1 tbsp oil and stir fry half of the chicken until cooked and lightly browned, around 5 minutes per side. Transfer chicken to a clean dish and repeat procedure to remaining batch of uncooked chicken. In same pan, add a tablespoon of oil and stir fry mushroom until liquid is evaporated and mushrooms are soft, around eight minutes. Stir occasionally. Add chicken back to the mushrooms along with cream and simmer for three minutes. Then add the remaining pepper and salt, parmesan cheese and ½ cup of Gorgonzola cheese. Cook until mixture is uniform. Turn off fire. Add pasta into the mixture, tossing to combine. Transfer to serving dish and garnish with remaining Gorgonzola cheese and serve.

Nutrition Info: Calories per Serving: 358; Carbs: 23.1g; Protein: 27.7g; Fat: 17.1g

673. Kefta Styled Beef Patties With Cucumber Salad

Servings: 4   Cooking Time: 10 Minutes

Ingredients:

2 pcs of 6-inch pita, quartered
½ tsp freshly ground black pepper
1 tbsp fresh lemon juice
½ cup plain Greek yogurt, fat free
2 cups thinly sliced English cucumber
½ tsp ground cinnamon
½ tsp salt
1 tsp ground cumin
2 tsp ground coriander
1 tbsp peeled and chopped ginger
¼ cup cilantro, fresh
¼ cup plus 2 tbsp fresh parsley, chopped and divided
1 lb. ground sirloin

Directions:

On medium high fire, preheat a grill pan coated with cooking spray.   In a medium bowl, mix together cinnamon, salt, cumin, coriander, ginger, cilantro, parsley and beef. Then divide the mixture equally into four parts and shaping each portion into a patty ½ inch thick.   Then place patties on pan cooking each side for three minutes or until desired doneness is achieved.   In a separate bowl, toss together vinegar and cucumber.   In a small bowl, whisk together pepper, juice, 2 tbsp parsley and yogurt.   Serve each patty on a plate with ½ cup cucumber mixture and 2 tbsp of the yogurt sauce.

Nutrition Info: Calories per serving: 313; Carbs: 11.7g; Protein: 33.9g; Fat: 14.1g

674. Italian Mac & Cheese

Servings: 4   Cooking Time: 6 Minutes

Ingredients:

1 lb whole grain pasta
2 tsp Italian seasoning
1 1/2 tsp garlic powder
1 1/2 tsp onion powder
1 cup sour cream
4 cups of water
4 oz parmesan cheese, shredded
12 oz ricotta cheese
Pepper
Salt

Directions:

Add all ingredients except ricotta cheese into the inner pot of instant pot and stir well.   Seal pot with lid and cook on high for 6 minutes.   Once done, allow to release pressure naturally for 5 minutes then release remaining using quick release. Remove lid.   Add ricotta cheese and stir well and serve.

Nutrition Info: Calories 388 Fat 25.8 g Carbohydrates 18.1 g Sugar 4 g Protein 22.8 g Cholesterol 74 mg

675. Saffron Green Bean-quinoa Soup

Servings: 6   Cooking Time: 20 Minutes

Ingredients:

2 tablespoons extra virgin olive oil
1 large leek, white and light green parts only, halved, washed, and sliced
2 cloves garlic, minced
8 ounces fresh green beans, trimmed and chopped into 1" pieces
freshly chopped basil, for serving
1 large carrot, chopped into 1/2"
2 large pinches saffron, or one capsule
15 ounces chickpeas and liquid (do not rinse!)
1 large tomato, seeded and chopped into 1" pieces
salt and freshly ground pepper, to taste
pieces
1 large celery stalk, chopped into 1/2" pieces
1 large zucchini, chopped into 1/2" pieces
1/2 cup quinoa, rinsed
4-5 cups vegetable stock

Directions:

Place a large pot on medium fire and heat olive oil for 2 minutes.   Stir in celery and carrots. Cook for 6 minutes or until soft.   Mix in garlic and leek. Sauté for 3 minutes.   Add the zucchini and green beans, and sauté 1 minute more.   Pour in broth and saffron. Bring to a boil. Stir in chickpeas and quinoa. Cook until quinoa is soft, around 11 minutes while covered.   Stir in the diced tomato and salt and pepper, to taste, and remove from heat. Serve the soup with the freshly chopped basil and enjoy!

Nutrition Info: Calories per serving: 196; Protein: 7.9g; Carbs: 26.6g; Fat: 7.5g

676. Pasta Shells Stuffed With Feta

Servings: 10   Cooking Time: 40 Minutes

Ingredients:

20 jumbo pasta shells, cooked and drained
2 garlic cloves, minced
5 oz frozen chopped spinach, thawed, drained and squeezed dry
1 9oz package frozen artichoke hearts, thawed and chopped
¼ tsp freshly ground black pepper
½ cup fat free cream cheese softened
Cooking spray
1 cup crumbled feta cheese
1 cup shredded provolone cheese, divided
1 8oz can no salt added tomato sauce
1 28oz can fire roasted crushed tomatoes with added puree
¼ cup chopped pepperoncini peppers
1 tsp dried oregano

Directions:

On medium fire, place a medium fry pan and for 12 minutes cook tomato sauce, crushed tomatoes, peppers and oregano. Put aside.   In a medium bowl, mix garlic, spinach, artichoke, black pepper, cream cheese, feta cheese and ½ cup provolone. Evenly stuff these to the cooked pasta shells. Grease a rectangular glass dish and arrange all the pasta shells within. Cover with tomato mixture and top with provolone.   Bake for 25 minutes in a preheated 375oF oven.

Nutrition Info: Calories per Serving: 284; Carbs: 38.5g; Protein: 15.9g; Fat: 8.3g

677. Italian Chicken Pasta

Servings: 8   Cooking Time: 9 Minutes

Ingredients:

1 lb chicken breast, skinless, boneless, and cut into chunks
1/2 cup cream cheese
1 cup mozzarella cheese, shredded
1 cup mushrooms, diced
1/2 onion, diced
2 tomatoes, diced
2 cups of water
16 oz whole wheat

1 1/2 tsp Italian seasoning
1 tsp garlic, minced
penne pasta
Pepper
Salt

Directions:
Add all ingredients except cheeses into the inner pot of instant pot and stir well. Seal pot with lid and cook on high for 9 minutes. Once done, allow to release pressure naturally for 5 minutes then release remaining using quick release. Remove lid. Add cheeses and stir well and serve.
Nutrition Info: Calories 328 Fat 8.5 g Carbohydrates 42.7 g Sugar 1.4 g Protein 23.7 g Cholesterol 55 mg

678. Black Bean Hummus

Servings: 8   Cooking Time: 0 Minutes
Ingredients:
10 Greek olives
¼ tsp paprika
¼ tsp cayenne pepper
½ tsp salt
¾ tsp ground cumin
1 ½ tbsp tahini
2 tbsp lemon juice
1 15-oz can black beans, drain and reserve liquid
1 clove garlic

Directions:
In food processor, mince garlic. Add cayenne pepper, salt, cumin, tahini, lemon juice, 2 tbsp reserved black beans liquid, and black beans. Process until smooth and creamy. Scrape the side of processor as needed and continue pureeing. To serve, garnish with Greek olives and paprika. Best eaten as a dip for pita bread or chips.
Nutrition Info: Calories per serving: 205; Protein: 12.1g; Carbs: 34.4g; Fat: 2.9g

679. White Bean And Tuna Salad

Servings: 4   Cooking Time: 8 Minutes
Ingredients:
1 (12 ounce) can solid white albacore tuna, drained
1 (16 ounce) can Great Northern beans, drained and rinsed
1 teaspoon dried oregano
1/2 teaspoon finely grated lemon zest
1/4 medium red onion, thinly sliced
3 tablespoons lemon juice
1 (2.25 ounce) can sliced black olives, drained
3/4-pound green beans, trimmed and snapped in half
4 large hard-cooked eggs, peeled and quartered
6 tablespoons extra-virgin olive oil
Salt and ground black pepper, to taste

Directions:
Place a saucepan on medium high fire. Add a cup of water and the green beans. Cover and cook for 8 minutes. Drain immediately once tender. In a salad bowl, whisk well oregano, olive oil, lemon juice, and lemon zest. Season generously with pepper and salt and mix until salt is dissolved. Stir in drained green beans, tuna, beans, olives, and red onion. Mix thoroughly to coat. Adjust seasoning to taste. Spread eggs on top. Serve and enjoy.
Nutrition Info: Calories per serving: 551; Protein: 36.3g; Carbs: 33.4g; Fat: 30.3g

680. Beans And Spinach Mediterranean Salad

Servings: 4   Cooking Time: 30 Minutes
Ingredients:
1 can (14 ounces) water-packed artichoke hearts, rinsed, drained and quartered
1 can (14-1/2 ounces) no-salt-added diced tomatoes, undrained
1 can (15 ounces) cannellini beans, rinsed and drained
1 small onion, chopped
1/4 teaspoon pepper
1 tablespoon olive oil
1/4 teaspoon salt
1/8 teaspoon crushed red pepper flakes
2 garlic cloves, minced
2 tablespoons Worcestershire sauce
6 ounces fresh baby spinach (about 8 cups)
Additional olive oil, optional

Directions:
Place a saucepan on medium high fire and heat for a minute. Add oil and heat for 2 minutes. Stir in onion and sauté for 4 minutes. Add garlic and sauté for another minute. Stir in seasonings, Worcestershire sauce, and tomatoes. Cook for 5 minutes while stirring continuously until sauce is reduced. Stir in spinach, artichoke hearts, and beans. Sauté for 3 minutes until spinach is wilted and other ingredients are heated through. Serve and enjoy.
Nutrition Info: Calories per serving: 187; Protein: 8.0g; Carbs: 30.0g; Fat: 4.0g

681. Grilled Veggie And Pasta With Marinara Sauce

Servings: 4   Cooking Time: 30 Minutes
Ingredients:
8 oz whole wheat spaghetti
1 sweet onion, sliced into ¼-inch wide rounds
1 zucchini, sliced lengthwise
1 yellow summer squash, sliced lengthwise
2 red peppers, sliced into chunks
1/8 tsp freshly ground black pepper
½ tsp dried oregano
1 tsp sugar
1 tbsp chopped fresh basil or 1 tsp dried basil
2 tbsp chopped onion
½ tsp minced garlic
salt
10 large fresh tomatoes, peeled and diced
2 tbsp extra virgin olive oil, divided

Directions:
Make the marinara sauce by heating on medium high fire a tablespoon of oil in a large fry pan. Sauté black pepper, oregano, sugar, basil, onions, garlic, salt and tomatoes. Once simmering, lower fire and allow to simmer for 30 minutes or until sauce has thickened. Meanwhile, preheat broiler and grease baking pan with cooking spray. Add sweet onion, zucchini, squash and red peppers in baking pan and brush with oil. Broil for 5 to 8 minutes or until vegetables are tender. Remove from oven and transfer veggies into a bowl. Bring a large pot of water to a boil. Once boiling, add pasta and cook following manufacturer's instructions. Once al dente, drain and divide equally into 4 plates. To serve, equally divide marinara sauce on to pasta, top with grilled veggies and enjoy.

Nutrition Info: Calories per Serving: ; Carbs: 41.9g; Protein: 8.3g; Fat: 6.2g

682.   Flavors Herb Risotto

Servings: 4   Cooking Time: 15 Minutes

Ingredients:

2 cups of rice
2 tbsp parmesan cheese, grated
1 tbsp fresh oregano, chopped
1 tbsp fresh basil, chopped
1/2 tbsp sage, chopped

3.5 oz heavy cream
1 onion, chopped
2 tbsp olive oil
1 tsp garlic, minced
4 cups vegetable stock
Pepper
Salt

Directions:

Add oil into the inner pot of instant pot and set the pot on sauté mode.   Add garlic and onion and sauté for 2-3 minutes.   Add remaining ingredients except for parmesan cheese and heavy cream and stir well.   Seal pot with lid and cook on high for 12 minutes.   Once done, allow to release pressure naturally for 10 minutes then release remaining using quick release. Remove lid. Stir in cream and cheese and serve.

Nutrition Info: Calories 514 Fat 17.6 g Carbohydrates 79.4 g Sugar 2.1 g Protein 8.8 g Cholesterol 36 mg

683.   Chicken And Sweet Potato Stir Fry

Servings: 6   Cooking Time: Minutes

Ingredients:

¼ tsp salt
½ cups quinoa, rinsed and drained
1 clove garlic, minced
1 cup frozen peas
1 cup water
1 jalapeno chili pepper, chopped
1 medium onion, chopped

1 medium-sized red bell pepper, chopped
1 tsp cumin, ground
1/8 tsp black pepper
12oz boneless chicken
1med sweet potatoes, cubed
3 tbsp fresh cilantro, chopped
4 tsp canola oil

Directions:

Bring to a boil water and quinoa over medium heat. Simmer until the quinoa has absorbed the water. In a small saucepan, put the sweet potatoes and enough water to cover the potatoes. Bring to a boil. Drain the potatoes and discard the water.   In a skillet, add the chicken and cook until brown. Transfer to a bowl.   Using the same skillet, heat 2 tablespoon of oil and sauté the onions and jalapeno pepper for one minute.   Add the bell pepper, cumin and garlic. Cook for three minutes until the vegetables have softened.   Add the peas and chicken. Cook for two minutes before adding the sweet potato and quinoa.   Stir cilantro and add salt and pepper to taste.   Serve and enjoy.

Nutrition Info: Calories per Serving: 187.6; Carbs: 18g; Protein: 16.3g; Fat: 5.6g

684.   Fasolakia – Potatoes & Green Beans In Olive Oil

Servings: 4   Cooking Time: 25 Minutes

Ingredients:

1 1/2 onion, sliced thin
1 bunch of dill, chopped

1/2 bunch parsley, chopped
1/2 cup extra virgin olive oil

1 cup water
1 large zucchini, quartered
1 lb. green beans frozen
1 tsp dried oregano

15 oz can diced tomatoes
2 potatoes, quartered
salt and pepper, to taste

Directions:

Place a pot on medium high fire and heat pot for 2 minutes.   Add oil and heat for 3 minutes.   Stir in onions and sauté for 2 minutes. Stir in dill, oregano, and potatoes. Cook for 3 minutes. Season with pepper and salt.   Add dice tomatoes and water. Cover and simmer for 10 minutes.   Stir in zucchini and green beans. Cook for 5 minutes. Adjust seasoning to taste, turn off fire, and stir in parsley.   Serve and enjoy.

Nutrition Info: Calories per serving: 384; Protein: 5.9g; Carbs: 30.6g; Fat: 27.9g

685.   Pesto Pasta And Shrimps

Servings: 4   Cooking Time: 15 Minutes

Ingredients:

¼ cup pesto, divided
¼ cup shaved Parmesan Cheese
1 ¼ lbs. large shrimp, peeled and deveined

1 cup halved grape tomatoes
4-oz angel hair pasta, cooked, rinsed and drained

Directions:

On medium high fire, place a nonstick large fry pan and grease with cooking spray.   Add tomatoes, pesto and shrimp. Cook for 15 minutes or until shrimps are opaque, while covered.   Stir in cooked pasta and cook until heated through. Transfer to a serving plate and garnish with Parmesan cheese.

Nutrition Info: Calories per Serving: 319; Carbs: 23.6g; Protein: 31.4g; Fat: 11g

686.   Tasty Greek Rice

Servings: 6   Cooking Time: 10 Minutes

Ingredients:

1 3/4 cup brown rice, rinsed and drained
3/4 cup roasted red peppers, chopped
1 cup olives, chopped
1 tsp dried oregano

1 tsp Greek seasoning
1 3/4 cup vegetable broth
2 tbsp olive oil
Salt

Directions:

Add oil into the inner pot of instant pot and set the pot on sauté mode.   Add rice and cook for 5 minutes.   Add remaining ingredients except for red peppers and olives and stir well.   Seal pot with lid and cook on high for 5 minutes.   Once done, allow to release pressure naturally for 10 minutes then release remaining using quick release. Remove lid.   Add red peppers and olives and stir well.   Serve and enjoy. Ingredients

Nutrition Info: Calories 285 Fat 9.1 g Carbohydrates 45.7 g Sugar 1.2 g Protein 6 g Cholesterol 0 mg

687.   Shrimp Paella Made With Quinoa

Servings: 7   Cooking Time: 40 Minutes

Ingredients:

1 lb. large shrimp, peeled, deveined and thawed
1 tsp seafood

½ tsp black pepper
½ tsp Spanish paprika

seasoning
1 cup frozen green peas
1 red bell pepper, cored, seeded & membrane removed, sliced into ½" strips
½ cup sliced sun-dried tomatoes, packed in olive oil
Salt to taste

½ tsp saffron threads (optional turmeric)
1 bay leaf
¼ tsp crushed red pepper flakes
3 cups chicken broth, fat free, low sodium
1 ½ cups dry quinoa, rinse well
1 tbsp olive oil
2 cloves garlic, minced
1 yellow onion, diced

Directions:
Season shrimps with seafood seasoning and a pinch of salt. Toss to mix well and refrigerate until ready to use.   Prepare and wash quinoa. Set aside. On medium low fire, place a large nonstick skillet and heat oil. Add onions and for 5 minutes sauté until soft and tender.   Add paprika, saffron (or turmeric), bay leaves, red pepper flakes, chicken broth and quinoa. Season with salt and pepper. Cover skillet and bring to a boil. Once boiling, lower fire to a simmer and cook until all liquid is absorbed, around ten minutes.   Add shrimp, peas and sun-dried tomatoes. For 5 minutes, cover and cook.   Once done, turn off fire and for ten minutes allow paella to set while still covered.   To serve, remove bay leaf and enjoy with a squeeze of lemon if desired.
Nutrition Info: Calories per Serving: 324.4; Protein: 22g; Carbs: 33g; Fat: 11.6g

688.   Seafood And Veggie Pasta
Servings: 4   Cooking Time: 20 Minutes
Ingredients:
¼ tsp pepper
¼ tsp salt
1 lb raw shelled shrimp
1 lemon, cut into wedges
1 tbsp butter
2 5-oz cans chopped clams, drained (reserve 2 tbsp clam juice)

1 tbsp olive oil
2 tbsp dry white wine
4 cloves garlic, minced
4 cups zucchini, spiraled (use a veggie spiralizer)
4 tbsp Parmesan Cheese
Chopped fresh parsley to garnish

Directions:
Ready the zucchini and spiralize with a veggie spiralizer. Arrange 1 cup of zucchini noodle per bowl. Total of 4 bowls.   On medium fire, place a large nonstick saucepan and heat oil and butter. For a minute, sauté garlic. Add shrimp and cook for 3 minutes until opaque or cooked.   Add white wine, reserved clam juice and clams. Bring to a simmer and continue simmering for 2 minutes or until half of liquid has evaporated. Stir constantly. Season with pepper and salt. And if needed add more to taste.   Remove from fire and evenly distribute seafood sauce to 4 bowls.   Top with a tablespoonful of Parmesan cheese per bowl, serve and enjoy.
Nutrition Info: Calories per Serving: 324.9; Carbs: 12g; Protein: 43.8g; Fat: 11.3g

689.   Cilantro-dijon Vinaigrette On Kidney Bean Salad
Servings: 4   Cooking Time: 0 Minutes
Ingredients:
1 15-oz. can kidney beans, drained and rinsed
1/2 English cucumbers, chopped
1 Medium-sized heirloom tomato, chopped
1 bunch fresh cilantro, stems removed, chopped (about 1 1/4 cup)
1 red onion, chopped (about 1 cup)

1 large lime or lemon, juice of
3 tbsp Private Reserve or Early Harvest Greek extra virgin olive oil
1 tsp Dijon mustard
½ tsp fresh garlic paste, or finely chopped garlic
1 tsp sumac
Salt and pepper, to taste

Directions:
In a small bowl, whisk well all vinaigrette ingredients.   In a salad bowl, combine cilantro chopped veggies, and kidney beans.   Add vinaigrette to salad and toss well to mix.   For 30 minutes allow for flavors to mix and set in the fridge.   Mix and adjust seasoning if needed before serving.
Nutrition Info: Calories per serving: 154; Protein: 5.5g; Carbs: 18.3g; Fat: 7.4g

690.   Tasty Mushroom Bolognese
Servings: 6   Cooking Time: 65 Minutes
Ingredients:
¼ cup chopped fresh parsley
1.5 oz Parmigiano-Reggiano cheese, grated
1 tbsp kosher salt
10-oz whole wheat spaghetti, cooked and drained
¼ cup milk
1 14-oz can whole peeled tomatoes
½ cup white wine
2 tbsp tomato paste

1 tbsp minced garlic
8 cups finely chopped cremini mushrooms
½ lb. ground pork
½ tsp freshly ground black pepper, divided
¾ tsp kosher salt, divided
2 ½ cups chopped onion
1 tbsp olive oil
1 cup boiling water
½-oz dried porcini mushrooms

Directions:
Let porcini stand in a boiling bowl of water for twenty minutes, drain (reserve liquid), rinse and chop. Set aside.   On medium high fire, place a Dutch oven with olive oil and cook for ten minutes cook pork, ¼ tsp pepper, ¼ tsp salt and onions. Constantly mix to break ground pork pieces.   Stir in ¼ tsp pepper, ¼ tsp salt, garlic and cremini mushrooms. Continue cooking until liquid has evaporated, around fifteen minutes.   Stirring constantly, add porcini and sauté for a minute. Stir in wine, porcini liquid, tomatoes and tomato paste. Let it simmer for forty minutes. Stir occasionally. Pour milk and cook for another two minutes before removing from fire.   Stir in pasta and transfer to a serving dish. Garnish with parsley and cheese before serving.
Nutrition Info: Calories per Serving: 358; Carbs: 32.8g; Protein: 21.1g; Fat: 15.4g

691. Delicious Chicken Pasta

Servings: 4   Cooking Time: 17 Minutes

Ingredients:

3 chicken breasts, skinless, boneless, cut into pieces
9 oz whole-grain pasta
1/2 cup olives, sliced
1/2 cup sun-dried tomatoes

1 tbsp roasted red peppers, chopped
14 oz can tomatoes, diced
2 cups marinara sauce
1 cup chicken broth
Pepper
Salt

Directions:

Add all ingredients except whole-grain pasta into the instant pot and stir well.   Seal pot with lid and cook on high for 12 minutes.   Once done, allow to release pressure naturally. Remove lid. Add pasta and stir well. Seal pot again and select manual and set timer for 5 minutes.   Once done, allow to release pressure naturally for 5 minutes then release remaining using quick release. Remove lid.   Stir well and serve.

Nutrition Info: Calories 615 Fat 15.4 g Carbohydrates 71 g Sugar 17.6 g Protein 48 g Cholesterol 100 mg

692. Tuna Pasta

Servings: 6   Cooking Time: 8 Minutes

Ingredients:

10 oz can tuna, drained
15 oz whole wheat rotini pasta
4 oz mozzarella cheese, cubed
1/2 cup parmesan cheese, grated
1 tsp dried basil
14 oz can tomatoes, diced

4 cups vegetable broth
1 tbsp garlic, minced
8 oz mushrooms, sliced
2 zucchini, sliced
1 onion, chopped
2 tbsp olive oil
Pepper
Salt

Directions:

Add oil into the inner pot of instant pot and set the pot on sauté mode.   Add mushrooms, zucchini, and onion and sauté until onion is softened.   Add garlic and sauté for a minute.   Add pasta, basil, tuna, tomatoes, and broth and stir well.   Seal pot with lid and cook on high for 4 minutes.   Once done, allow to release pressure naturally for 5 minutes then release remaining using quick release. Remove lid.   Add remaining ingredients and stir well and serve.

Nutrition Info: Calories 346 Fat 11.9 g Carbohydrates 31.3 g Sugar 6.3 g Protein 6.3 g Cholesterol 30 mg

693. Garlicky Lemon-parsley Hummus

Servings: 8   Cooking Time: 0 Minutes

Ingredients:

1/4 cup tahini
1/4 teaspoon fine grain sea salt
1/3 cup fresh lemon juice
3/4 cup chopped parsley
1 tablespoon olive oil, plus more for

1 1/2 cans (15 ounces each) chickpeas, rinsed and drained
5 cloves garlic, peeled and roughly chopped
Dash freshly ground black pepper

drizzling

Directions:

Place all ingredients in a blender and puree until smooth and creamy.   Transfer to a bowl and adjust seasoning if needed.   If dip dries up, just add more olive oil and mix well.   Serve and enjoy with carrot sticks.

Nutrition Info: Calories per serving: 131; Protein: 4.9g; Carbs: 13.8g; Fat: 7.0g

694. Black Eyed Peas Stew

Servings: 4   Cooking Time: 20 Minutes

Ingredients:

1/2 cup extra virgin olive oil, divided
1 cup fresh dill, stems removed, chopped
1 cup fresh parsley, stems removed, chopped
1 cup water
2 bay leaves
2 carrots, peeled and sliced

2 cups black eyed beans, drained and rinsed
2 slices orange with peel and flesh
2 Tablespoons tomato paste
4 green onions, thinly sliced
Salt and pepper, to taste

Directions:

Place a pot on medium high fire and heat. Add 1/4 cup oil and heat for 3 minutes.   Stir in bay leaves and tomato paste. Sauté for 2 minutes.   Stir in carrots and a up of water. Cover and simmer for 5 minutes.   Stir in dill, parsley, beans, and orange. Cover and cook for 3 minutes or until heated through.   Season with pepper and salt to taste. Stir in remaining oil and green onions cook for 2 minutes.   Serve and enjoy.

Nutrition Info: Calories per serving: 376; Protein: 8.8g; Carbs: 25.6g; Fat: 27.8g

695. Cheese Basil Tomato Rice

Servings: 8   Cooking Time: 26 Minutes

Ingredients:

1 1/2 cups brown rice
1 cup parmesan cheese, grated
1/4 cup fresh basil, chopped
2 cups grape tomatoes, halved
8 oz can tomato sauce

1 3/4 cup vegetable broth
1 tbsp garlic, minced
1/2 cup onion, diced
1 tbsp olive oil
Pepper
Salt

Directions:

Add oil into the inner pot of instant pot and set the pot on sauté mode.   Add garlic and onion and sauté for 4 minutes.   Add rice, tomato sauce, broth, pepper, and salt and stir well.   Seal pot with lid and cook on high for 22 minutes.   Once done, allow to release pressure naturally for 10 minutes then release remaining using quick release. Remove lid.   Add remaining ingredients and stir well.   Serve and enjoy.

Nutrition Info: Calories 208 Fat 5.6 g Carbohydrates 32.1 g Sugar 2.8 g Protein 8.3 g Cholesterol 8 mg

696. Pasta Primavera Without Cream

Servings: 6   Cooking Time: 30 Minutes

Ingredients:

1/2 cup grated Romano cheese
3 tbsp balsamic

1/4 tsp salt
1/4 cup olive oil,

vinegar
1/3 cup chopped fresh parsley
1/3 cup chopped fresh basil
2 tsp lemon zest
2 cloves garlic, sliced thinly
¼ large yellow onion, sliced thinly
1 tbsp butter
1 tbsp Italian seasoning
¼ tsp coarsely ground black pepper

divided
5 spears asparagus, trimmed and cut into 1-inch pieces
1 cup fresh green beans, trimmed and cut into 1-inch pieces
½ pint grape tomatoes
½ red bell pepper, julienned
1 carrot, julienned
1 zucchini, chopped
1 package 12-oz penne pasta

Directions:
Cook pasta according to manufacturer's instructions, drain and rinse in running cold water. Line baking sheet with aluminum foil and preheat oven to 4500F. Mix thoroughly together in a bowl Italian seasoning, lemon juice, pepper, salt, 2 tbsp olive oil, asparagus, green beans, tomatoes, red bell pepper, carrot, zucchini and squash. Arrange veggies in baking sheet and bake until tender for 15 minutes. Remove from oven. In a large skillet, heat butter and stir fry garlic and onion until soft. Add balsamic vinegar, parsley, basil, lemon zest and pasta. Continue cooking until heated through while gently tossing around the pasta. Remove from fire and transfer to a large serving bowl and mix in the roasted veggies. Serve and enjoy.
Nutrition Info: Calories per Serving: 406; Carbs: 54.4g; Protein: 15.4g; Fat: 13.6g

697.	**Spicy Sweet Red Hummus**

Servings: 8   Cooking Time: 0 Minutes
Ingredients:

1 (15 ounce) can garbanzo beans, drained
1 (4 ounce) jar roasted red peppers
1 1/2 tablespoons tahini
1 clove garlic, minced

1 tablespoon chopped fresh parsley
1/2 teaspoon cayenne pepper
1/2 teaspoon ground cumin
1/4 teaspoon salt
3 tablespoons lemon juice

Directions:
In a blender, add all ingredients and process until smooth and creamy. Adjust seasoning to taste if needed. Can be stored in an airtight container for up to 5 days.
Nutrition Info: Calories per serving: 64; Protein: 2.5g; Carbs: 9.6g; Fat: 2.2g

698.	**Veggies And Sun-dried Tomato Alfredo**

Servings: 4   Cooking Time: 30 Minutes
Ingredients:

2 tsp finely shredded lemon peel
½ cup finely shredded Parmesan cheese
1 ¼ cups milk
2 tbsp all-purpose

4 oz fresh trimmed and quartered Brussels sprouts
4 oz trimmed fresh asparagus spears
1 tbsp olive oil
4 tbsp butter

flour
8 fresh mushrooms, sliced
1 ½ cups fresh broccoli florets

½ cup chopped dried tomatoes
8 oz dried fettuccine

Directions:
In a boiling pot of water, add fettuccine and cook following manufacturer's instructions. Two minutes before the pasta is cooked, add the dried tomatoes. Drain pasta and tomatoes and return to pot to keep warm. Set aside. On medium high fire, in a big fry pan with 1 tbsp butter, fry mushrooms, broccoli, Brussels sprouts and asparagus. Cook for eight minutes while covered, transfer to a plate and put aside. Using same fry pan, add remaining butter and flour. Stirring vigorously, cook for a minute or until thickened. Add Parmesan cheese, milk and mix until cheese is melted around five minutes. Toss in the pasta and mix. Transfer to serving dish. Garnish with Parmesan cheese and lemon peel before serving.
Nutrition Info: Calories per Serving: 439; Carbs: 52.0g; Protein: 16.3g; Fat: 19.5g

699.	**Delicious Greek Chicken Pasta**

Servings: 6   Cooking Time: 10 Minutes
Ingredients:

2 chicken breasts, skinless, boneless, and cut into chunks
1/2 cup olives, sliced
2 cups vegetable stock

12 oz Greek vinaigrette dressing
1 lb whole grain pasta
Pepper
Salt

Directions:
Add all ingredients into the inner pot of instant pot and stir well. Seal pot with lid and cook on high for 10 minutes. Once done, release pressure using quick release. Remove lid. Stir well and serve.
Nutrition Info: Calories 325 Fat 25.8 g Carbohydrates 10.5 g Sugar 4 g Protein 15.6 g Cholesterol 43 mg

700.	**Breakfast Salad From Grains And Fruits**

Servings: 6   Cooking Time: 20 Minutes
Ingredients:

¼ tsp salt
¾ cup bulgur
¾ cup quick cooking brown rice
1 8-oz low fat vanilla yogurt

1 cup raisins
1 Granny Smith apple
1 orange
1 Red delicious apple
3 cups water

Directions:
On high fire, place a large pot and bring water to a boil. Add bulgur and rice. Lower fire to a simmer and cook for ten minutes while covered. Turn off fire, set aside for 2 minutes while covered. In baking sheet, transfer and evenly spread grains to cool. Meanwhile, peel oranges and cut into sections. Chop and core apples. Once grains are cool, transfer to a large serving bowl along with fruits. Add yogurt and mix well to coat. Serve and enjoy.
Nutrition Info: Calories per Serving: 48.6; Carbs: 23.9g; Protein: 3.7g; Fat: 1.1g

Salads & Side Dishes

701. Vinegar Cucumber Mix

Servings: 6   Cooking Time: 0 Minutes

Ingredients:

1 tablespoon olive oil
4 cucumbers, sliced
Salt and black pepper to the taste
1 red onion, chopped
3 tablespoons red wine vinegar
1 bunch basil, chopped
1 teaspoon honey

Directions:

In a bowl, mix the vinegar with the basil, salt, pepper, the oil and the honey and whisk well. In a bowl, mix the cucumber with the onion and the vinaigrette, toss and serve as a side salad.

Nutrition Info: calories 182, fat 7.8, fiber 2.1, carbs 4.3, protein 4.1

702. Crispy Fennel Salad

Servings: 2   Cooking Time: 15 Minutes

Ingredients:

1 fennel bulb, finely sliced
1 grapefruit, cut into segments
1 orange, cut into segments
2 tablespoons almond slices, toasted
1 teaspoon chopped mint
1 tablespoon chopped dill
Salt and pepper to taste
1 tablespoon grape seed oil

Directions:

Mix the fennel bulb with the grapefruit and orange segments on a platter. Top with almond slices, mint and dill then drizzle with the oil and season with salt and pepper. Serve the salad as fresh as possible.

Nutrition Info: Per Serving:Calories:104 Fat:0.5g Protein:3.1g Carbohydrates:25.5g

703. Red Beet Feta Salad

Servings: 4   Cooking Time: 15 Minutes

Ingredients:

6 red beets, cooked and peeled
3 oz. feta cheese, cubed
2 tablespoons extra virgin olive oil
2 tablespoons balsamic vinegar

Directions:

Combine the beets and feta cheese on a platter. Drizzle with oil and vinegar and serve right away.

Nutrition Info: Per Serving:Calories: 230 Fat: 12.0g Protein: 7.3g Carbohydrates: 26.3g

704. Cheesy Potato Mash

Servings: 8   Cooking Time: 20 Minutes

Ingredients:

2 pounds gold potatoes, peeled and cubed
1 and ½ cup cream cheese, soft
Sea salt and black pepper to the taste
½ cup almond milk
2 tablespoons chives, chopped

Directions:

Put potatoes in a pot, add water to cover, add a pinch of salt, bring to a simmer over medium heat, cook for 20 minutes, drain and mash them. Add the rest of the ingredients except the chives and whisk well. Add the chives, stir, divide between plates and serve as a side dish.

Nutrition Info: calories 243, fat 14.2, fiber 1.4, carbs 3.5, protein 1.4

705. Provencal Summer Salad

Servings: 4   Cooking Time: 25 Minutes

Ingredients:

1 zucchini, sliced
1 eggplant, sliced
2 red onions, sliced
2 tomatoes, sliced
2 garlic cloves, minced
1 teaspoon dried mint
2 tablespoons balsamic vinegar
Salt and pepper to taste

Directions:

Season the zucchini, eggplant, onions and tomatoes with salt and pepper. Cook the vegetable slices on the grill until browned. Transfer the vegetables in a salad bowl then add the mint, garlic and vinegar. Serve the salad right away.

Nutrition Info: Per Serving:Calories: 74 Fat: 0.5g Protein: 3.0g Carbohydrates: 16.5g

706. Sunflower Seeds And Arugula Garden Salad

Servings: 6   Cooking Time: 0 Minutes

Ingredients:

¼ tsp black pepper
¼ tsp salt
1 tsp fresh thyme, chopped
2 tbsp sunflower seeds, toasted
2 cups red grapes, halved
7 cups baby arugula, loosely packed
1 tbsp coconut oil
2 tsp honey
3 tbsp red wine vinegar
½ tsp stone-ground mustard

Directions:

In a small bowl, whisk together mustard, honey and vinegar. Slowly pour oil as you whisk. In a large salad bowl, mix thyme, seeds, grapes and arugula. Drizzle with dressing and serve.

Nutrition Info: Calories per serving: 86.7; Protein: 1.6g; Carbs: 13.1g; Fat: 3.1g

707. Ginger Pumpkin Mash

Servings: 4   Cooking Time: 30 Minutes

Ingredients:

10 oz pumpkin, peeled
¾ teaspoon ground ginger
½ teaspoon butter
1/3 teaspoon salt

Directions:

Chop the pumpkin into the cubes and bake in the preheated to the 360F oven for 30 minutes or until the pumpkin is soft. After this, transfer the pumpkin cubes in the food processor. Add butter, salt, and ground ginger. Blend the vegetable until you get puree or use the potato masher for this step.

Nutrition Info: Per Serving:calories 30, fat 0.7, fiber 2.1, carbs 6, protein 0.8

708. Yogurt Peppers Mix

Servings: 4   Cooking Time: 15 Minutes

Ingredients:

2 red bell peppers, cut into thick strips
2 tablespoons olive
3 shallots, chopped
Salt and black pepper to the taste

oil
3 garlic cloves, minced

½ cup Greek yogurt
1 tablespoon cilantro, chopped

Directions:
Heat up a pan with the oil over medium heat, add the shallots and garlic, stir and cook for 5 minutes. Add the rest of the ingredients, toss, cook for 10 minutes more, divide the mix between plates and serve as a side dish.
Nutrition Info:calories 274, fat 11, fiber 3.5, protein 13.3, carbs 6.5

709. Lemony Carrots

Servings: 4   Cooking Time: 40 Minutes
Ingredients:

3 tablespoons olive oil
2 pounds baby carrots, trimmed
Salt and black pepper to the taste
½ teaspoon lemon zest, grated
1/3 cup Greek yogurt

1 tablespoon lemon juice
1 garlic clove, minced
1 teaspoon cumin, ground
1 tablespoon dill, chopped

Directions:
In a roasting pan, combine the carrots with the oil, salt, pepper and the rest of the ingredients except the dill, toss and bake at 400 degrees F for 20 minutes.   Reduce the temperature to 375 degrees F and cook for 20 minutes more.   Divide the mix between plates, sprinkle the dill on top and serve.
Nutrition Info:calories 192, fat 5.4, fiber 3.4, carbs 7.3, protein 5.6

710. Roasted Vegetable Salad

Servings: 6   Cooking Time: 30 Minutes
Ingredients:

½ pound baby carrots
2 red onions, sliced
1 zucchini, sliced
2 eggplants, cubed
1 cauliflower, cut into florets
1 sweet potato, peeled and cubed
1 endive, sliced

3 tablespoons extra virgin olive oil
1 teaspoon dried basil
Salt and pepper to taste
1 lemon, juiced
1 tablespoon balsamic vinegar

Directions:
Combine the vegetables with the oil, basil, salt and pepper in a deep dish baking pan and cook in the preheated oven at 350F for 25-30 minutes. When done, transfer in a salad bowl and add the lemon juice and vinegar.   Serve the salad fresh.
Nutrition Info: Per Serving:Calories:164 Fat:7.6g Protein:3.7g Carbohydrates:24.2g

711. Chicken Kale Soup

Servings: 6   Cooking Time: 6 Hours 10 Minutes
Ingredients:

2poundschicken breast, skinless
1/3cuponion
1tablespoonolive oil
14ounceschicken bone broth

½ cup olive oil
4 cups chicken stock
¼ cup lemon juice
5ouncesbaby kale leaves
Salt, to taste

Directions:

Season chicken with salt and black pepper.   Heat olive oil over medium heat in a large skillet and add seasoned chicken.   Reduce the temperature and cook for about 15 minutes.   Shred the chicken and place in the crock pot.   Process the chicken broth and onions in a blender and blend until smooth.   Pour into crock pot and stir in the remaining ingredients.   Cook on low for about 6 hours, stirring once while cooking.
Nutrition Info: Calories: 261 Carbs: 2g Fats: 21g Proteins: 14.1g Sodium: 264mg Sugar: 0.3g

712. Mozzarella Pasta Mix

Servings: 2   Cooking Time: 15 Minutes
Ingredients:

2 oz whole grain elbow macaroni
1 tablespoon fresh basil
¼ cup cherry size Mozzarella
½ cup cherry tomatoes, halved

1 tablespoon olive oil
1 teaspoon dried marjoram
1 cup water, for cooking

Directions:
Boil elbow macaroni in water for 15 minutes. Drain water and chill macaroni little.   Chop fresh basil roughly and place it in the salad bowl.   Add Mozzarella, cherry tomatoes, dried marjoram, olive oil, amd macaroni.   Mix up salad well.
Nutrition Info: Per Serving:calories 170, fat 9.7, fiber 1.1, carbs 15, protein 6

713. Quinoa Salad

Servings: 2 Cups   Cooking Time: 20 Minutes
Ingredients:

2 cups red quinoa
1 (15-oz.) can chickpeas, drained
1 medium red onion, chopped (1/2 cup)
3 TB. fresh mint leaves, finely chopped

4 cups water
1/4 cup extra-virgin olive oil
3 TB. fresh lemon juice
1/2 tsp. salt
1/2 tsp. fresh ground black pepper

Directions:
In a medium saucepan over medium-high heat, bring red quinoa and water to a boil. Cover, reduce heat to low, and cook for 20 minutes or until water is absorbed and quinoa is tender. Let cool.   In a large bowl, add quinoa, chickpeas, red onion, and mint.   In a small bowl, whisk together extra-virgin olive oil, lemon juice, salt, and black pepper.   Pour dressing over quinoa mixture, and stir well to combine.   Serve immediately, or refrigerate and enjoy for up to 2 or 3 days.

714. Couscous And Toasted Almonds

Servings: 4   Cooking Time: 10 Minutes
Ingredients:

1 cup (about 200 g) whole-grain couscous
1 tablespoon extra-virgin olive oil
1/2 red onion, chopped
1/2 teaspoon ground ginger,

400 ml boiling water
1/2 teaspoon ground cinnamon and
1/2 teaspoon ground coriander
2 tablespoons blanched almonds, toasted, and chopped

Directions:
Preheat the oven to 110C.   In a casserole, toss the couscous with the olive oil, onion, spices, salt and

pepper. Stir in the boiling water, cover, and bake for 10 minutes. Fluff using a fork. Scatter the nuts over the top and then serve. Pair with harira.
Nutrition Info: Per Serving:261.23 cal,8 g total fat (1 g sat. fat), 37 g carb, 7 g protein, 1 g sugar, and 6.85 mg sodium.

715.Spanish Tomato Salad

Servings: 4   Cooking Time: 15 Minutes
Ingredients:

1 pound tomatoes, cubed	2 anchovy fillets
2 cucumbers, cubed	1 tablespoon balsamic vinegar
2 garlic cloves, chopped	1 pinch chili powder
1 red onion, sliced	Salt and pepper to taste

Directions:
Combine the tomatoes, cucumbers, garlic and red onion in a bowl.   In a mortar, mix the anchovy fillets, vinegar, chili powder, salt and pepper. Drizzle the mixture over the salad and mix well. Serve the salad fresh.
Nutrition Info: Per Serving:Calories: 61 Fat: 0.6g Protein: 3.0g Carbohydrates: 13.0g

716.Chickpeas And Beets Mix

Servings: 4   Cooking Time: 25 Minutes
Ingredients:

3 tablespoons capers, drained and chopped	14 ounces canned chickpeas, drained
Juice of 1 lemon	8 ounces beets, peeled and cubed
Zest of 1 lemon, grated	1 tablespoon parsley, chopped
1 red onion, chopped	Salt and pepper to the taste
3 tablespoons olive oil	

Directions:
Heat up a pan with the oil over medium heat, add the onion, lemon zest, lemon juice and the capers and sauté fro 5 minutes.   Add the rest of the ingredients, stir and cook over medium-low heat for 20 minutes more.   Divide the mix between plates and serve as a side dish.
Nutrition Info:calories 199, fat 4.5, fiber 2.3, carbs 6.5, protein 3.3

717. Roasted Bell Pepper Salad With Anchovy Dressing

Servings: 4   Cooking Time: 20 Minutes
Ingredients:

8 roasted red bell peppers, sliced	4 anchovy fillets
2 tablespoons pine nuts	1 lemon, juiced
	1 garlic clove
1 cup cherry tomatoes, halved	1 tablespoon extra-virgin olive oil
2 tablespoons chopped parsley	Salt and pepper to taste

Directions:
Combine the anchovy fillets, lemon juice, garlic and olive oil in a mortar and mix them well.   Mix the rest of the ingredients in a salad bowl then drizzle in the dressing.   Serve the salad as fresh as possible.
Nutrition Info: Per Serving: Calories: 81 Fat: 7.0g Protein: 2.4g Carbohydrates: 4.0g

718.   Warm Shrimp And Arugula Salad

Servings: 4   Cooking Time: 20 Minutes
Ingredients:

2 tablespoons extra virgin olive oil	2 garlic cloves, minced
1 red pepper, sliced	1 orange, juiced
1 pound fresh shrimps, peeled and deveined	Salt and pepper to taste
	3 cups arugula

Directions:
Heat the oil in a frying pan and stir in the garlic and red pepper. Cook for 1 minute then add the shrimps. Cook for 5 minutes then add the orange juice and cook for another 5 more minutes.   When done, spoon the shrimps and the sauce over the arugula. Serve the salad fresh.
Nutrition Info: Per Serving:Calories:232 Fat:9.2g Protein:27.0g Carbohydrates:10.0g

719.Cheesy Tomato Salad

Servings: 4   Cooking Time: 0 Minutes
Ingredients:

2 pounds tomatoes, sliced	1 red onion, chopped
Sea salt and black pepper to the taste	2 tablespoons mint, chopped
4 ounces feta cheese, crumbled	A drizzle of olive oil

Directions:
In a salad bowl, mix the tomatoes with the onion and the rest of the ingredients, toss and serve as a side salad.
Nutrition Info:calories 190, fat 4.5, fiber 3.4, carbs 8.7, protein 3.3

720.   Garlic Cucumber Mix

Servings: 4   Cooking Time: 0 Minutes
Ingredients:

2 cucumbers, sliced	1 tablespoon thyme, chopped
2 spring onions, chopped	Salt and black pepper to the taste
2 tablespoons olive oil	
3 garlic cloves, grated	3 and ½ ounces goat cheese, crumbled

Directions:
In a salad bowl, mix the cucumbers with the onions and the rest of the ingredients, toss and serve after keeping it in the fridge for 15 minutes.
Nutrition Info:calories 140, fat 5.4, fiber 4.3, carbs 6.5, protein 4.8

721.Cucumber Salad Japanese Style

Servings: 5   Cooking Time: 0 Minutes
Ingredients:

1 ½ tsp minced fresh ginger root	2 large cucumbers, ribbon cut
1 tsp salt	4 tsp white sugar
1/3 cup rice vinegar	

Directions:
Mix well ginger, salt, sugar and vinegar in a small bowl.   Add ribbon cut cucumbers and mix well. Let stand for at least one hour in the ref before serving.
Nutrition Info: Calories per Serving: 29; Fat: .2g; Protein: .7g; Carbs: 6.1g

722. Cheesy Keto Zucchini Soup

Servings: 2   Cooking Time: 20 Minutes

Ingredients:

½ medium onion, peeled and chopped
1 cup bone broth
1 tablespoon coconut oil
1½ zucchinis, cut into chunks

½ tablespoon nutrition al yeast
Dash of black pepper
½ tablespoon parsley, chopped, for garnish
½ tablespoon coconut cream, for garnish

Directions:

Melt the coconut oil in a large pan over medium heat and add onions.   Sauté for about 3 minutes and add zucchinis and bone broth.   Reduce the heat to simmer for about 15 minutes and cover the pan.   Add nutrition al yeast and transfer to an immersion blender.   Blend until smooth and season with black pepper.   Top with coconut cream and parsley to serve.

Nutrition Info: Calories: 154 Carbs: 8.9g Fats: 8.1g Proteins: 13.4g Sodium: 93mg Sugar: 3.9g

723. Grilled Salmon Summer Salad

Servings: 4   Cooking Time: 30 Minutes

Ingredients:

Salmon fillets - 2
Salt and pepper - to taste
Vegetable stock - 2 cups
Bulgur - 1 2 cup
Cherry tomatoes - 1 cup, halved
Sweet corn - 1 2 cup
Lemon - 1, juiced

Green olives - 1 2 cup, sliced
Cucumber - 1, cubed
Green onion - 1, chopped
Red pepper - 1, chopped
Red bell pepper - 1, cored and diced

Directions:

Heat a grill pan on medium and then place salmon on, seasoning with salt and pepper. Grill both sides of salmon until brown and set aside.   Heat stock in sauce pan until hot and then add in bulgur and cook until liquid is completely soaked into bulgur. Mix salmon, bulgur and all other Ingredients in a salad bowl and again add salt and pepper, if desired, to suit your taste.   Serve salad as soon as completed.

724. Dill Beets Salad

Servings: 6   Cooking Time: 0 Minutes

Ingredients:

2 tablespoons olive oil
1 tablespoon lemon juice
2 tablespoons balsamic vinegar
1 cup feta cheese, crumbled
3 small garlic cloves, minced

2 pounds beets, cooked, peeled and cubed
4 green onions, chopped
5 tablespoons parsley, chopped
Salt and black pepper to the taste

Directions:

In a bowl, mix the beets with the oil, lemon juice and the rest of the ingredients, toss and serve as a side dish.

Nutrition Info:calories 268, fat 15.5, fiber 5.1, carbs 25.7, protein 9.6

725. Green Couscous With Broad Beans, Pistachio, And Dill

Servings: 4   Cooking Time: 8 Minutes

Ingredients:

200 g fresh or frozen broad beans, podded
2 teaspoons ground ginger
2 tablespoons spring onion, thinly sliced
2 tablespoons pistachio kernels, roughly chopped
2 tablespoons lemon juice, and wedges to serve
Olive oil, extra-virgin - 1/4 cup (about 60 ml)

Dill, chopped - 1/4 cup
1/2 onion, thinly sliced
Watercress, leaves picked - 1/2 bunch
1/2 avocado, chopped
1 green bell pepper, thinly sliced
1 garlic clove, crushed
1 cup (about 200 g) whole-grain couscous
1 1/2 cups boiling water

Directions:

In a heat-safe bowl, toss the couscous with the ginger and the onion. Stir in the boiling water, cover and let stand for 5 minutes.   Meanwhile, cook the beans for about 3 minutes in boiling salted water, drain, and refresh under running cold water; discard the outer skins.   With a fork, fluff the couscous. Add the beans, avocado, bell pepper, spring onion, and dill.   In a bowl, whisk the olive oil, lemon juice, and garlic; toss with the couscous. Scatter the pistachio over the mix, serve with cress and the lemon wedges.

Nutrition Info: Per Serving:608 cal, 25.40 g total fat (4 g sat. fat), 51.50 g carb, 18.10 g protein, 45 mg sodium, and 11 g fiber.

726. Bell Peppers Salad

Servings: 6   Cooking Time: 0 Minutes

Ingredients:

2 green bell peppers, cut into thick strips
2 red bell peppers, cut into thick strips
2 tablespoons olive oil

1 garlic clove, minced
½ cup goat cheese, crumbled
A pinch of salt and black pepper

Directions:

In a bowl, mix the bell peppers with the garlic and the other ingredients, toss and serve.

Nutrition Info:calories 193, fat 4.5, fiber 2, carbs 4.3, protein 3

727. Thyme Corn And Cheese Mix

Servings: 4   Cooking Time: 0 Minutes

Ingredients:

1 tablespoon olive oil
1 teaspoon thyme, chopped
1 cup scallions, sliced
2 cups corn

Salt and black pepper to the taste
2 tablespoons blue cheese, crumbled
1 tablespoon chives, chopped

Directions:

In a salad bowl, combine the corn with scallions, thyme and the rest of the ingredients, toss, divide between plates and serve.

Nutrition Info:calories 183, fat 5.5, fiber 7.5, carbs 14.5

728. Garden Salad With Oranges And Olives

Servings: 4   Cooking Time: 15 Minutes
Ingredients:

½ cup red wine vinegar
1 tbsp extra virgin olive oil
1 tbsp finely chopped celery
1 tbsp finely chopped red onion
16 large ripe black olives
2 garlic cloves
2 navel oranges, peeled and segmented
4 boneless, skinless chicken breasts, 4-oz each
4 garlic cloves, minced
8 cups leaf lettuce, washed and dried
Cracked black pepper to taste

Directions:
Prepare the dressing by mixing pepper, celery, onion, olive oil, garlic and vinegar in a small bowl. Whisk well to combine.   Lightly grease grate and preheat grill to high.   Rub chicken with the garlic cloves and discard garlic.   Grill chicken for 5 minutes per side or until cooked through. Remove from grill and let it stand for 5 minutes before cutting into ½-inch strips.   In 4 serving plates, evenly arrange two cups lettuce, ¼ of the sliced oranges and 4 olives per plate.   Top each plate with ¼ serving of grilled chicken, evenly drizzle with dressing, serve and enjoy.
Nutrition Info: Calories per serving: 259.8; Protein: 48.9g; Carbs: 12.9g; Fat: 1.4g

729. Smoked Salmon Lentil Salad

Servings: 4   Cooking Time: 25 Minutes
Ingredients:

1 cup green lentils, rinsed
2 cups vegetable stock
½ cup chopped parsley
2 tablespoons chopped cilantro
1 red pepper, chopped
1 red onion, chopped
Salt and pepper to taste
4 oz. smoked salmon, shredded
1 lemon, juiced

Directions:
Combine the lentils and stock in a saucepan. Cook on low heat for 15-20 minutes or until all the liquid has been absorbed completely.   Transfer the lentils in a salad bowl and add the parsley, cilantro, red pepper and onion. Season with salt and pepper. Add the smoked salmon and lemon juice and mix well.   Serve the salad fresh.
Nutrition Info: Per Serving: Calories:233 Fat:2.0g Protein:18.7g Carbohydrates:35.5g

730. Salmon & Arugula Salad

Servings: 2   Cooking Time: 12 Minutes
Ingredients:

¼ cup red onion, sliced thinly
1 ½ tbsp fresh lemon juice
1 ½ tbsp olive oil
1 tbsp extra-virgin olive oil
1 tbsp red-wine vinegar
2 center cut salmon fillets (6-oz each)
2/3 cup cherry tomatoes, halved
3 cups baby arugula leaves
Pepper and salt to taste

Directions:
In a shallow bowl, mix pepper, salt, 1 ½ tbsp olive oil and lemon juice. Toss in salmon fillets and rub with the marinade. Allow to marinate for at least 15 minutes.   Grease a baking sheet and preheat oven to 350oF.   Bake marinated salmon fillet for 10 to 12 minutes or until flaky with skin side touching the baking sheet.   Meanwhile, in a salad bowl mix onion, tomatoes and arugula.   Season with pepper and salt. Drizzle with vinegar and oil. Toss to combine and serve right away with baked salmon on the side.
Nutrition Info: Calories per serving: 400; Protein: 36.6g; Carbs: 5.8g; Fat: 25.6g

731. Keto Bbq Chicken Pizza Soup

Servings: 6   Cooking Time: 1 Hour 30 Minutes
Ingredients:

6 chicken legs
1 medium red onion, diced
4 garlic cloves
1 large tomato, unsweetened
4 cups green beans
1½ cups mozzarella cheese, shredded
¾ cup BBQ Sauce
¼ cup ghee
2 quarts water
2 quarts chicken stock
Salt and black pepper, to taste
Fresh cilantro, for garnishing

Directions:
Put chicken, water and salt in a large pot and bring to a boil.   Reduce the heat to medium-low and cook for about 75 minutes.   Shred the meat off the bones using a fork and keep aside.   Put ghee, red onions and garlic in a large soup and cook over a medium heat.   Add chicken stock and bring to a boil over a high heat.   Add green beans and tomato to the pot and cook for about 15 minutes. AddBBQ Sauce, shredded chicken, salt and black pepper to the pot.   Ladle the soup into serving bowls and top with shredded mozzarella cheese and cilantro to serve.
Nutrition Info: Calories: 449 Carbs: 7.1g Fats: 32.5g Proteins: 30.8g Sodium: 252mg Sugar: 4.7g

732. Mediterranean Garden Salad

Servings: 2 Cups   Cooking Time: 5 Minutes
Ingredients:

6 cups mixed greens
2 cups cherry tomatoes, halved
1 medium red onion, sliced (1/2 cup)
3 TB. fresh lemon juice
3 TB. balsamic vinegar
3 TB. tahini paste
3 TB. plus 1 tsp. extra-virgin olive oil
3 TB. water
1/2 tsp. salt
1/2 tsp. fresh ground black pepper
1/2 cup pine nuts

Directions:
In a large bowl, add mixed greens, cherry tomatoes, and red onion.   In a small bowl, whisk together tahini paste, lemon juice, balsamic vinegar, 3 tablespoons extra-virgin olive oil, water, salt, and black pepper.   Preheat a small skillet over medium-low heat for 1 minute. Add remaining 1 teaspoon extra-virgin olive oil and pine nuts, and cook, stirring to toast evenly on all sides, for 4 minutes. Transfer pine nuts to a plate, and let cool for 2 minutes.   Pour dressing over vegetables, and toss to coat evenly. Top with toasted pine nuts, and serve immediately.

733. Buttery Millet

Servings: 3   Cooking Time: 15 Minutes

Ingredients:

¼ cup mushrooms, sliced
¾ cup onion, diced
1 tablespoon olive oil
1 teaspoon salt
3 tablespoons milk
½ cup millet
1 cup of water
1 teaspoon butter

Directions:

Pour olive oil in the skillet and add the onion. Add mushrooms and roast the vegetables for 10 minutes over the medium heat. Stir them from time to time.   Meanwhile, pour water in the pan. Add millet and salt.   Cook the millet with the closed lid for 15 minutes over the medium heat. Then add the cooked mushroom mixture in the millet.   Add milk and butter. Mix up the millet well.

Nutrition Info: Per Serving:calories 198, fat 7.7, fiber 3.5, carbs 27.9, protein 4.7

734. Delicata Squash Soup

Servings: 5   Cooking Time: 45minutes

Ingredients:

1½ cups beef bone broth
1small onion, peeled and grated.
½ teaspoon sea salt
¼ teaspoon poultry seasoning
2small Delicata Squash, chopped
2 garlic cloves, minced
2tablespoons olive oil
¼ teaspoon black pepper
1 small lemon, juiced
5 tablespoons sour cream

Directions:

Put Delicata Squash and water in a medium pan and bring to a boil.   Reduce the heat and cook for about 20 minutes.   Drain and set aside.   Put olive oil, onions, garlic and poultry seasoning in a small sauce pan.   Cook for about 2 minutes and add broth.   Allow it to simmer for 5 minutes and remove from heat.   Whisk in the lemon juice and transfer the mixture in a blender.   Pulse until smooth and top with sour cream.

Nutrition Info: Calories: 109 Carbs: 4.9g Fats: 8.5g Proteins: 3g Sodium: 279mg Sugar: 2.4g

735. Parsley Couscous And Cherries Salad

Servings: 6   Cooking Time: 0 Minutes

Ingredients:

2 cups hot water
½ cup walnuts, roasted and chopped
½ cup cherries, pitted
½ cup parsley, chopped
1 cup couscous
A pinch of sea salt and black pepper
1 tablespoon lime juice
2 tablespoons olive oil

Directions:

Put the couscous in a bowl, add the hot water, cover, leave aside for 10 minutes, fluff with a fork and transfer to a bowl.   Add the rest of the ingredients, toss and serve.

Nutrition Info:calories 200, fat 6.71, fiber 7.3, carbs 8.5, protein 5

736. Mint Quinoa

Servings: 8   Cooking Time: 10 Minutes

Ingredients:

1 cup quinoa
1 ¼ cup water
4 teaspoons lemon juice
¼ teaspoon garlic clove, diced
5 tablespoons sesame oil
2 cucumbers, chopped
1/3 teaspoon ground black pepper
1/3 cup tomatoes, chopped
½ oz scallions, chopped
¼ teaspoon fresh mint, chopped

Directions:

Pour water in the pan. Add quinoa and boil it for 10 minutes.   Then close the lid and let it rest for 5 minutes more.   Meanwhile, in the mixing bowl mix up together lemon juice, diced garlic, sesame oil, cucumbers, ground black pepper, tomatoes, scallions, and fresh mint.   Then add cooked quinoa and carefully mix the side dish with the help of the spoon.   Store tabbouleh up to 2 days in the fridge.

Nutrition Info: Per Serving:calories 168, fat 9.9, fiber 2, carbs 16.9, protein 3.6

737. Spicy Halibut Tomato Soup

Servings: 8   Cooking Time: 1 Hour 5minutes

Ingredients:

2garliccloves, minced
1tablespoonolive oil
¼ cup fresh parsley, chopped
10anchoviescanned in oil, minced
6cupsvegetable broth
1teaspoonblack pepper
1poundhalibut fillets, chopped
3tomatoes, peeled and diced
1teaspoonsalt
1teaspoonred chili flakes

Directions:

Heat olive oil in a large stockpot over medium heat and add garlic and half of the parsley.   Add anchovies, tomatoes, vegetable broth, red chili flakes, salt and black pepper and bring to a boil. Reduce the heat to medium-low and simmer for about 20 minutes.   Add halibut fillets and cook for about 10 minutes.   Dish out the halibut and shred into small pieces.   Mix back with the soup and garnish with the remaining fresh parsley to serve.

Nutrition Info: Calories: 170 Carbs: 3g Fats: 6.7g Proteins: 23.4g Sodium: 2103mg Sugar: 1.8g

738. Beans With Pancetta, Sage, And Vinegar

Servings: 6   Cooking Time: 15 Minutes

Ingredients:

1 red onion, finely chopped
1/4 cup fresh continental parsley, chopped
2 cans (400 g each) borlotti beans, rinsed, and drained
2 garlic cloves, finely chopped
3 anchovy fillets, drained, finely chopped
3 fresh sage leaves, chopped
50 g pancetta, finely chopped
60 ml (about 1/4 cup) red wine vinegar
60 ml (about 1/4 cup) water
80 ml (about 1/3 cup) extra-virgin olive oil
Fresh continental parsley leaves, plus more to serve
Red wine vinegar, plus more, to serve

Directions:
In a heavy-bottomed saucepan, heat the oil over medium-low heat. Add the garlic, onion, pancetta, and the anchovy; cook for about 8 minutes, stirring often, until the onion is soft.   Add the water, vinegar, and the sage. Adjust the heat to medium-high; bring to a simmer, cooking for about 3 minutes or until the liquid is slightly reduced. Transfer into a bowl. Stir in the beans and set aside; letting the mixture cool completely.   Season the mixture with more salt, pepper, and vinegar. Stir in the parsley, transfer into a serving bowl, top with the parsley, and serve.   Make-ahead: Prepare the ingredients up to step 2 up to 1 day ahead before serving day; cover and store in the refrigerator. Four hours before serving, remove from the fridge. Continue from step 3 thirty minutes before serving.
Nutrition Info: Per Serving:245 cal, 14 g total fat (1 g sat. fat), 19 g carb, 9 g protein, 579.84 mg sodium, 1 g sugar, 6 mg chol., and 6 g fiber.

739. Mediterranean-style Vegetable Stew

Servings: 4   Cooking Time: 15 Minutes
Ingredients:

1 can (14 ounces) cannelini beans, rinsed, drained	2 tablespoons olive oil, divided
1 red onion, peeled, chopped	4 cups vegetable stock
1 tablespoon cilantro, chopped	5 ounces carrots, peeled, cut into ribbons using a vegetable peeler
2 cloves garlic, peeled, crushed	8 ounces turnips, peeled, chopped
2 small zucchini, thinly sliced	Crusty whole-wheat bread, to serve
2 tablespoons lemon juice	Lemon wedges, to serve
3 tomatoes, quartered	

Directions:
In a large-sized pot, heat 1 tablespoons of the olive oil. Add the garlic, onion, and turnip; sauté for 5 minutes. Add the carrots, tomatoes, zucchini; sauté for 2 minutes.   Add the stock, the lemon juice, the beans, and the remaining oil; season to taste. Bring to a boil; simmer for 3 to 4 minutes. Sprinkle with cilantro. Serve with the bread and the lemon wedges.
Nutrition Info: Per Serving:190 cal., 11 g total fat (1 g sat. fat), 0 mg chol., 1020 mg sodium, 1000 mg potassium, 29 g carb, 9 g fiber, 16 g sugar, 5 g protein, 160% vitamin A, 140% vitamin C, 10% calcium, and 8% iron.

740.   Cheesy Potatoes

Servings: 4   Cooking Time: 20 Minutes
Ingredients:

4 sweet potatoes	1 tablespoon fresh parsley, chopped
¼ cup Cheddar cheese, shredded	½ teaspoon salt
2 teaspoons butter	

Directions:
Make the lengthwise cut in every sweet potato and bake them for 10 minutes at 360F.   After this, scoop ½ part of every sweet potato flesh.   Fill the vegetables with salt, parsley, butter, and shredded cheese.   Return the sweet potatoes in the oven back and bake them for 10 minutes more at 355F.

Nutrition Info: Per Serving:calories 47, fat 4.3, fiber 0.1, carbs 0.4, protein 1.8

741.Greek Beets

Servings: 2   Cooking Time: 25 Minutes
Ingredients:

1 beet, trimmed	2 tablespoons walnuts
1/3 teaspoon minced garlic	2 tablespoons Greek yogurt

Directions:
Preheat the oven to 360F.   Place the beet in the tray and bake it for 25 minutes. The baked beet should be tender.   Let the beet chill little. Peel it. After this, grate it with the help of the grated and transfer in the bowl.   Add walnuts, Greek yogurt, and minced garlic. Mix up the mixture well. Place it in the fridge for at least 10 minutes before serving.
Nutrition Info: Per Serving:calories 79, fat 4.8, fiber 1.5, carbs 6.4, protein 3.9

742.   Snow Peas Salad

Servings: 4   Cooking Time: 10 Minutes
Ingredients:

3 cups snow peas, trimmed	1 teaspoon ginger, grated
1 and ¼ cup bean sprouts	2 spring onions, chopped
1 tablespoon basil, chopped	2 garlic cloves, minced
1 tablespoon lime juice	

Directions:
Put the snow peas in a pot, add water to cover, bring to a simmer and cook over medium heat for 10 minutes.   Drain the peas, transfer them to a bowl, add the sprouts and the rest of the ingredients, toss and keep in the fridge for 6 hours before serving.
Nutrition Info:calories 200, fat 8.6, fiber 3, carbs 5.4, protein 3.4

743.   Beans And Rice

Servings: 6   Cooking Time: 55 Minutes
Ingredients:

1 tablespoon olive oil	2 cups brown rice
1 yellow onion, chopped	1 and ½ cup canned black beans, rinsed and drained
2 celery stalks, chopped	4 cups water
2 garlic cloves, minced	Salt and black pepper to the taste

Directions:
Heat up a pan with the oil over medium heat, add the celery, garlic and the onion, stir and cook for 10 minutes.   Add the rest of the ingredients, stir, bring to a simmer and cook over medium heat for 45 minutes.   Divide between plates and serve.
Nutrition Info:calories 224, fat 8.4, fiber 3.4, carbs 15.3, protein 6.2

744.   Parsley Tomato Mix

Servings: 4   Cooking Time: 10 Minutes
Ingredients:

4 medium tomatoes, roughly cubed	½ teaspoon sweet paprika
1 garlic clove, minced	Salt and black pepper

1 tablespoon olive oil   to the taste
                          ½ bunch parsley,
                          chopped

Directions:
Heat up a pot with the olive oil over medium heat, add the tomatoes and the garlic and sauté for 5 minutes.   Add the rest of the ingredients, toss, cook for 3-4 minutes more, divide into bowls and serve.
Nutrition Info:calories 220, fat 9.4, fiber 5.3, carbs 6.5, protein 4.6

---

745.   Lemon Chili Cucumbers

Servings: 3   Cooking Time: 30 Minutes
Ingredients:

3 cucumbers   ¾ teaspoon lemon
3 tablespoons lemon   zest
juice   1 tablespoon olive oil
3 teaspoons dill,   ¾ teaspoon chili
chopped   flakes

Directions:
Peel the cucumbers and chop them roughly. Place the cucumbers in the big glass jar.   Add lemon zest, lemon juice, dill, olive oil, and chili flakes.   Close the lid and shake well.   Marinate the cucumbers for 30 minutes.
Nutrition Info: Per Serving:calories 92, fat 5.2, fiber 1.8, carbs 11.9, protein 2.3

---

746.   Tuna-dijon Salad

Servings: 6   Cooking Time: Minutes
Ingredients:

5 whole small   1/2 English
radishes, stems   cucumber, chopped
removed and   1/2 medium-sized red
chopped   onion, finely chopped
3 stalks green onions,   3 5-ounce cans
chopped   Genova tuna in olive
1 cup chopped   oil
parsley leaves   1 1/2 limes, juice of
½ cup chopped fresh   1/2 tsp crushed red
mint leaves, stems   pepper flakes,
removed   optional
Six slices heirloom   1/2 tsp sumac
tomatoes for serving   1/3 cup Early Harvest
Pita chips or pita   extra virgin olive oil
pockets for serving   2 1/2 tsp good quality
2 1/2 celery stalks,   Dijon mustard
chopped   Pinch of salt and
1/2 cup pitted   pepper
Kalamata olives,   Zest of 1 lime
halved

Directions:
Make the dressing by mixing all ingredients in a small bowl until thoroughly blended. Set aside to allow flavors to mix.   In a large salad bowl, make the salad.   Mix well mint leaves, parsley. Olives, chopped veggies, and tuna.   Drizzle with vinaigrette and toss well to coat.   Put in the fridge for at least half an hour to allow flavors to mix. Toss again. Top with tomatoes.   Serve with pita chips on the side and enjoy.
Nutrition Info: Calories per Serving: 299; Carbs: 6.6g; Protein: 25.7g; Fats: 19.2g

---

747.   Grilled Chicken Salad

Servings: 4   Cooking Time: 30 Minutes

Ingredients:
2 chicken fillets   2 cups arugula leaves
1 teaspoon dried   ¼ cup green olives
oregano   1 cucumber, sliced
1 teaspoon dried basil   1 lemon, juiced
2 tablespoons olive   2 tablespoons extra
oil   virgin olive oil
1 cup cherry   Salt and pepper to
tomatoes, halved   taste

Directions:
Season the chicken with salt, pepper, oregano and basil then drizzle it with olive oil.   Heat a grill pan over medium flame then place the chicken on the grill. Cook on each side until browned then cut into thin strips.   Combine the chicken with the rest of the ingredients and mix gently.   Adjust the taste with salt and pepper and serve the salad as fresh as possible.
Nutrition Info: Per Serving:Calories: 280 Fat: 19.5g Protein: 21.6g Carbohydrates: 6.4g

---

748.   Chili Cabbage And Coconut

Servings: 4   Cooking Time: 20 Minutes
Ingredients:

3 tablespoons olive   4 green chili peppers,
oil   chopped
1 spring curry leaves,   ½ cup coconut flesh,
chopped   grated
1 teaspoon mustard   Salt and black pepper
seeds, crushed   to the taste
1 green cabbage head,
shredded

Directions:
Heat up a pan with the oil over medium heat, add the curry leaves, mustard seeds and the chili peppers and cook for 5 minutes.   Add the rest of the ingredients, toss and cook for 15 minutes more. Divide the mix between plates and serve as a side dish.
Nutrition Info:calories 221, fat 5.5, fiber 11.1, carbs 22.1, protein 6.7

---

749.   Spinach And Cranberry Salad

Servings: 4   Cooking Time: 5 Minutes
Ingredients:

¼ cup cider vinegar   1 cup dried
¼ cup honey   cranberries
¼ cup white wine   1 lb spinach, rinsed
vinegar   and torn into bite
¼ tsp paprika   sized pieces
½ cup olive oil   2 tsp minced onion
½ cup pumpkin
seeds

Directions:
Toast pumpkin seeds by placing in a nonstick saucepan on medium fire. Stir frequently and toast for at least 3 to 5 minutes. Remove from fire and set aside.   In a medium bowl, mix well olive oil, cider vinegar, white wine vinegar, paprika, onion, and honey. Whisk well until mixture is uniform. In a large salad bowl, add torn spinach.   Drizzle with dressing and toss well to coat.   Garnish with cooled and toasted pumpkin seeds and dried cranberries.   Serve and enjoy.
Nutrition Info: Calories per Serving: 531.3; Fat: 34.9g; Protein: 9.1g; Carbs: 45.2g

750.   Dill Cucumber Salad

Servings: 8   Cooking Time: 0 Minutes
Ingredients:

1 cup white wine
vinegar
2 white onions, sliced

4 cucumbers, sliced
1 tablespoon dill,
chopped

Directions:
In a bowl, mix the cucumber with the onions, vinegar and the dill, toss well and keep in the fridge for 1 hour before serving as a side salad.
Nutrition Info:calories 182, fat 3.5, fiber 4.5, carbs 8.5, protein 4.5

751. Nutty, Curry-citrus Garden Salad

Servings: 2   Cooking Time: 0 Minutes
Ingredients:

¼ tsp curry powder
1 medium carrot,
shredded
1 tsp Balsamic
vinegar
2 cups spring mix
salad greens

2 tbsp orange juice
2 tsp extra virgin
olive oil
8 pecan halves,
chopped
Pepper and salt to
taste

Directions:
In a small bowl, whisk well curry powder, balsamic vinegar, olive oil, and orange juice.   Season with pepper and salt to taste. Mix well.   In a salad bowl, mix shredded carrot and salad greens. Pour in dressing, toss well to coat.   To serve, top with chopped pecans and enjoy.
Nutrition Info: Calories per serving: 117; Protein: 2.39g; Carbs: 10.2g; Fat: 7.4g

752.   Mouthwatering Steakhouse Salad

Servings: 4   Cooking Time: 30 Minutes
Ingredients:

½ tsp pepper
½ tsp salt
1 lb. green beans,
trimmed
10oz timed filet
mignon
2 garlic cloves
2 tsp extra virgin
olive oil

3 tbsp balsamic
vinegar
4 medium red bell
peppers, seeded and
halved
6 medium tomatoes
cut into ¼ wedges
8 cups mesclun

Directions:
Preheat the grill or the broiler. Put the red peppers on the grill and cook until the skin blisters and chars. Peel away blackened skins and cut into chunks.   Meanwhile, lay the filet mignon on a cutting board and slit it lengthwise until it opens like a book when pressed flat. Sprinkle with ¼ teaspoon salt and ¼ teaspoon pepper. Cut 1 garlic clove and rub the cut sides all over the steak. Grill the beef until done. Slice it thinly and set aside. In a saucepan, cook the beans in the boiling water until tender. Drain and rinse with cold water. Set aside.   Mince the remaining garlic and add to vinegar, oil and shallot. Season with salt and pepper.   In a plate, prepare a mesclun bead and arrange the steak, beans, tomatoes and red peppers on top. Drizzle with the dressing. Serve warm.
Nutrition Info: Calories per serving 220.3; Protein: 21.6g; Carbs: 21.1g; Fat: 5.5g

753.   Green Beans With Pomegranate Dressing

Servings: 8   Cooking Time: 30 Minutes
Ingredients:

1 small red onion,
sliced into half moons
1 teaspoon cinnamon
2 red pepper, cut into
quarters
200 g green beans,
blanched (frozen
beans preferred)
3 medium aubergine
or eggplant, cut into
chunks, or 15 small,
halved
6 tablespoons
extra-virgin olive oil

200 g feta cheese,
drained, crumbled
Handful parsley,
roughly chopped
Seeds of 1
pomegranate
5 tablespoons
extra-virgin olive oil
2 tablespoons
pomegranate
molasses
1 tablespoon lemon
juice
1 small garlic clove,
crushed

Directions:
Heat the oven to 200C, gas to 6, or fan to 180C. Preheat the grill to the highest setting.   With the skin side up, place them in a baking sheet; grill until blackened. Place in a plastic bag, seal, and let rest for 5 minutes. When cool enough to handle, scrape the blackened skins off, discard, the set aside the peppers.   Place the aubergine chunks into a baking tray; drizzle with the olive oil, sprinkle with the cinnamon, and season with the salt and pepper. Roast for about 25 minutes, or until softened and golden.   Meanwhile, in a bowl, combine all the dressing ingredients until well mixed.   To serve: Place the green beans, aubergine chunks, peppers, and onion into a large-sized serving platter. Scatter the feta and the pomegranate seeds over the vegetables. Drizzle the dressing and top with parsley.
Nutrition Info: Per Serving:258 cal, 21 g fat (5 g sat. fat), 12 g carbs, 11 g sugars, 0 g fiber, 6 g protein, and 0.94 g sodium.

754.   Cauliflower And Thyme Soup

Servings: 6   Cooking Time: 30 Minutes
Ingredients:

2teaspoonsthyme
powder
1head cauliflower
3cupsvegetable stock
½ teaspoon matcha
green tea powder

3tablespoonsolive oil
Salt and black
pepper, to taste
5garlic
cloves,chopped

Directions:
Put the vegetable stock, thyme and matcha powder to a large pot over medium-high heat and bring to a boil.   Add cauliflower and cook for about 10 minutes.   Meanwhile, put the olive oil and garlic in a small sauce pan and cook for about 1 minute. Add the garlic, salt and black pepper and cook for about 2 minutes.   Transfer into an immersion blender and blend until smooth.   Dish out and serve immediately.
Nutrition Info: Calories: 79 Carbs: 3.8g Fats: 7.1g Proteins: 1.3g Sodium: 39mg Sugar: 1.5g

755.   Turkey Magiritsa

Servings: 6   Cooking Time: 20 Minutes
Ingredients:

1 1/2 cups leftover
cooked turkey,

1/2 teaspoon freshly
squeezed lemon juice

shredded (lean meat preferred, but you can use light and dark meat)
1 cup cooked whole-grain rice
1 cup romaine lettuce, shredded
1 tablespoon fresh dill, chopped
1/2 cup sliced green onions
1/2 teaspoon whole-wheat flour
1/4 teaspoon freshly ground black pepper
1/4 teaspoon salt
2 1/2 cups onion, finely chopped
2 large eggs
2 tablespoons freshly squeezed lemon juice
2 tablespoons olive oil
7 cups chicken broth, fat-free, less-sodium divided
Dash of salt

Directions:
In a bowl, whisk the flour and 2 tablespoons lemon juice until smooth. Add the eggs; whisk until smooth. In a medium-sized saucepan, bring 1 cup of the broth into a simmer over medium-high heat. Gradually add the hot broth into the egg mixture, constantly stirring with a whisk. Return the egg mixture into the saucepan; cook for 2 minutes, constantly whisking, until slightly thick. Remove from the heat and set aside. In a large-sized saucepan, heat the olive oil over medium-high heat. Add the onion and the dash of salt; sauté for about 8 minutes or until tender. Add the remaining 6 cups of broth; bring to a boil. When boiling, reduce the heat to a simmer; cook for 5 minutes more. Add the turkey; simmer for 2 minutes. Add the rice and slowly whisk in the egg mixture. Keep the soup warm over low heat. When ready to serve, add the remaining ingredients.

Nutrition Info: Per Serving:232 Cal, 9.1 g total fat (1.9 g sat. fat, 4.9 g mono fat, 1.3 g poly fat), 18 g protein, 17g carb, 2 g fiber, 98 g chol., 1.5 mg iron, 697 mg sodium, and 34 mg calcium.

756. Quinoa And Greens Salad

Servings: 4   Cooking Time: 0 Minutes
Ingredients:
1 cup quinoa, cooked
1 medium bunch collard greens, chopped
4 tablespoons walnuts, chopped
2 tablespoons balsamic vinegar
4 tablespoons tahini paste
4 tablespoons cold water
A pinch of salt and black pepper
1 tablespoon olive oil

Directions:
In a bowl, mix the tahini with the water and vinegar and whisk. In a bowl, mix the quinoa with the rest of the ingredients and the tahini dressing, toss, divide the mix between plates and serve as a side dish.

Nutrition Info:calories 175, fat 3, fiber 3, carbs 5, protein 3

757. Mushroom Spinach Soup

Servings: 4   Cooking Time: 25 Minutes
Ingredients:
1cupspinach,cleaned and chopped
100gmushrooms,chopped
1onion
6 garlic cloves
½ teaspoon red chili powder
Salt and black pepper, to
3 tablespoons buttermilk
1 teaspoon almond flour
2 cups chicken broth
3 tablespoons butter
¼ cup fresh cream,for garnish

taste
Directions:
Heat butter in a pan and add onions and garlic. Sauté for about 3 minutes and add spinach, salt and red chili powder. Sauté for about 4 minutes and add mushrooms. Transfer into a blender and blend to make a puree. Return to the pan and add buttermilk and almond flour for creamy texture. Mix well and simmer for about 2 minutes. Garnish with fresh cream and serve hot.
Nutrition Info: Calories: 160 Carbs: 7g Fats: 13.3g Proteins: 4.7g Sodium: 462mg Sugar: 2.7g

758. Spicy Herb Potatoes (batata Harra)

Servings: 1 Cup   Cooking Time: 25 Minutes
Ingredients:
15 small new red potatoes (11/2 lb.), scrubbed and dried
1 tsp. salt
4 TB. extra-virgin olive oil
3 TB. minced garlic
1 cup fresh cilantro, finely chopped
1/2 tsp. cayenne
1/2 tsp. black pepper

Directions:
Preheat the oven to 425°F. Cut red potatoes into 1-inch pieces. Add potatoes to a large bowl, and toss with salt and 3 tablespoons extra-virgin olive oil. Spread potatoes in an even layer on a baking sheet, and bake for 20 to 25 minutes or until golden. Remove from the oven, and let stand for 5 minutes. Using a spatula, transfer potatoes to a large serving bowl. Heat a small saucepan over low heat. Add remaining 1 tablespoon extra-virgin olive oil and garlic, and sauté for 3 minutes. Add garlic to potatoes. Add cilantro, cayenne, and black pepper to potatoes, and gently toss to combine. Serve warm or at room temperature.

759. Orange Couscous

Servings: 2   Cooking Time: 15 Minutes
Ingredients:
1/3 cup couscous
¼ cup of water
4 tablespoons orange juice
¼ orange, chopped
1 teaspoon Italian seasonings
1/3 teaspoon salt
½ teaspoon butter

Directions:
Pour water and orange juice in the pan. Add orange, Italian seasoning, and salt. Bring the liquid to boil and remove it from the heat. Add butter and couscous. Stir well and close the lid. Leave the couscous rest for 10 minutes.
Nutrition Info: Per Serving:calories 149, fat 1.9, fiber 2.1, carbs 28.5, protein 4.1

760. Walnuts Cucumber Mix

Servings: 2   Cooking Time: 0 Minutes
Ingredients:
1 tablespoon olive oil
Salt and black pepper to the taste
1 red chili pepper, dried
1 tablespoon lemon juice
2 cucumbers, chopped
3 tablespoons walnuts, chopped
1 tablespoon balsamic vinegar
1 teaspoon chives, chopped

Directions:

In a bowl, mix the cucumbers with the oil and the rest of the ingredients, toss and serve as a side dish.
Nutrition Info:calories 121, fat 2.3, fiber 2.0, carbs 6.7, protein 2.4

761. Red Beet Spinach Salad

Servings: 4   Cooking Time: 20 Minutes
Ingredients:

3 cups baby spinach	1 tablespoon apple
2 red beets, cooked	cider vinegar
and diced	¼ cup Greek yogurt
1 tablespoon	Salt and pepper to
prepared horseradish	taste

Directions:
Combine the baby spinach and red beets in a salad bowl.   Add the horseradish, vinegar and yogurt and mix well then season with salt and pepper. Serve the salad as fresh as possible.
Nutrition Info: Per Serving:Calories:64 Fat:1.2g Protein:6.4g Carbohydrates:7.5g

762.   Broccoli Spaghetti

Servings: 2   Cooking Time: 10 Minutes
Ingredients:

1/3 cup broccoli	½ teaspoon ground
7 oz whole grain	black pepper
spaghetti	1 cup water, for
2 oz Parmesan,	cooking
shaved	

Directions:
Chop the broccoli into the small florets.   Pour water in the pan. Bring it to boil.   Add broccoli florets and spaghetti.   Close the lid and cook the ingredients for 10 minutes.   Then drain water. Add ground black pepper and shaved Parmesan. Shake the spaghetti well.
Nutrition Info: Per Serving:calories 430, fat 8.8, fiber 9.3, carbs 72.4, protein 23.6

763.   Leeks Sauté

Servings: 4   Cooking Time: 15 Minutes
Ingredients:

2 pounds leeks, sliced	1 tablespoon olive oil
2 tablespoons	2 tablespoons thyme,
chicken stock	chopped
2 tablespoons tomato	Salt and black pepper
paste	to the taste

Directions:
Heat up a pan with the oil over medium heat, add the leeks and brown for 5 minutes.   Add the rest of the ingredients, toss, increase the heat to medium-high and cook for 10 minutes more. Divide everything between plates and serve as a side dish.
Nutrition Info:calories 200, fat 11.4, fiber 5.6, carbs 16.4, protein 3.6

764.   Whole-wheat Soft Dinner Dough And Rolls

Servings: 5   Cooking Time: 20-25 Minutes
Ingredients:

2 tablespoons yeast	1 cup warm
1/2 cup warm	buttermilk (or milk)
1/2 cup softened	4 1/2 cups
butter	whole-wheat flour
1/4 cup honey	1 1/2 teaspoons salt
3 eggs	

Directions:

Dissolve the yeast in the warm water in a bowl or a glass measuring cup, stirring with a whisk, then set aside.   In the bowl of a stand mixer, put the softened butter. Add the honey; cream together using the paddle attachment.   Add the eggs; beat, scraping the butter from the bowl sides. Add the warm buttermilk and then the yeast mixture. The mixture will not be smooth and you'll see butter lumps floating. Add the whole-wheat flour and the salt; mix well.   Change to the dough hook; knead for a couple of minutes. You just need to lose the extreme stickiness of the dough, but not to develop the gluten. If needed, add a couple of tablespoons of flour. To test, touch the dough surface with a finger. No dough should stick on your finger even though it will look sticky. The dough should still be sticking to the bowl, but should not stick on our finger.   When you achieved the correct texture, cover the bowl with towel, and let sit for 1 hour at room temperature. The dough will rise, but it will not double.   Transfer the dough onto a floured surface. Knead with your hands a few times, cover with a towel, and let rest for 3 minutes. Meanwhile, generously butter the sides and the bottom of a 9x13-inch pan.   Flatten it into an even rectangle shape, roughly about the size of the pan. With a knife, cut the dough into 24 pieces. Now shape them into dinner rolls. If you are right-handed, form your left hand into a circle, the tipoff the thumb almost touching the pointing the middle finger. With your right hand, take a dough and push it up through the hand circle, forming the rounded top. Now turn the ball over and pinch the ends to come together. With the round side up, place the seam side down in the prepared dish - six balls down and fur balls across. The doughs should be touching the pan. Cover with the towel and let rise for 1 more hour. Set a timer for 45 minutes. Start preheating the oven to 350F during the last 15 minutes of letting the dough rise. After 1 hour, the dough will rise and they will be touching each other. Bake for about 20 to 25 minutes or until golden brown. Rotate the pan 180 degrees for an even browning. As soon as they come out from the oven, brush thee tops with softened butter. As soon as they are cooled to warm, pull the rolls out of the pan and pull them apart to serve.
Nutrition Info: Per Serving:135 cal., 4.7 g fat (2.7 g sat. fat), 32 mg chol., 194 mg sodium, 68 mg pot., 19.7 total carb., 0.8 fiber, 3.5 g sugar, and 3.6 g protein.

765.   Peppers And Lentils Salad

Servings: 4   Cooking Time: 0 Minutes
Ingredients:

2 spring onions,	14 ounces canned
chopped	lentils, drained and
1 red bell pepper,	rinsed
chopped	1/3 cup coriander,
1 green bell pepper,	chopped
chopped	2 teaspoon balsamic
1 tablespoon fresh	vinegar
lime juice	

Directions:
In a salad bowl, combine the lentils with the onions, bell peppers and the rest of the ingredients, toss and serve.
Nutrition Info:calories 200, fat 2.45, fiber 6.7, carbs 10.5, protein 5.6

766. Avocado And Onion Mix

Servings: 4   Cooking Time: 0 Minutes

Ingredients:

4 avocados, pitted, peeled and sliced
1 red onion, sliced
2 tablespoons olive oil
2 tablespoons lime juice
¼ cup dill, chopped
Sea salt and black pepper to the taste

Directions:

In a salad bowl, mix the avocados with the onion and the rest of the ingredients, toss and serve as a side dish.

Nutrition Info:calories 465, fat 23.5, fiber 14.3, carbs 21.4, protein 5.4

767. Lemony Barley And Yogurt

Servings: 4   Cooking Time: 30 Minutes

Ingredients:

½ cup barley
1 and ½ cup veggie stock
Salt and black pepper to the taste
2 tablespoons olive oil
½ cup Greek yogurt
1 tablespoon lemon juice
¼ cup mint, chopped
1 apple, cored and chopped

Directions:

Put barley in a pot, add the stock and salt, bring to a boil and simmer for 30 minutes.   Drain, transfer the barley to a bowl, add the rest of the ingredients, toss, divide between plates and serve as a side dish.

Nutrition Info:calories 263, fat 9, fiber 11.4, carbs 17.4, protein 6.5

768. Chives Quinoa Mix

Servings: 4   Cooking Time: 10 Minutes

Ingredients:

1 cup quinoa
2 cups chicken stock
1 tablespoon butter
4 teaspoons chives, chopped
½ teaspoon salt

Directions:

Pour chicken stock in the pan.   Add quinoa and salt.   Close the lid and boil the mixture for 10 minutes or until quinoa will soak all liquid.   After this, add chives and butter. Mix up the quinoa well.

Nutrition Info: Per Serving:calories 187, fat 5.8, fiber 3, carbs 27.7, protein 6.4

769. Beef soup With Mushrooms

Servings: 2   Cooking Time: 1 Hour 40 Minutes

Ingredients:

3 1/2 cups (about 8 ounces) mushrooms, halved
2 tablespoons red wine vinegar
2 garlic cloves, minced
2 cups carrot, diagonally cut
2 bay leaves
2 cans (14.5-ounce each) stewed tomatoes, no-salt-added, undrained
1/4 teaspoon black
1/2 teaspoon dried thyme
1 cup cabernet sauvignon or other dry red wine
1 1/4 teaspoons kosher salt
1 1/2 teaspoons olive oil
1 1/2 pounds beef stew meat, cut into 1-inch pieces
1 1/2 cups water
1 1/2 cups celery, sliced
1 1/2 cups onion,

pepper, coarsely ground
1/4 cup fresh flat-leaf parsley, chopped
coarsely chopped
1 can (2 1/4-ounce) ripe olives, sliced, drained

Directions:

Over medium heat, heat the olive oil in a large-sized Dutch oven. Add the beef; cook for about 5 minutes, or until all sides are browned.   Remove the beef. Add the mushrooms, carrots, onion, celery, and garlic cloves; cook for about 5 minutes, occasionally stirring.   Return the beef. Stir in the water, wine, salt, black pepper, tomatoes, thyme, and bay leaves; bring to a boil. Cover, reduce the heat, and simmer for about1 hour. Stir in the olives; cook for 30 more minutes or until the beef is tender. Discard the bay leaves. Stir in the vinegar and sprinkle with the parsley.

Nutrition Info: Per Serving:288 cal, 10.3 g total fat (3.3 g sat. fat, 5 g mono fat, 0.6 g poly fat), 25.2 g protein, 20.1 g carb, 5.7 g fiber, 71 g chol., 5.5 mg iron, 584 mg sodium, and 100 mg calcium.

770. Chickpea Arugula Salad

Servings: 4   Cooking Time: 15 Minutes

Ingredients:

1 can chickpeas, drained
1 cup cherry tomatoes, halved
1/2cup sun-dried tomatoes, chopped
2 cups arugula
1 pita bread, cubed
½ cup black olives, pitted
½ teaspoon cumin seeds
1 shallot, sliced
½ teaspoon coriander seeds
¼ teaspoon chili powder
1 teaspoon chopped mint
Salt and pepper to taste
4 oz. goat cheese, crumbled

Directions:

Combine the chickpeas, tomatoes, arugula, pita bread, olives, shallot, spices and mint in a salad bowl.   Add salt and pepper to taste and mix well then stir in the cheese.   Serve the salad fresh.

Nutrition Info: Per Serving:Calories:385 Fat:15.3g Protein:20.6g Carbohydrates:43.2g

771. Balsamic Mushrooms

Servings: 4-6   Cooking Time: 7 Minutes

Ingredients:

1 pound white mushroom, halved (or quartered if they are very large)
1 teaspoon salt
1/4 cup olive oil
1/4 teaspoon red pepper flakes
3 tablespoons balsamic vinegar
Pepper, to taste

Directions:

In a medium-sized skillet, heat the oil over medium high-heat. Add the mushrooms; cook for about 5 minutes or until golden.   Stir in the vinegar, red pepper flakes, and the salt, then season with pepper; cook for 1 minute more. Transfer into a serving bowl.   Notes: Serve this dish with your favorite steak. You can also add this to spinach salad to give it a different spin.

Nutrition Info: Per Serving:155.3 cal., 13.9 g fat (1.9 g sat. fat), 0 mg chol., 590.1 mg sodium, 5.8 g total carb., 1.2 g fiber, 4.1 g sugar, and 3.6 g protein.

772. Greek Potato And Corn Salad

Servings: 2   Cooking Time: 20 Minutes

Ingredients:

2 medium potatoes, peeled and cubed
2 shallots, chopped
1 tablespoon olive oil
2 cups corn
1 tablespoon dill, chopped
1 tablespoon balsamic vinegar
Salt and black pepper to the taste

Directions:
Put the potatoes in a pot, add water to cover, bring to a simmer over medium heat, cook for 20 minutes, drain and transfer to a bowl. Add the shallots and the other ingredients, toss and serve cold.
Nutrition Info:calories 198, fat 5.3, fiber 6.5, carbs 11.6, protein 4.5

773. Mint Avocado Chilled Soup

Servings: 2   Cooking Time: 15 Minutes
Ingredients:

2 romaine lettuce leaves
1 Tablespoon lime juice
1 medium ripe avocado
1 cup coconut milk, chilled
20 fresh mint leaves
Salt to taste

Directions:
Put all the ingredients in a blender and blend until smooth. Refrigerate for about 10 minutes and serve chilled.
Nutrition Info: Calories: 432 Carbs: 16.1g Fats: 42.2g Proteins: 5.2g Sodium: 33mg Sugar: 4.5g

774. Amazingly Fresh Carrot Salad

Servings: 4   Cooking Time: 0 Minutes
Ingredients:

¼ tsp chipotle powder
1 bunch scallions, sliced
1 cup cherry tomatoes, halved
1 large avocado, diced
1 tbsp chili powder
1 tbsp lemon juice
2 tbsp olive oil
3 tbsp lime juice
4 cups carrots, spiralized
salt to taste

Directions:
In a salad bowl, mix and arrange avocado, cherry tomatoes, scallions and spiralized carrots. Set aside. In a small bowl, whisk salt, chipotle powder, chili powder, olive oil, lemon juice and lime juice thoroughly. Pour dressing over noodle salad. Toss to coat well. Serve and enjoy at room temperature.
Nutrition Info: Calories per Serving: 243.6; Fat: 14.8g; Protein: 3g; Carbs: 24.6g

775. Feta And Almond Pasta

Servings: 4   Cooking Time: 25 Minutes
Ingredients:

5 oz whole grain macaroni
4 oz Feta cheese, crumbled
½ teaspoon chili pepper
2 eggs, beaten
1 teaspoon almond butter
1 cup water, for cooking

Directions:
Mix up together water and macaroni and boil according to the directions of the manufacturer. Then drain water. Add almond butter, chili pepper, and Feta cheese. Mix up well. Transfer the mixture in the casserole mold and flatten well.

Pour beaten eggs over the macaroni and bake for 10 minutes at 355F.
Nutrition Info: Per Serving:calories 262, fat 11.4, fiber 4.2, carbs 27.2, protein 13.9

776. Italian-style Butter Beans

Servings: 4   Cooking Time: 15 Minutes
Ingredients:

1 can (400 g) chopped tomato
2 cans (400 g) butter beans, rinsed, drained
2 teaspoons sugar
1 tablespoon olive oil
4 garlic cloves, crushed
Small bunch basil, chopped

Directions:
In a medium-sized saucepan, heat the olive oil. Add the garlic; cook for 1 minute. Add the tomatoes, sugar, and a bit of seasoning. Add the beans and a splash of water. Cover and let simmer for 5 minutes. Stir in the basil; serve.
Nutrition Info: Per Serving:140 cal, 4 g fat (1 g sat. fat), 20 g carbs, 6 g sugars, 6 g fiber, 8 g protein, and 1.41 g sodium.

777. Leeks Salad

Servings: 4   Cooking Time: 0 Minutes
Ingredients:

1 tablespoon olive oil
4 leeks, sliced
3 garlic cloves, grated
A pinch of sea salt and white pepper
½ teaspoon apple cider vinegar
A drizzle of olive oil
1 tablespoon dill, chopped

Directions:
In a salad bowl, combine the leeks with the garlic and the rest of the ingredients, toss and serve cold.
Nutrition Info:calories 71, fat 2.1, fiber 1.1, carbs 1.3, protein 2.4

778. Tomato Greek Salad

Servings: 4   Cooking Time: 15 Minutes
Ingredients:

1 pound tomatoes, cubed
1 cucumber, sliced
½ cup black olives
¼ cup sun-dried tomatoes, chopped
¼ cup parsley, chopped
1 red onion, sliced
Salt and pepper to taste
1 tablespoon balsamic vinegar
2 tablespoons extra virgin olive oil

Directions:
Combine the tomatoes, cucumber, black olives, sun-dried tomatoes, onion and parsley in a bowl. Add salt and pepper to taste then stir in the vinegar and olive oil. Mix well and serve the salad fresh.
Nutrition Info: Per Serving:Calories: 126 Fat: 9.2g Protein: 2.1g Carbohydrates: 11.5g

779. Broccoli And Mushroom Salad

Servings: 4   Cooking Time: 0 Minutes
Ingredients:

½ pound white mushrooms, sliced
1 broccoli head, florets separated and steamed
1 garlic clove, minced
1 tablespoon balsamic
1 yellow onion, chopped
1 tablespoon olive oil
A pinch of sea salt and black pepper
A pinch of red pepper flakes

vinegar
Directions:
In a bowl, mix the broccoli with the mushrooms and the other ingredients, toss and serve cold.
Nutrition Info:calories 183, fat 6.5, fiber 4.2, carbs 8.5, protein 4

780. Saffron Zucchini Mix
Servings: 4   Cooking Time: 10 Minutes
Ingredients:

2 zucchinis, sliced	1 tablespoon olive oil
A pinch of sea salt and black pepper	1 teaspoon saffron powder
1 tablespoon white vinegar	

Directions:
Heat up a pan with the oil over medium heat, add the zucchinis and sauté for 8 minutes.   Add the rest of the ingredients, toss, cook for 2 minutes more, divide between plates and serve.
Nutrition Info:calories 150, fat 5.2, fiber 4.3, carbs 5, protein 4

781. Thai Salad With Cilantro Lime Dressing
Servings: 2   Cooking Time: 20 Minutes
Ingredients:

¼ cup cashews	1 loose handful fresh cilantro
¼ cup fresh mint leaves	1 tablespoon lime juice
¼ cup fresh Thai basil leaves	1 teaspoon coconut aminos
¼ teaspoon fish sauce	3 tablespoon olive oil
½ cup green papaya, julienned	3 tangerines, peeled and segmented
½ teaspoon honey	
1 head green leaf lettuce, chopped	

Directions:
Prepare the lime cilantro dressing by mixing honey, fresh cilantro, fish sauce, coconut aminos, lime juice and oil in a mixing bowl. Mix then set aside. Prepare the salad by mixing the remaining six ingredients. Toss everything to distribute the ingredients.   Toss the salad dressing into the vegetables.   Serve chilled.
Nutrition Info: Calories per Serving: 649.8; Fat: 57.4 g; Protein: 7.5 g; Carbs: 25.8 g;

782. Green Mediterranean Salad
Servings: 4   Cooking Time: 15 Minutes
Ingredients:

2 cups arugula leaves	½ cup chopped parsley
2 cups baby spinach	1 lemon, juiced
2 cucumbers, sliced	1 tablespoon balsamic vinegar
2 celery stalks, sliced	Salt and pepper to taste
¼ cup chopped cilantro	

Directions:
Combine the arugula and spinach with the rest of the ingredients in a salad bowl.   Add salt and pepper to taste and season well with salt and pepper.   Serve the salad fresh.
Nutrition Info: Per Serving:Calories: 38 Fat: 0.4g Protein: 2.1g Carbohydrates: 8.5g

783. Salad Greens With Pear And Persimmon
Servings: 2   Cooking Time: 0 Minutes
Ingredients:

½ cup chopped pecans, toasted	1 tsp whole grain mustard
1 ripe persimmon, sliced	2 tbsp fresh lemon juice
1 ripe red pear, sliced	3 tbsp extra virgin olive oil
1 shallot, minced	6 cups baby spinach
1 tsp minced garlic	

Directions:
In a big mixing bowl, mix garlic, olive oil, lemon juice and mustard.   Once thoroughly mixed, add remaining ingredients.   Toss to coat.   Equally divide into two bowls, serve and enjoy.
Nutrition Info: Calories per serving: 429.1; Protein: 6.2g; Carbs: 39.2g; Fat: 27.5g

784. Easy Eggplant Salad
Servings: 4   Cooking Time: 30 Minutes
Ingredients:

Salt and pepper - to taste	Eggplant - 2, sliced
Smoked paprika - 1 tsp.	Garlic cloves - 2, minced
Extra virgin olive oil - 2 tbsp.	Mixed greens - 2 cups
	Sherry vinegar - 2 tbsp.

Directions:
Mix together garlic, paprika and oil in a small bowl. Place eggplant on a plate and sprinkle with salt and pepper to suit your taste. Next, brush oil mixture onto the eggplant.   Cook eggplant on a medium heated grill pan until brown on both sides. Once cooked, put eggplant into a salad bowl.   Top with greens and vinegar and greens, serve and eat.

785. Wheatberry And Walnuts Salad
Servings: 2   Cooking Time: 50 Minutes
Ingredients:

¼ cup of wheat berries	¼ cup fresh parsley, chopped
1 cup of water	2 oz pomegranate seeds
1 teaspoon salt	1 tablespoon canola oil
2 tablespoons walnuts, chopped	1 teaspoon chili flakes
1 tablespoon chives, chopped	

Directions:
Place wheat berries and water in the pan.   Add salt and simmer the ingredients for 50 minutes over the medium heat.   Meanwhile, mix up together walnuts, chives, parsley, pomegranate seeds, and chili flakes.   When the wheatberry is cooked, transfer it in the walnut mixture.   Add canola oil and mix up the salad well.
Nutrition Info: Per Serving:calories 160, fat 11.8, fiber 1.2, carbs 12, protein 3.4

786. Lemony Butter Beans With Parsley
Servings: 4   Cooking Time: 20 Minutes
Ingredients:

1 garlic clove, crushed	1 large onion, sliced
1 large bunch parsley, chopped (or 2 small bunches)	2 cans (400 g or 14 ounces) butter beans, rinsed, drained

1 tablespoon olive oil   Zest and juice 1
                          lemon

Directions:
In a pan, heat the olive oil. Add the onion; cook for about 10 to 15 minutes or until soft   Add the garlic; cook for 1 minute. Stir in the beans, cooking until heated through. Add the lemon juice and zest. Stir in the parsley; serve.
Nutrition Info: Per Serving:134 cal, 4 g fat (0 g sat. fat), 19 g carbs, 4 g sugars, 6 g fiber, 8 g protein, and 1.29 g sodium.

787.   Sautéed Zucchini And Mushrooms

Servings: 1 Cup   Cooking Time: 12 Minutes
Ingredients:

3 TB. extra-virgin   1 tsp. salt
olive oil   1 TB. minced garlic
1 large white onion,   2 medium zucchini,
chopped   chopped
2 cups crimini   2 TB. fresh thyme
mushrooms, rinsed   1/2 tsp. ground black
and chopped   pepper

Directions:
In a large skillet over medium heat, heat extra-virgin olive oil. Add white onion, crimini mushrooms, and salt, and toss. Cook for 5 minutes. Stir in garlic, and cook for another 2 minutes. Add zucchini, thyme, and black pepper, and stir to combine. Cook for 5 minutes.   Serve warm.

788.   Spring Soup Recipe With Poached Egg

Servings: 2   Cooking Time: 20 Minutes
Ingredients:

2 eggs   1 head of romaine
2 tablespoons butter   lettuce, chopped
4 cups chicken broth   Salt, to taste

Directions:
Boil the chicken broth and lower heat.   Poach the eggs in the broth for about 5 minutes and remove the eggs.   Place each egg into a bowl and add chopped romaine lettuce into the broth.   Cook for about 10 minutes and ladle the broth with the lettuce into the bowls.
Nutrition Info: Calories: 264 Carbs: 7g Fats: 18.9g Proteins: 16.1g Sodium: 1679mg Sugar: 3.4g

789.   Eggplant Ragoût With Chickpeas, Tomatoes, And Peppers

Servings: 4-6   Cooking Time: 45 Minutes
Ingredients:

5 plum tomatoes;   1 1/4 cups water
peel, quarter in a   1 teaspoons ground
lengthwise direction,   cumin
seed   1/4 cup fresh flat-leaf
1 can (15-ounces)   parsley, coarsely
chickpeas (preferably   chopped
organic), rinsed,   2 plump cloves garlic,
drained   sliced to thin pieces
1 1/2 pounds   2 tablespoons olive
eggplant, use plump   oil; plus more for
round ones   brushing the eggplant
1 large bell pepper,   2 tablespoons tomato
yellow or red, cored,   paste
seeded, cut to 1-inch   2 teaspoons paprika
pieces   Black pepper, freshly

1 large red onion, cut   ground, to taste
into 1/2-inch dices   Generous pinch
1 teaspoon salt, plus   cayenne
more to taste

Directions:
Preheat the broiler. In crosswise direction, cut the eggplant to 3/4-inch rounds; brush each side with the olive oil and broil for 2 minutes each side, or until both sides are light gold. Cool; cut to 1-inch pieces.   Over medium-high heat, heat 2 tablespoons olive oil in a medium-sized Dutch oven. Add the onion and the bell pepper and sauté for about 12 to 15 minutes or until the onions are slightly browned.   About 1-2 minutes before the onion browning is finished, add garlic, cumin, paprika, and the cayenne. Stir in the tomato paste; cook for 1 minutes, stirring.   Stir in the 1/4 cup water; boil. With wooden spoon, scrape the juices that stuck on the pan bottom.   Add the eggplant, tomatoes, chickpeas, remaining water, and salt; bring to boil. Simmer covered for about 25 minutes or until the veggies are tender, stirring one or 2 times. Stir the parsley in the pot, adjust seasoning, and serve.
Nutrition Info: Per Serving:220 cal., 8 g fat (1 g sat. fat, 1 g poly fat, 5 g mono fat), 0 mg chol., 550 mg sodium, 32 g carbs., 8 g fiber, and 6 g protein.

790.   Crispy Watermelon Salad

Servings: 4   Cooking Time: 20 Minutes
Ingredients:

2 flat breads, sliced   1 cucumber, sliced
10 oz. watermelon,   2 tablespoons extra
cubed   virgin olive oil
4 oz. feta cheese,   2 tablespoons mixed
cubed   seeds

Directions:
Combine flat bread, watermelon, cheese, cucumber, oil and seeds in a salad bowl and mix gently. Serve the salad fresh.
Nutrition Info: Per Serving:Calories: 167 Fat: 13.2g Protein: 4.9g Carbohydrates: 9.2g

791. White Bean Soup And Gremolata

Servings: 4   Cooking Time: 15 Minutes
Ingredients:

For the soup: 1/2 cup pancetta,
2 teaspoons olive oil   finely chopped
2 teaspoons garlic,   1/2 cup celery,
minced   pre-chopped
2 cups chicken broth,   1 cup onion,
fat-free, less-sodium   pre-chopped
2 cans (19-ounce   1 bay leaf
each) cannellini   2 teaspoons lemon
beans, rinsed,   rind, freshly grated
drained   1 tablespoon fresh
1/4 teaspoon black   parsley, chopped
pepper   1 teaspoon garlic,
1/2 cup water   minced

Directions:
For the soup: In a large-sized saucepan, heat the oil over medium-high heat.   Add the pancetta and cook for 2 minutes.   Stir in the onion, the celery, and the garlic; sauté for about 3 minutes or until almost tender.   Stir in the broth, the water, black pepper, the beans, and the bay leaf; bring the mixture to a boil. Reduce the heat; simmer, stirring occasionally, for 8 minutes.   For the gremolata:

Combine all of the ingredients; sprinkle over the soup.

Nutrition Info: Per Serving:227 cal, 7.6 g total fat (2.4 g sat. fat, 3.2 g mono fat, 1.4 g poly fat), 9.8 g protein, 28.7 g carb, 7.7 g fiber, 10 g chol., 2.6 mg iron, 710 mg sodium, and 75 mg calcium.

---

792.   Artichoke Farro Salad

Servings: 6   Cooking Time: 30 Minutes
Ingredients:

1 cup faro	2 garlic cloves, chopped
2 cups vegetable stock	2 tablespoons extra virgin olive oil
6 artichoke hearts, chopped	Salt and pepper to taste
½ cup chopped parsley	4 oz. feta cheese, crumbled
2 tablespoons chopped cilantro	

Directions:
Combine the faro and stock in a saucepan and cook on low heat until all the liquid has been absorbed. When done, transfer the faro in a salad bowl then stir in the rest of the ingredients.   Adjust the taste with salt and pepper and mix well.   Serve the salad fresh.

Nutrition Info: Per Serving:Calories:171 Fat:9.0g Protein:8.3g Carbohydrates:18.8g

---

793.   Balsamic Tomato Mix

Servings: 4   Cooking Time: 0 Minutes
Ingredients:

2 pounds cherry tomatoes, halved	1 garlic clove, minced
2 tablespoons olive oil	1 tablespoon chives, chopped
2 tablespoons balsamic vinegar	Salt and black pepper to the taste
1 cup basil, chopped	

Directions:
In a bowl, combine the tomatoes with the garlic, basil and the rest of the ingredients, toss and serve as a side salad.

Nutrition Info:calories 200, fat 5.6, fiber 4.5, carbs 15.1, protein 4.3

---

794.   Red Wine Dressed Arugula Salad

Servings: 2   Cooking Time: 12 Minutes
Ingredients:

¼ cup red onion, sliced thinly	2 center cut salmon fillets (6-oz each)
1 ½ tbsp fresh lemon juice	2/3 cup cherry tomatoes, halved
1 ½ tbsp olive oil	3 cups baby arugula leaves
1 tbsp extra-virgin olive oil	Pepper and salt to taste
1 tbsp red-wine vinegar	

Directions:
In a shallow bowl, mix pepper, salt, 1 ½ tbsp olive oil and lemon juice. Toss in salmon fillets and rub with the marinade. Allow to marinate for at least 15 minutes.   Grease a baking sheet and preheat oven to 350oF.   Bake marinated salmon fillet for 10 to 12 minutes or until flaky with skin side touching the baking sheet.   Meanwhile, in a salad bowl mix onion, tomatoes and arugula.   Season with pepper and salt. Drizzle with vinegar and oil.

Toss to combine and serve right away with baked salmon on the side.

Nutrition Info: Calories per serving: 400; Protein: 36.6g; Carbs: 5.8g; Fat: 25.6g

---

795.   Gigantes Plaki

Servings: 4   Cooking Time: 2 Hour
Ingredients:

1 Spanish onion, finely chopped	1 teaspoon sugar
1 teaspoon dried oregano	3 tablespoons extra-virgin olive oil, plus more to serve
2 garlic cloves, finely chopped	400 g dried butter beans
2 tablespoons flat-leaf parsley, chopped, plus more to serve	800 g ripe tomatoes, skinned, roughly chopped
2 tablespoons tomato purée	Pinch ground cinnamon

Directions:
In water, soak the beans overnight, drain, rinse, and then place in a pan filled with water; bring to a boil. When boiling, reduce the heat to a simmer, cooking for about 50 minutes or until the beans are slightly tender but still not soft. Drain and set aside. Preheat the oven to 180C, gas to 4, or fan to 160C. In a large-sized frying pan, heat the olive oil. Add the onion and the garlic; cook for 10 minutes over medium heat or until soft but not browned.   Add the tomato puree, cook for 1 minute more. Add the rest of the ingredients; simmer for about 2 to 3 minutes, season generously, then stir in the beans. Pour the mixture into an oven-safe dish; bake for 1 hour, uncovered, without stirring, or until the beans are tender.

Nutrition Info: Per Serving:431 cal, 11 g fat (1 g sat. fat), 66 g carbs, 15 g sugars, 19 g fiber, 22 g protein, and 0.2 g sodium.

---

796.   Squash And Tomatoes Mix

Servings: 6   Cooking Time: 20 Minutes
Ingredients:

5 medium squash, cubed	¼ cup goat cheese, crumbled
A pinch of salt and black pepper	½ yellow onion, chopped
3 tablespoons olive oil	2 tablespoons cilantro, chopped
1 cup pine nuts, toasted	2 tablespoons lemon juice
6 tomatoes, cubed	

Directions:
Heat up a pan with the oil over medium heat, add the onion and pine nuts and cook for 3 minutes. Add the squash and the rest of the ingredients, cook everything for 15 minutes, divide between plates and serve as a side dish.

Nutrition Info:calories 200, fat 4.5, fiber 3.4, carbs 6.7, protein 4

---

797.   Chickpeas, Corn And Black Beans Salad

Servings: 4   Cooking Time: 0 Minutes
Ingredients:

1 and ½ cups canned black beans, drained and rinsed	1 avocado, pitted, peeled and chopped
½ teaspoon garlic	1 cup corn kernels, chopped

powder
2 teaspoons chili powder
A pinch of sea salt and black pepper
1 and ½ cups canned chickpeas, drained and rinsed
1 cup baby spinach

2 tablespoons lemon juice
1 tablespoon olive oil
1 tablespoon apple cider vinegar
1 teaspoon chives, chopped

Directions:
In a salad bowl, combine the black beans with the garlic powder, chili powder and the rest of the ingredients, toss and serve cold.
Nutrition Info:calories 300, fat 13.4, fiber 4.1, carbs 8.6, protein 13

798. Eggplant And Bell Pepper Mix

Servings: 4   Cooking Time: 45 Minutes
Ingredients:
2 green bell peppers, cut into strips
2 eggplants, sliced
2 tablespoons tomato paste
Salt and black pepper to the taste

4 garlic cloves, minced
¼ cup olive oil
1 tablespoon cilantro, chopped
1 tablespoon chives, chopped

Directions:
In a roasting pan, combine the bell peppers with the eggplants and the rest of the ingredients, introduce in the oven and cook at 380 degrees F for 45 minutes.   Divide the mix between plates and serve as a side dish.
Nutrition Info:calories 207, fat 13.3, fiber 10.5, carbs 23.4, protein 3.8

799. Broccoli Salad With Caramelized Onions

Servings: 4   Cooking Time: 25 Minutes
Ingredients:
Extra virgin olive oil - 3 tbsp.
Red onions - 2, sliced
Balsamic vinegar - 2 tbsp. vinegar

Dried thyme - 1 tsp.
Broccoli - 1 lb., cut into florets
Salt and pepper - to taste

Directions:
Heat extra virgin olive oil in a pan over high heat and add in sliced onions. Cook for approximately 10 minutes or until the onions are caramelized. Stir in vinegar and thyme and then remove from stove. Mix together the broccoli and onion mixture in a bowl, adding salt and pepper if desired. Serve and eat salad as soon as possible.

800. Easy Butternut Squash Soup

Servings: 4   Cooking Time: 1 Hour 45 Minutes
Ingredients:
1 small onion, chopped
4 cups chicken broth
3 tablespoons coconut oil

1 butternut squash
Salt, to taste
Nutmeg and pepper, to taste

Directions:
Put oil and onions in a large pot and add onions. Sauté for about 3 minutes and add chicken broth and butternut squash.   Simmer for about 1 hour on medium heat and transfer into an immersion blender.   Pulse until smooth and season with salt, pepper and nutmeg.   Return to the pot and cook for about 30 minutes.   Dish out and serve hot.
Nutrition Info: Calories: 149 Carbs: 6.6g Fats: 11.6g Proteins: 5.4g Sodium: 765mg Sugar: 2.2g

Dessert Recipes

801. Soothing Red Smoothie

Servings: 2   Cooking Time: 3 Minutes

Ingredients:

4 plums, pitted
¼ cup raspberry
1 tablespoon lemon juice
¼ cup blueberry
1 tablespoon linseed oil

Directions:

Place all Ingredients: in a blender.   Blend until smooth.   Pour in a glass container and allow to chill in the fridge for at least 30 minutes.

Nutrition Info: Calories per serving: 201; Carbs: 36.4g; Protein: 0.8g; Fat: 7.1g

802. Minty Orange Greek Yogurt

Servings: 1   Cooking Time: 5 Minutes

Ingredients:

6 tablespoons Greek yogurt, fat-free
4 fresh mint leaves, thinly sliced
1 1/2 teaspoons honey
1 large orange, peeled, quartered, and then sliced crosswise

Directions:

Stir together the honey and the yogurt.   Place the orange slices into a dessert glass. Spoon the honeyed yogurt over the orange slices in the glass and scatter the mint on top of the yogurt.

Nutrition Info: Per Serving:171 cal., 34 g total carbs, 5 g fiber, and 11 g protein.

803. Yogurt Mousse With Sour Cherry Sauce

Servings: 6   Cooking Time: 1 Hour

Ingredients:

1 ½ cups Greek yogurt
1 teaspoon vanilla extract
1 ½ cups heavy cream, whipped
4 tablespoons honey
2 cups sour cherries
¼ cup white sugar
1 cinnamon stick

Directions:

Combine the yogurt with vanilla and honey in a bowl.   Fold in the whipped cream then spoon the mousse into serving glasses and refrigerate.   For the sauce, combine the cherries, sugar and cinnamon in a saucepan. Allow to rest for 10 minutes then cook on low heat for 10 minutes. Cool the sauce down then spoon it over the mousse. Serve it right away.

Nutrition Info: Per Serving:Calories:245 Fat:12.1g Protein:5.8g Carbohydrates:29.7g

804. Vanilla Apple Pie

Servings: 8   Cooking Time: 50 Minutes

Ingredients:

3 apples, sliced
½ teaspoon ground cinnamon
1 teaspoon vanilla extract
1 tablespoon Erythritol
7 oz yeast roll dough
1 egg, beaten

Directions:

Roll up the dough and cut it on 2 parts.   Line the springform pan with baking paper.   Place the first dough part in the springform pan.   Then arrange the apples over the dough and sprinkle it with Erythritol, vanilla extract, and ground cinnamon.   Then cover the apples with remaining dough and secure the edges of the pie with the help of the fork.   Make the small cuts in the surface of the pie.   Brush the pie with beaten egg and bake it for 50 minutes at 375F.   Cool the cooked pie well and then remove from the springform pan.   Cut it on the servings.

Nutrition Info: Per Serving:calories 139, fat 3.6, fiber 3.1, carbs 26.1, protein 2.8

805. Spinach Pancake Cake

Servings: 6   Cooking Time: 15 Minutes

Ingredients:

1 cup heavy cream
¼ cup Erythritol
1 cup fresh spinach, chopped
½ cup skim milk
1 teaspoon vanilla extract
1 cup all-purpose flour
½ cup of rice flour
1 teaspoon baking powder
1 teaspoon olive oil
1 egg, beaten
¼ teaspoon ground clove
1 teaspoon butter

Directions:

Blend the spinach until you get puree mixture. After this, add skim milk, vanilla extract, all-purpose flour, and rice flour.   Add baking powder, egg, and ground clove.   Blend the ingredients until you get a smooth and thick batter. Then add olive oil and pulse the batter for 30 seconds more.   Heat up butter in the skillet. Ladle 1 ladle of the crepe batter in the skillet and flatten it in the shape of crepe.   Cook it for 1.5 minutes from one side and them flip into another side and cook for 20 seconds more.   Place the cooked crepe in the plate.   Repeat the same steps will all crepe batter.   Make the cake filling: whip the heavy cream with Erythritol.   Spread every crepe with sweet whipped cream.   Store the cake in the fridge for up to 2 days.

Nutrition Info: Per Serving:calories 228, fat 10, fiber 1, carbs 38.8, protein 5.1

806. Fruit Salad With Orange Blossom Water

Servings: 8   Cooking Time: 3 Minutes

Ingredients:

4 oranges, peeled and cut into bite-sized pieces
8 dried figs, quartered
2 Medjool dates, pitted then chopped
2 tablespoons honey
½ cup pomegranate seeds
2 tablespoons orange blossom water
2 bananas, peeled and sliced
¼ cup pistachio nuts, shelled and chopped

Directions:

In a large mixing bowl, toss in all the ingredients except for the pistachio nuts.   Let the fruits rest in the fridge for at least 8 hours before serving. Garnish with chopped pistachios before serving.

Nutrition Info: Calories per serving: 185; Carbs: 43g; Protein: 3g; Fat: 2g

807. Blueberry Frozen Yogurt

Servings: 6   Cooking Time: 30 Minutes
Ingredients:

1-pint blueberries, fresh
2/3 cup honey
2 cups yogurt, chilled
1 small lemon, juiced and zested

Directions:

In a saucepan, combine the blueberries, honey, lemon juice, and zest.   Heat over medium heat and allow to simmer for 15 minutes while stirring constantly.   Once the liquid has reduced, transfer the fruits in a bowl and allow to cool in the fridge for another 15 minutes.   Once chilled, mix together with the chilled yogurt.
Nutrition Info: Calories per serving: 233; Carbs:52.2 g; Protein:3.5 g; Fat: 2.9g

808. Apple Pear Compote

Servings: 6   Cooking Time: 45 Minutes
Ingredients:

4 apples, cored and cubed
2 pears, cored and cubed
1 cinnamon stick
1 star anise
2 whole cloves
1 orange peel
4 cups water
2 tablespoons lemon juice

Directions:

Combine all the ingredients in a saucepan.   Place over low heat and cook for 25 minutes.   Serve the compote chilled.
Nutrition Info: Per Serving:Calories:110 Fat:0.5g Protein:0.8g Carbohydrates:28.6g

809. Cream Cheese Cake

Servings: 2   Cooking Time: 60 Minutes
Ingredients:

2 teaspoons cream cheese
1 cup Erythritol
½ teaspoon lemon juice
2 egg whites
½ teaspoon vanilla extract
2 strawberries, sliced

Directions:

Whisk the egg whites until you get soft peaks. Keep whisking and gradually add Erythritol and lemon juice.   Whisk the egg whites till you get strong peak mass.   After this, mix up together cream cheese and vanilla extract.   Line the baking tray with baking paper.   With the help of the spoon make egg white nests in the tray.   Bake the egg white nests for 60 minutes at 205F. When the "nests' are cooked, fill them with vanilla cream cheese and top with sliced strawberries.
Nutrition Info: Per Serving:calories 36, fat 1.3, fiber 0.3, carbs 121.4, protein 3.9

810. Nutmeg Lemon Pudding

Servings: 6   Cooking Time: 20 Minutes
Ingredients:

2 tablespoons lemon marmalade
4 eggs, whisked
2 tablespoons stevia
3 cups almond milk
4 allspice berries, crushed
¼ teaspoon nutmeg, grated

Directions:

In a bowl, mix the lemon marmalade with the eggs and the other ingredients and whisk well.   Divide the mix into ramekins, introduce in the oven and bake at 350 degrees F for 20 minutes.   Serve cold.
Nutrition Info:calories 220, fat 6.6, fiber 3.4, carbs 12.4, protein 3.4

811.Yogurt Panna Cotta With Fresh Berries

Servings: 6   Cooking Time: 1 Hour
Ingredients:

2 cups Greek yogurt
1 cup milk
1 cup heavy cream
2 teaspoons gelatin powder
4 tablespoons cold water
4 tablespoons honey
1 teaspoon vanilla extract
1 teaspoon lemon zest
1 pinch salt
2 cups mixed berries for serving

Directions:

Combine the milk and cream in a saucepan and heat them up.   Bloom the gelatin in cold water for 10 minutes.   Remove the milk off heat and stir in the gelatin until dissolved.   Add the vanilla, lemon zest and salt and allow to cool down.   Stir in the yogurt then pour the mixture into serving glasses.   When set, top with fresh berries and serve.
Nutrition Info: Per Serving:Calories:219 Fat:9.7g Protein:10.8g Carbohydrates:22.6g

812. Flourless Chocolate Cake

Servings: 8   Cooking Time: 1 Hour
Ingredients:

8 oz. dark chocolate, chopped
4 oz. butter, cubed
1 teaspoon vanilla extract
6 eggs, separated
1 pinch salt
4 tablespoons white sugar
Berries for serving

Directions:

Combine the chocolate and butter in a heatproof bowl and melt them together until smooth. When smooth, remove off heat and place aside. Separate the eggs.   Mix the egg yolks with the chocolate mixture.   Whip the egg whites with a pinch of salt until puffed up. Add the sugar and mix for a few more minutes until glossy and stiff. Fold the meringue into the chocolate mixture then pour the batter in a 9-inch round cake pan lined with baking paper.   Bake in the preheated oven at 350F for 25 minutes.   Serve the cake chilled.
Nutrition Info: Per Serving:Calories:324 Fat:23.2g Protein:6.4g Carbohydrates:23.2g

813. Strawberry And Avocado Medley

Servings: 4   Cooking Time: 5 Minutes
Ingredients:

2 cups strawberry, halved
1 avocado, pitted and sliced
2 tablespoons slivered almonds

Directions:

Place all Ingredients: in a mixing bowl.   Toss to combine.   Allow to chill in the fridge before serving.
Nutrition Info: Calories per serving: 107; Carbs: 9.9g; Protein: 1.6g; Fat: 7.8g

814. Creamy Mint Strawberry Mix

Servings: 6   Cooking Time: 30 Minutes

Ingredients:

Cooking spray	2 cups strawberries,
¼ cup stevia	sliced
1 and ½ cup almond	1 tablespoon mint,
flour	chopped
1 teaspoon baking	1 teaspoon lime zest,
powder	grated
1 cup almond milk	½ cup whipping
1 egg, whisked	cream

Directions:
In a bowl, combine the almond with the strawberries, mint and the other ingredients except the cooking spray and whisk well. Grease 6 ramekins with the cooking spray, pour the strawberry mix inside, introduce in the oven and bake at 350 degrees F for 30 minutes. Cool down and serve.
Nutrition Info:calories 200, fat 6.3, fiber 2, carbs 6.5, protein 8

815. Creamy Pie

Servings: 6   Cooking Time: 30 Minutes
Ingredients:

¼ cup lemon juice	4 egg yolks
1 cup cream	1 teaspoon vanilla
4 tablespoons	extract
Erythritol	3 tablespoons butter
1 tablespoon	6 oz wheat flour,
cornstarch	whole grain

Directions:
Mix up together wheat flour and butter and knead the soft dough. Put the dough in the round cake mold and flatten it in the shape of pie crust. Bake it for 15 minutes at 365F. Meanwhile, make the lemon filling: Mix up together cream, egg yolks, and lemon juice. When the liquid is smooth, start to heat it up over the medium heat. Stir it constantly. When the liquid is hot, add vanilla extract, cornstarch, and Erythritol. Whisk well until smooth. Brin the lemon filling to boil and remove it from the heat. Cool it to the room temperature. Cook the pie crust to the room temperature. Pour the lemon filling over the pie crust, flatten it well and leave to cool in the fridge for 25 minutes.
Nutrition Info: Per Serving:calories 225, fat 11.4, fiber 0.8, carbs 34.8, protein 5.2

816. Watermelon Ice Cream

Servings: 2   Cooking Time: 5 Minutes
Ingredients:

1 tablespoon gelatin	8 oz watermelon
powder	

Directions:
Make the juice from the watermelon with the help of the fruit juicer. Combine together 5 tablespoons of watermelon juice and 1 tablespoon of gelatin powder. Stir it and leave for 5 minutes. Then preheat the watermelon juice until warm, add gelatin mixture and heat it up over the medium heat until gelatin is dissolved. Then remove the liquid from the heat and pout it in the silicone molds. Freeze the jelly for 30 minutes in the freezer or for 4 hours in the fridge.
Nutrition Info: Per Serving:calories 46, fat 0.2, fiber 0.4, carbs 8.5, protein 3.7

817. Hazelnut Pudding

Servings: 8   Cooking Time: 40 Minutes
Ingredients:

2 and ¼ cups almond	1 and 1/3 cups Greek
flour	yogurt
3 tablespoons	1 teaspoon baking
hazelnuts, chopped	powder
5 eggs, whisked	1 teaspoon vanilla
1 cup stevia	extract

Directions:
In a bowl, combine the flour with the hazelnuts and the other ingredients, whisk well, and pour into a cake pan lined with parchment paper, Introduce in the oven at 350 degrees F, bake for 30 minutes, cool down, slice and serve.
Nutrition Info:calories 178, fat 8.4, fiber 8.2, carbs 11.5, protein 1.4

818. Mediterranean Cheesecakes

Servings: 1 Cheesecake   Cooking Time: 20 Minutes
Ingredients:

4 cups shredded	1 cup Greek yogurt
phyllo (kataifi dough)	1 TB. vanilla extract
1/2 cup butter,	2 TB. orange blossom
melted	water
12 oz. cream cheese	1 TB. orange zest
3/4 cup	2 large eggs
confectioners' sugar	1 cup coconut flakes

Directions:
Preheat the oven to 450°F. In a large bowl, and using your hands, combine shredded phyllo and melted butter, working the two together and breaking up phyllo shreds as you work. Using a 12-cup muffin tin, add 1/3 cup shredded phyllo mixture to each tin, and press down to form crust on the bottom of the cup. Bake crusts for 8 minutes, remove from the oven, and set aside. In a large bowl, and using an electric mixer on low speed, blend cream cheese and Greek yogurt for 1 minute. Add confectioners' sugar, vanilla extract, orange blossom water, and orange zest, and blend 1 minute. Add eggs, and blend for about 30 seconds or just until eggs are incorporated. Lightly coat the sides of each muffin tin with cooking spray. Pour about 1/3 cup cream cheese mixture over crust in each tin. Do not overflow. Bake for 12 minutes. Spread shredded coconut on a baking sheet, and place in the oven with cheesecakes to toast for 4 or 5 minutes or until golden brown. Remove from the oven, and set aside. Remove cheesecakes from the oven, and cool for 1 hour on the countertop. Place the tin in the refrigerator, and cool for 1 more hour. To serve, dip a sharp knife in warm water and then run it along the sides of cheesecakes to loosen from the tin. Gently remove cheesecakes and place on a serving plate. Sprinkle with toasted coconut flakes, and serve.

819. Melon Cucumber Smoothie

Servings: 2   Cooking Time: 5 Minutes
Ingredients:

½ cucumber	1 pear, peeled and
2 slices of melon	sliced
2 tablespoons lemon	3 fresh mint leaves
juice	½ cup almond milk

Directions:

Place all Ingredients: in a blender. Blend until smooth. Pour in a glass container and allow to chill in the fridge for at least 30 minutes.

Nutrition Info: Calories per serving: 253; Carbs: 59.3g; Protein: 5.7g; Fat: 2.1g

820. Mediterranean Style Fruit Medley

Servings: 7   Cooking Time: 5 Minutes

Ingredients:

4 fuyu persimmons, sliced into wedges
1 ½ cups grapes, halved
8 mint leaves, chopped

1 tablespoon lemon juice
1 tablespoon honey
½ cups almond, toasted and chopped

Directions:
Combine all Ingredients: in a bowl. Toss then chill before serving.

Nutrition Info: Calories per serving:159; Carbs: 32g; Protein: 3g; Fat: 4g

821. White Wine Grapefruit Poached Peaches

Servings: 6   Cooking Time: 40 Minutes

Ingredients:

4 peaches
2 cups white wine
1 grapefruit, peeled and juiced
¼ cup white sugar

1 cinnamon stick
1 star anise
1 cardamom pod
1 cup Greek yogurt for serving

Directions:
Combine the wine, grapefruit, sugar and spices in a saucepan. Bring to a boil then place the peaches in the hot syrup. Lower the heat and cover with a lid. Cook for 15 minutes then allow to cool down. Carefully peel the peaches and place them in a small serving bowl. Top with yogurt and serve right away.

Nutrition Info: Per Serving:Calories:157 Fat:0.9g Protein:4.2g Carbohydrates:20.4g

822. Cinnamon Stuffed Peaches

Servings: 4   Cooking Time: 5 Minutes

Ingredients:

4 peaches, pitted, halved
2 tablespoons ricotta cheese
2 tablespoons of liquid honey
¾ cup of water

½ teaspoon vanilla extract
¾ teaspoon ground cinnamon
1 tablespoon almonds, sliced
¾ teaspoon saffron

Directions:
Pour water in the saucepan and bring to boil. Add vanilla extract, saffron, ground cinnamon, and liquid honey. Cook the liquid until the honey is melted. Then remove it from the heat. Put the halved peaches in the hot honey liquid. Meanwhile, make the filling: mix up together ricotta cheese, vanilla extract, and sliced almonds. Remove the peaches from honey liquid and arrange in the plate. Fill 4 peach halves with ricotta filling and cover them with remaining peach halves. Sprinkle the cooked dessert with liquid honey mixture gently.

Nutrition Info: Per Serving:calories 113, fat 1.8, fiber 2.8, carbs 23.9, protein 2.7

823. Eggless Farina Cake (namoura)

Servings: 1 Piece   Cooking Time: 40 Minutes

Ingredients:

2 cups farina
1/2 cup semolina
1/2 cup all-purpose flour
1 TB. baking powder
1 tsp. active dry yeast
1/2 cup sugar
1/2 cup plain Greek yogurt

1 cup whole milk
3/4 cup butter, melted
1/4 cup water
2 TB. tahini paste
15 almonds
2 cups Simple Syrup (recipe in Chapter 21)

Directions:
In a large bowl, combine farina, semolina, all-purpose flour, baking powder, yeast, sugar, Greek yogurt, whole milk, butter, and water. Set aside for 15 minutes. Preheat the oven to 375°F. Spread tahini paste evenly in the bottom of a 9×13-inch baking pan, and pour in the cake batter. Arrange almonds on top of batter, about where each slice will be. Bake for 45 minutes or until golden brown. Remove cake from the oven, and using a toothpick, poke holes throughout cake for Simple Syrup to seep into. Pour syrup over cake, and let cake sit for 1 hour to absorb syrup. Cool cake completely before cutting and serving.

824. Mixed Berry Sorbet

Servings: 8   Cooking Time: 2 ½ Hours

Ingredients:

2 cups water
½ cup white sugar
1 tablespoon lemon juice

2 cups mixed berries
2 tablespoons honey
1 teaspoon lemon zest
1 mint sprig

Directions:
Combine the water, sugar, berries, lemon juice, honey and lemon zest in a saucepan. Bring to a boil and cook on low heat for 5 minutes. Add the mint sprig and remove off heat. Allow to infuse for 10 minutes then remove the mint. Pour the syrup into a blender and puree until smooth and creamy. Pour the smooth syrup into an airtight container and freeze for at least 2 hours. Serve the sorbet chilled.

Nutrition Info: Per Serving:Calories:84 Fat:0.1g Protein:0.4g Carbohydrates:21.3g

825. Almonds And Oats Pudding

Servings: 4   Cooking Time: 15 Minutes

Ingredients:

1 tablespoon lemon juice
1 and ½ cups almond milk
1 teaspoon almond extract

Zest of 1 lime
½ cup oats
2 tablespoons stevia
½ cup silver almonds, chopped

Directions:
In a pan, combine the almond milk with the lime zest and the other ingredients, whisk, bring to a simmer and cook over medium heat for 15 minutes. Divide the mix into bowls and serve cold.

Nutrition Info:calories 174, fat 12.1, fiber 3.2, carbs 3.9, protein 4.8

826. Banana And Berries Trifle

Servings: 10   Cooking Time: 5 Minutes

Ingredients:

8 oz biscuits, chopped
¼ cup strawberries, chopped
1 banana, chopped
1 peach, chopped
½ mango, chopped
1 cup grapes, chopped

1 tablespoon liquid honey
1 cup of orange juice
½ cup Plain yogurt
¼ cup cream cheese
1 teaspoon coconut flakes

Directions:
Bring the orange juice to boil and remove it from the heat. Add liquid honey and stir until it is dissolved. Cool the liquid to the room temperature. Add chopped banana, peach, mango, grapes, and strawberries. Shake the fruits gently and leave to soak the orange juice for 15 minutes. Meanwhile, with the help of the hand mixer mix up together Plain yogurt and cream cheese. Then separate the chopped biscuits, yogurt mixture, and fruits on 4 parts. Place the first part of biscuits in the big serving glass in one layer. Spread it with yogurt mixture and add fruits. Repeat the same steps till you use all ingredients. Top the trifle with coconut flakes.
Nutrition Info: Per Serving:calories 164, fat 6.2, fiber 1.3, carbs 24.8, protein 3.2

827.   Chocolate Rice
Servings: 4   Cooking Time: 20 Minutes
Ingredients:
1 cup of rice
1 tbsp cocoa powder
2 tbsp maple syrup
2 cups almond milk
Directions:
Add all ingredients into the inner pot of instant pot and stir well. Seal pot with lid and cook on high for 20 minutes. Once done, allow to release pressure naturally for 10 minutes then release remaining using quick release. Remove lid. Stir and serve.
Nutrition Info: Calories 474 Fat 29.1 g Carbohydrates 51.1 g Sugar 10 g Protein 6.3 g Cholesterol 0 mg

828.   Lemon And Semolina Cookies
Servings: 6   Cooking Time: 20 Minutes
Ingredients:
½ teaspoon lemon zest, grated
4 tablespoons Erythritol
4 tablespoons semolina
2 tablespoons olive oil
8 tablespoons wheat flour, whole grain

1 teaspoon vanilla extract
½ teaspoon ground clove
3 tablespoons coconut oil
¼ teaspoon baking powder
¼ cup of water

Directions:
Make the dough: in the mixing bowl combine together lemon zest, semolina, olive oil, wheat flour, vanilla extract, ground clove, coconut oil, and baking powder. Knead the soft dough. Make the small cookies in the shape of walnuts and press them gently with the help of the fork. Line the baking tray with the baking paper. Place the cookies in the tray and bake them for 20 minutes at 375F. Meanwhile, bring the water to boil. Add Erythritol and simmer the liquid for 2 minutes over the medium heat. Cool it. Pour the cooled sweet

water over the hot baked cookies and leave them for 10 minutes. When the cookies soak all liquid, transfer them in the serving plates.
Nutrition Info: Per Serving:calories 165, fat 11.7, fiber 0.6, carbs 23.7, protein 2

829.   Strawberry Sorbet
Servings: 2   Cooking Time: 20 Minutes
Ingredients:
1 cup strawberries, chopped
1 tablespoon of liquid honey
2 tablespoons water
1 tablespoon lemon juice
Directions:
Preheat the water and liquid honey until you get homogenous liquid. Blend the strawberries until smooth and combine them with honey liquid and lemon juice. Transfer the strawberry mixture in the ice cream maker and churn it for 20 minutes or until the sorbet is thick. Scoop the cooked sorbet in the ice cream cups.
Nutrition Info: Per Serving:calories 57, fat 0.3, fiber 1.5, carbs 14.3, protein 0.6

830.   Halva (halawa)
Servings: ¼ Cup   Cooking Time: 10 Minutes
Ingredients:
1 1/2 cups honey
1 1/2 cups tahini paste
1 cup pistachios, coarsely chopped
Directions:
Pour honey into a saucepan, set over low heat, and bring to 240ºF. In another saucepan over low heat, bring tahini paste to 120ºF. In a bowl, whisk together heated honey and tahini paste until smooth. Fold in pistachios. Line a loaf pan with parchment paper and spray with cooking spray. Pour tahini mixture into the loaf pan, and refrigerate for 2 days to set. Cut halva into bite-size pieces, and serve.

831.   Semolina Cake
Servings: 6   Cooking Time: 30 Minutes
Ingredients:
½ cup wheat flour, whole grain
½ cup semolina
1 teaspoon baking powder
1 teaspoon vanilla extract
4 tablespoons Erythritol

½ cup Plain yogurt
1 teaspoon lemon rind
2 tablespoons olive oil
1 tablespoon almond flakes
4 teaspoons liquid honey
½ cup of orange juice

Directions:
Mix up together wheat flour, semolina, baking powder, Plain yogurt, vanilla extract, Erythritol, and olive oil. Then add lemon rind and mix up the ingredients until smooth. Transfer the mixture in the non-sticky cake mold, sprinkle with almond flakes, and bake for 30 minutes at 365F. Meanwhile, bring the orange juice to boil. Add liquid honey and stir until dissolved. When the cake is cooked, pour the hot orange juice mixture over it and let it rest for at least 10 minutes. Cut the cake into the servings.
Nutrition Info: Per Serving:calories 179, fat 6.1, fiber 1.1, carbs 36.3, protein 4.5

832. Shredded Phyllo And Sweet Cheese Pie (knafe)

Servings: 1/8 Pie   Cooking Time: 30 Minutes

Ingredients:

1 lb. pkg. shredded phyllo (kataifi dough)
1 cup butter, melted
1/2 cup whole milk
2 TB. semolina flour
1 lb. ricotta cheese

2 cups mozzarella cheese, shredded
2 TB. sugar
1 cup Simple Syrup (recipe later in this chapter)

Directions:

1 cup Simple Syrup (recipe later in this chapter) In a food processor fitted with a chopping blade, pulse shredded phyllo and butter 10 times. Transfer mixture to a bowl.   In a small saucepan over low heat, warm whole milk.   Stir in semolina flour, and cook for 1 minute.   Rinse the food processor, and to it, add ricotta cheese, mozzarella cheese, sugar, and semolina mixture. Blend for 1 minute. Preheat the oven to 375°F.   In a 9-inch-round baking dish, add 1/2 of shredded phyllo mixture, and press down to compress. Add cheese mixture, and spread out evenly. Add rest of shredded phyllo mixture, spread evenly, and gently press down. Bake for 40 minutes or until golden brown.   Let pie rest for 10 minutes before serving with Simple Syrup drizzled over top.

833. Lemon Pear Compote

Servings: 6   Cooking Time: 15 Minutes

Ingredients:

3 cups pears, cored and cut into chunks
1 tsp vanilla
1 tsp liquid stevia

1 tbsp lemon zest, grated
2 tbsp lemon juice

Directions:

Add all ingredients into the inner pot of instant pot and stir well.   Seal pot with lid and cook on high for 15 minutes.   Once done, allow to release pressure naturally for 10 minutes then release remaining using quick release. Remove lid.   Stir and serve.

Nutrition Info: Calories 50 Fat 0.2 g Carbohydrates 12.7 g Sugar 8.1 g Protein 0.4 g Cholesterol 0 mg

834. Cinnamon Pear Jam

Servings: 12   Cooking Time: 4 Minutes

Ingredients:

8 pears, cored and cut into quarters
1 tsp cinnamon

1/4 cup apple juice
2 apples, peeled, cored and diced

Directions:

Add all ingredients into the inner pot of instant pot and stir well.   Seal pot with lid and cook on high for 4 minutes.   Once done, allow to release pressure naturally. Remove lid.   Blend pear apple mixture using an immersion blender until smooth. Serve and enjoy.

Nutrition Info: Calories 103 Fat 0.3 g Carbohydrates 27.1 g Sugar 18 g Protein 0.6 g Cholesterol 0 mg

835. Apple And Walnut Salad

Servings: 6   Cooking Time: 5 Minutes

Ingredients:

Juice from ½ orange
Zest from ½ orange,

4 medium Gala apples, cubed

grated
2 tablespoons honey
1 tablespoon olive oil

8 dried apricots, chopped
¼ cup walnuts, toasted and chopped

Directions:

In a small bowl, whisk together the orange juice, zest, honey, and olive oil. Set aside.   In a larger bowl, toss the apples, apricots, and walnuts. Drizzle with the vinaigrette and toss to coat all Ingredients.   Serve chilled.

Nutrition Info: Calories per serving: 178; Carbs: 30g; Protein: 1g; Fat: 6g

836. Banana Kale Smoothie

Servings: 3   Cooking Time: 5 Minutes

Ingredients:

2 cups kale leaves
1 cup almond milk
½ cup crushed ice
1 banana, peeled

1 apple, peeled and cored
A dash of cinnamon

Directions:

Place all Ingredients: in a blender.   Blend until smooth.   Pour in a glass container and allow to chill in the fridge for at least 30 minutes.

Nutrition Info: Calories per serving: 165; Carbs: 32.1g; Protein: 2.3g; Fat: 4.2g

837. Phyllo Custard Pockets (shaabiyat)

Servings: 1 Pocket   Cooking Time: 10 Minutes

Ingredients:

8 phyllo sheets
1/2 cup butter, melted
21/4 cups Ashta Custard (recipe later in this chapter)

1 cup Simple Syrup (recipe later in this chapter)
1/2 cup pistachios, ground

Directions:

Preheat the oven to 450°F.   Lay out a sheet of phyllo dough, brush with butter, and layer another sheet of phyllo dough on top. Cut sheets into 3 equal-size columns, each about 3 or 4 inches wide. Place 3 tablespoons Ashta Custard at one end of each column, and fold the bottom-right corner up and over custard. Pull up bottom-left corner, and repeat folding each corner up to the opposite corner, forming a triangle as you fold.   Place triangle pockets on a baking sheet, brush with butter, and bake for 10 minutes or until golden brown.   Serve warm or cold, drizzled with Simple Syrup and sprinkled with pistachios.

838. Chocolate Baklava

Servings: 4   Cooking Time: 35 Minutes

Ingredients:

24 sheets (14 x 9-inch) frozen whole-wheat phyllo (filo) dough, thawed
1/3 cup toasted walnuts, chopped coarsely
1/3 cup almonds, blanched toasted, chopped coarsely
1/2 teaspoon ground cinnamon
1/2 cup hazelnuts,

1/8 teaspoon salt
1/2 cup water
1/2 cup pistachios, roasted, chopped coarsely
3/4 cup honey
1/2 cup of butter, melted
1 cup chocolate-hazelnut spread (I used Nutella)
1 piece (3-inch)

toasted, chopped coarsely
cinnamon stick
Cooking spray

Directions:
Into medium-sized saucepan, combine the water, honey, and the cinnamon stick; stir until the honey is dissolved. Increase the heat/flame to medium; continue cooking for about 10 minutes without stirring. A candy thermometer should read 230F. Remove the saucepan from the heat and then keep warm. Remove and discard the cinnamon stick. Preheat the oven to 350F. Put the chocolate-hazelnut spread into microwavable bowl; microwave the spread for about 30 seconds on HIGH or until the spread is melted. In a bowl, combine the hazelnuts, pistachios, almonds, walnuts, ground cinnamon, and the salt. Lightly grease with the cooking spray a 9x13-inch ceramic or glass baking dish. Put 1 sheet lengthwise into the bottom of the prepared baking dish, extending the ends of the sheet over the edges of the dish. Lightly brush the sheet with the butter. Repeat the process with 5 sheets phyllo and a light brush of butter. Drizzle 1/3 cup of the melted chocolate-hazelnut spread over the buttered phyllo sheets. Sprinkle about 1/3 of the nut mixture (1/2 cup) over the spread. Repeat the process, layering phyllo sheet, brush of butter, spread, and with nut mixture. For the last, nut mixture top layer, top with 6 phyllo sheets, pressing each phyllo gently into the dish and brushing each sheet with butter. Slice the layers into 24 portions by making 3 cuts lengthwise and then 5 cuts crosswise with a sharp knife; bake for about 35 minutes at 350F or until the phyllo sheets are golden. Remove the dish from the oven, drizzle the honey sauce over the baklava. Pace the dish on a wire rack and let cool. Cover and store the baklavas at normal room temperature if not serving right away.
Nutrition Info: Per Serving:238 Cal, 13.4 g total fat (4.3 g sat. fat, 5.6 g mono fat, 2 g poly fat), 4 g protein, 27.8 g total carbs., 1.6 g fiber, 10 mg chol., 1.3 mg iron, 148 mg sodium, and 29 mg calcium.

839. Apricot Rosemary Muffins

Servings: 12   Cooking Time: 1 Hour
Ingredients:
2 eggs
1/3 cup white sugar
1 teaspoon vanilla extract
1 cup buttermilk
¼ cup olive oil
1 ½ cups all-purpose flour
¼ teaspoon salt

1 teaspoon baking powder
¼ teaspoon baking soda
4 apricots, pitted and diced
1 teaspoon dried rosemary

Directions:
Combine the eggs, sugar and vanilla in a bowl and mix until double in volume. Stir in the oil and buttermilk and mix well. Fold in the flour, salt, baking powder and baking soda then add the apricots and rosemary and mix gently. Spoon the batter in a muffin tin lined with muffin papers and bake in the preheated oven at 350F for 20-25 minutes or until the muffins pass the toothpick test. Serve the muffins chilled.
Nutrition Info: Per Serving:Calories:140 Fat:5.4g Protein:3.4g Carbohydrates:20.1g

840. Blueberry Yogurt Mousse

Servings: 4   Cooking Time: 0 Minutes
Ingredients:
2 cups Greek yogurt
¼ cup stevia

¾ cup heavy cream
2 cups blueberries

Directions:
In a blender, combine the yogurt with the other ingredients, pulse well, divide into cups and keep in the fridge for 30 minutes before serving.
Nutrition Info:calories 141, fat 4.7, fiber 4.7, carbs 8.3, protein 0.8

841. Pistachio Cheesecake

Servings: 6   Cooking Time: 10 Minutes
Ingredients:
½ cup pistachio, chopped
4 teaspoons butter, softened

4 teaspoon Erythritol
2 cups cream cheese
½ cup cream, whipped

Directions:
Mix up together pistachios, butter, and Erythritol. Put the mixture in the baking mold and bake for 10 minutes at 355F. Meanwhile, whisk together cream cheese and whipped cream. When the pistachio mixture is baked, chill it well. After this, transfer the pistachio mixture in the round cake mold and flatten in one layer. Then put the cream cheese mixture over the pistachio mixture, flatten the surface until smooth. Cool the cheesecake in the fridge for 1 hour before serving.
Nutrition Info: Per Serving:calories 332, fat 33, fiber 0.5, carbs 7.4, protein 7

842. Almond Citrus Muffins

Servings: 6   Cooking Time: 30 Minutes
Ingredients:
2 eggs, beaten
1 ½ cup whole wheat flour
½ cup almond meal
1 teaspoon vanilla extract
1 tablespoon butter, softened
1 teaspoon orange zest, grated

1 tablespoon orange juice
¾ cup Erythritol
1 oz orange pulp
1 teaspoon baking powder
½ teaspoon lime zest, grated
Cooking spray

Directions:
Make the muffin batter: combine together almond meal, eggs, whole wheat flour, vanilla extract, butter, orange zest, orange juice, and orange pulp. Add lime zest and baking powder. Then add Erythritol. With the help of the hand mixer mix up the ingredients. When the mixture is soft and smooth, it is done. Spray the muffin molds with cooking spray from inside and preheat the oven to 365F. Fill ½ part of every muffin mold with muffin batter and transfer them in the oven. Cook the muffins for 30 minutes. Then check if the muffins are cooked by piercing them with a toothpick (if it is dry, the muffins are cooked; if it is not dry, bake the muffins for 5-7 minutes more.)
Nutrition Info: Per Serving:calories 204, fat 7.7, fiber 1.9, carbs 57.1, protein 6.8

843. Mediterranean Bread Pudding (aish El Saraya)ad

Servings: 1/9 Of Pudding   Cooking Time: 20 Minutes

Ingredients:

8 slices white bread, crust removed
1 cup sugar
1/2 cup water
1 TB. fresh lemon juice
2 cups Simple Syrup (recipe later in this chapter)
4 cups Ashta Custard (recipe later in this chapter)
1/2 cup coconut flakes, toasted
1/2 cup pistachios, ground
1 strawberry, sliced

Directions:

Preheat the oven to 450°F.   Place slices of bread on a baking sheet, and toast for 10 minutes or until bread is golden brown and dry.   In a small saucepan over medium-low heat, combine sugar, water, and lemon juice. Simmer for 5 to 7 minutes or until sugar reaches a dark golden brown color. Carefully pour hot dark brown syrup into an 8×8-inch baking dish, shifting the dish from side to side to spread syrup around bottom of dish. Place 4 slices of bread on top of brown syrup. Pour 1 cup of Simple Syrup over bread, spread 2 cups Ashta Custard over bread, and add another layer of 4 slices of bread. Pour remaining 1 cup Simple Syrup over bread, and spread remaining 2 cups Ashta Custard over top bread layer.   Cover the dish with plastic wrap, and refrigerate for 4 hours. Decorate top of dish with toasted coconut, pistachios, and strawberry slices, and serve.

844. Cinnamon Apple Rice Pudding

Servings: 8   Cooking Time: 15 Minutes

Ingredients:

1 cup of rice
1 tsp vanilla
1/4 apple, peeled and chopped
1/2 cup water
1 1/2 cup almond milk
1 tsp cinnamon
1 cinnamon stick

Directions:

Add all ingredients into the instant pot and stir well. Seal pot with lid and cook on high for 15 minutes. Once done, release pressure using quick release. Remove lid.   Stir and serve.

Nutrition Info: Calories 206 Fat 11.5 g Carbohydrates 23.7 g Sugar 2.7 g Protein 3 g Cholesterol 0 mg

845. Custard-filled Pancakes (atayef)

Servings: 1 Pancake   Cooking Time: 15 Minutes

Ingredients:

1 cup all-purpose flour
1/2 cup whole-wheat flour
1 cup whole milk
1/2 cup water
1 tsp. active dry yeast
1 tsp. baking powder
1/2 tsp. salt
2 TB. sugar
2 cups Ashta Custard (recipe later in this chapter)
1/2 cup ground pistachios
1 cup Simple Syrup (recipe later in this chapter)

Directions:

In a large bowl, whisk together all-purpose flour, whole-wheat flour, whole milk, water, yeast, baking powder, salt, and sugar. Set aside for 30 minutes. Preheat a nonstick griddle over low heat.   Spoon 3 tablespoons batter onto the griddle, and cook pancake for about 30 seconds or until bubbles form along entire top of pancake. Do not flip over pancake. You're only browning the bottom. Transfer pancake to a plate, and let cool while cooking remaining pancakes. Do not overlap the pancakes while letting them cool.   Form pancake into a pocket by folding pancake into a half-moon, and pinch together the edges, but only halfway up. Spoon Ashta Custard into a piping bag or a zipper-lock plastic bag, snip off the corner, and squeeze about 2 tablespoons custard into each pancake pocket. Sprinkle custard with pistachios. Serve pancakes chilled with Simple Syrup drizzled on top.

846. Pomegranate Granita With Lychee

Servings: 7   Cooking Time: 5 Minutes

Ingredients:

500 millimeters pomegranate juice, organic and sugar-free
1 cup water
1/2 cup lychee syrup
2 tablespoons lemon juice
4 mint leaves
1 cup fresh lychees, pitted and sliced

Directions:

Place all Ingredients: in a large pitcher.   Place inside the fridge to cool before serving.

Nutrition Info: Calories per serving: 96; Carbs: 23.8g; Protein: 0.4g; Fat: 0.4g

847. Lime Grapes And Apples

Servings: 2   Cooking Time: 25 Minutes

Ingredients:

1/2 cup red grapes
2 apples
1 teaspoon lime juice
1 teaspoon Erythritol
3 tablespoons water

Directions:

Line the baking tray with baking paper.   Then cut the apples on the halves and remove the seeds with the help of the scooper.   Cut the apple halves on 2 parts more.   Arrange all fruits in the tray in one layer, drizzle with water, and bake for 20 minutes at 375F.   Flip the fruits on another side after 10 minutes of cooking.   Then remove them from the oven and sprinkle with lime juice and Erythritol. Return the fruits back in the oven and bake for 5 minutes more.   Serve the cooked dessert hot or warm.

Nutrition Info: Per Serving:calories 142, fat 0.4, fiber 5.7, carbs 40.1, protein 0.9

848. Mediterranean Baked Apples

Servings: 4   Cooking Time: 25 Minutes

Ingredients:

1.5 pounds apples, peeled and sliced
Juice from 1/2 lemon
A dash of cinnamon

Directions:

Preheat the oven to 250F.   Line a baking sheet with parchment paper then set aside.   In a medium bowl, apples with lemon juice and cinnamon.   Place the apples on the parchment paper-lined baking sheet.   Bake for 25 minutes until crisp.

Nutrition Info: Calories per serving: 90; Carbs: 23.9g; Protein: 0.5g; Fat: 0.3g

849. Poached Cherries

Servings: 5   Cooking Time: 10 Minutes

Ingredients:

1 pound fresh and sweet cherries, rinsed, pitted	3 strips (1x3 inches each) lemon zest,
3 strips (1x3 inches each) orange zest,	15 peppercorns
2/3 cup sugar	1/4 vanilla bean, split but not scraped
	1 3/4 cups water

Directions:

In a saucepan, mix the water, citrus zest, sugar, peppercorns, and vanilla bean; bring to a boil, stirring until the sugar is dissolved. Add the cherries; simmer for about 10 minutes until the cherries are soft, but not falling apart. Skim any foam from the surface and let the poached cherries cool. Refrigerate with the poaching liquid. Before serving, strain the cherries.

Nutrition Info: Per Serving:170 cal., 1 g total fat (0 g sat. fat, 0 g mono fat, 0.5 g poly fat), 0 mg chol., 0 mg sodium, 42 g total carbs., and 2 g fiber.

850. Watermelon Salad

Servings: 6   Cooking Time: 0 Minutes

Ingredients:

14 oz watermelon	1 teaspoon Erythritol
1 oz dark chocolate	2 kiwi, chopped
3 tablespoons coconut cream	1 oz Feta cheese, crumbled

Directions:

Peel the watermelon and remove the seeds from it. Chop the fruit and place in the salad bowl.   Add chopped kiwi and crumbled Feta. Stir the salad well. Then mix up together coconut cream and Erythritol. Pour the cream mixture over the salad.   Then shave the chocolate over the salad with the help of the potato peeler.   The salad should be served immediately.

Nutrition Info: Per Serving:calories 90, fat 4.4, fiber 1.4, carbs 12.9, protein 1.9

851. Easy Fruit Compote

Servings: 2   Cooking Time: 15 Minutes

Ingredients:

1-pound fresh fruits of your choice	2 tablespoons maple syrup
A dash of salt	

Directions:

Slice the fruits thinly and place them in a saucepan. Add the honey and salt.   Heat the saucepan over medium low heat and allow the fruits to simmer for 15 minutes or until the liquid has reduced.   Make sure that you stir constantly to prevent the fruits from sticking at the bottom of your pan and eventually burning.   Transfer in a lidded jar. Allow to cool.   Serve with slices of whole wheat bread or vegan ice cream.

Nutrition Info: Calories per serving:218; Carbs: 56.8g; Protein: 0.9g; Fat: 0.2g

852. Papaya Cream

Servings: 2   Cooking Time: 0 Minutes

Ingredients:

1 cup papaya, peeled and chopped	1 tablespoon stevia
1 cup heavy cream	1/2 teaspoon vanilla

extract

Directions:

In a blender, combine the cream with the papaya and the other ingredients, pulse well, divide into cups and serve cold.

Nutrition Info:calories 182, fat 3.1, fiber 2.3, carbs 3.5, protein 2

853. Minty Tart

Servings: 6   Cooking Time: 30 Minutes

Ingredients:

1 cup tart cherries, pitted	1/2 teaspoon baking powder
1 cup wheat flour, whole grain	1 tablespoon Erythritol
1/3 cup butter, softened	1/4 teaspoon dried mint
	3/4 teaspoon salt

Directions:

Mix up together wheat flour and cutter.   Add baking powder and salt. Knead the soft dough. Then place the dough in the freezer for 10 minutes. When the dough is solid, remove it from the freezer and grate with the help of the grater. Place 1/4 part of the grated dough in the freezer.   Sprinkle the springform pan with remaining dough and place tart cherries on it.   Sprinkle the berries with Erythritol and dried mint and cover with 1/4 part of dough from the freezer.   Bake the cake for 30 minutes at 365F. The cooked tart will have a golden brown surface.

Nutrition Info: Per Serving:calories 177, fat 10.4, fiber 0.9, carbs 21, protein 2.4

854. Orange-sesame Almond Tuiles

Servings: 20   Cooking Time: 45 Minutes

Ingredients:

3/4 cup unblanched or blanched sliced almonds	3 tablespoons (about 1 1/2 ounce) unsalted or salted butter
3 tablespoons orange juice, freshly squeezed	1/8 cup all-purpose flour
2 tablespoons white sesame seeds	1 tablespoon toasted sesame oil
10 tablespoons granulated sugar	1 1/2 teaspoons black sesame seeds
1/8 cup whole-wheat flour	Grated zest of 1 orange, preferably organic

Directions:

In a small-sized saucepan, warm the butter, sesame oil, orange zest, orange juice, and sugar over low heat until the mixture is smooth. Remove from the heat, Stir the flour, almonds and the sesame seeds; let the batter rest for 1 hour at normal room temperature.   Preheat the oven to 375F. Line 2 pieces baking sheet with parchment paper.   Set a rolling pin on a folded dishtowel. Ready a wire rack. Measuring by level tablespoons, drop batter into the prepared baking sheets, placing only 4 on each sheet and spacing them apart evenly.   With dampened fingers, slightly flatten the batter. Place one baking sheet in the oven, bake the tuiles for about 8 to 9 minutes, rotating the baking sheet halfway through baking, until the cookies are evenly browned. Let the cookies cool slightly for1

minute.   With a metal spatula, lift each cookie of the baking sheet and then drape them over the rolling pin. Let them cool in the rolling pin and then transfer to a wire rack. Repeat the process with the remaining batter. Serve the tuiles a few hours after baking.
Nutrition Info: Per Serving:78 cal., 4.7 g total fat (1.4 g sat. fat), 5 mg chol., 13 mg sodium, 39 mg pto., 8.6 g total carbs., 0.7 g fiber, 6.4 g sugar, and 1.1 g protein.

855.   Strawberry Ice Cream

Servings: 6   Cooking Time: 1 ¼ Hours
Ingredients:

1 pound strawberries, hulled	1 cup heavy cream
1 cup Greek yogurt	3 tablespoons honey
	1 teaspoon lime zest

Directions:
Combine all the ingredients in a blender and pulse until well mixed and smooth.   Pour the mixture into your ice cream machine and churn for 1 hour or according to your machine's instructions. Serve the ice cream right away.
Nutrition Info: Per Serving:Calories:150 Fat:8.3g Protein:4.3g Carbohydrates:16.4g

856.   Creamy Strawberries

Servings: 4   Cooking Time: 5 Minutes
Ingredients:

6 tablespoons almond butter	1 teaspoon vanilla extract
1 tablespoon Erythritol	1 cup strawberries, sliced
1 cup milk	

Directions:
Pour milk in the saucepan.   Add Erythritol, vanilla extract, and almond butter.   With the help of the hand mixer mix up the liquid until smooth and bring it to boil.   Then remove the mixture from the heat and let it cool.   The cooled mixture will be thick.   Put the strawberries in the serving glasses and top with the thick almond butter dip.
Nutrition Info: Per Serving:calories 192, fat 14.9, fiber 3.1, carbs 10.4, protein 7.3

857.   Greek Yogurt Pie

Servings: 8   Cooking Time: 1 Hour
Ingredients:

1 package phyllo dough sheets	1 teaspoon vanilla extract
4 cups plain yogurt	1 teaspoon lemon zest
4 eggs	1 teaspoon orange zest
½ cup white sugar	

Directions:
Mix the yogurt, eggs, sugar, vanilla and citrus zest in a bowl.   Layer 2 phyllo sheets in a deep dish baking pan then pour a few tablespoons of yogurt mixture over the dough.   Continue layering the phyllo dough and yogurt in the pan.   Bake in the preheated oven at 350F for 40 minutes.   Allow the pie to cool down before serving.
Nutrition Info: Per Serving:Calories:175 Fat:3.8g Protein:9.9g Carbohydrates:22.7g

858.   Five Berry Mint Orange Infusion

Servings: 12   Cooking Time: 10 Minutes
Ingredients:

½ cup water	1 cup blackberries
3 orange pekoe tea bags	1 cup fresh blueberries
3 sprigs of mint	1 cup pitted fresh cherries
1 cup fresh strawberries	1 bottle Sauvignon Blanc
1 cup fresh golden raspberries	½ cup pomegranate juice, natural
1 cup fresh raspberries	1 teaspoon vanilla

Directions:
In a saucepan, bring water to a boil over medium heat. Add the tea bags, mint and stir. Let it stand for 10 minutes.   In a large bowl, combine the rest of the ingredients.   Put in the fridge to chill for at least 3 hours.
Nutrition Info: Calories per serving: 140; Carbs: 32.1g; Protein: 1.2g; Fat: 1.5g

859.   Cocoa Yogurt Mix

Servings: 2   Cooking Time: 0 Minutes
Ingredients:

1 tablespoon cocoa powder	¾ cup Greek yogurt
¼ cup strawberries, chopped	5 drops vanilla stevia

Directions:
In a bowl, mix the yogurt with the cocoa, strawberries and the stevia and whisk well. Divide the mix into bowls and serve.
Nutrition Info:calories 200, fat 8, fiber 3.4, carbs 7.6, protein 4.3

860.   Almond Rice Dessert

Servings: 4   Cooking Time: 20 Minutes
Ingredients:

1 cup white rice	1 tablespoon cinnamon powder
2 cups almond milk	
1 cup almonds, chopped	½ cup pomegranate seeds
½ cup stevia	

Directions:
In a pot, mix the rice with the milk and stevia, bring to a simmer and cook for 20 minutes, stirring often. Add the rest of the ingredients, stir, divide into bowls and serve.
Nutrition Info:calories 234, fat 9.5, fiber 3.4, carbs 12.4, protein 6.5

861.   Frozen Strawberry Greek Yogurt

Servings: 16   Cooking Time: 15 Minutes
Ingredients:

3 cups Greek yogurt, plain, low-fat (2%)	1/8 teaspoon salt
2 teaspoons vanilla	1 cup sugar
1/4 cup freshly squeezed lemon juice	1 cup strawberries, sliced

Directions:
In a medium-sized bowl, except for the strawberries, combine the rest of the ingredients; whisking until the mixture is smooth.   Transfer the yogurt into a 1 1/2 or 2-quart ice cream make and freeze according to the manufacturer's direction, adding the strawberry slices for the last minute. Transfer into an airtight container and freeze for about 2-4 hours. Before serving, let stand for 15 minutes at room temperature.

Nutrition Info: Per Serving:86 cal., 1 g total fat (1 g sat. fat), 3 mg chol., 16g carbs., 0 g fiber, 15 g sugar, and 4 g protein.

---

862.   Almond Peaches Mix

Servings: 4   Cooking Time: 10 Minutes
Ingredients:

1/3 cup almonds, toasted	½ cup coconut water
1/3 cup pistachios, toasted	1 teaspoon lemon zest, grated
1 teaspoon mint, chopped	4 peaches, halved
	2 tablespoons stevia

Directions:
In a pan, combine the peaches with the stevia and the rest of the ingredients, simmer over medium heat for 10 minutes, divide into bowls and serve cold.
Nutrition Info:calories 135, fat 4.1, fiber 3.8, carbs 4.1, protein 2.3

---

863.   Raisin Pecan Baked Apples

Servings: 6   Cooking Time: 4 Minutes
Ingredients:

6 apples, cored and cut into wedges	1/4 cup raisins
1 cup red wine	1/4 tsp nutmeg
1/4 cup pecans, chopped	1 tsp cinnamon
	1/3 cup honey

Directions:
Add all ingredients into the instant pot and stir well. Seal pot with lid and cook on high for 4 minutes. Once done, allow to release pressure naturally for 10 minutes then release remaining using quick release. Remove lid.   Stir well and serve.
Nutrition Info: Calories 229 Fat 0.9 g Carbohydrates 52.6 g Sugar 42.6 g Protein 1 g Cholesterol 0 mg

---

864.   Walnuts Cake

Servings: 4   Cooking Time: 40 Minutes
Ingredients:

½ pound walnuts, minced	1 teaspoon almond extract
Zest of 1 orange, grated	1 and ½ cup almond flour
1 and ¼ cups stevia eggs, whisked	1 teaspoon baking soda

Directions:
In a bowl, combine the walnuts with the orange zest and the other ingredients, whisk well and pour into a cake pan lined with parchment paper. Introduce in the oven at 350 degrees F, bake for 40 minutes, cool down, slice and serve.
Nutrition Info:calories 205, fat 14.1, fiber 7.8, carbs 9.1, protein 3.4

---

865.   Spiced Cookies

Servings: 6   Cooking Time: 30 Minutes
Ingredients:

1 teaspoon vanilla extract	1 egg, beaten
½ teaspoon ground cinnamon	1 cup wheat flour
1 teaspoon ground turmeric	1 teaspoon baking powder
1 tablespoon butter, softened	4 tablespoons pumpkin puree
	1 tablespoon Erythritol

Directions:
Put all ingredients in the mixing bowl and knead the soft and non-sticky dough.   After this, line the baking tray with baking paper.   Make 6 balls from the dough and press them gently with the help of the spoon.   Arrange the dough balls in the tray. Bake the cookies for 30 minutes at 355F.   Chill the cooked cookies well and store them in the glass jar.
Nutrition Info: Per Serving:calories 111, fat 2.9, fiber 1.1, carbs 20.2, protein 3.2

---

866.   Scrumptious Cake With Cinnamon

Servings: 8   Cooking Time: 40 Minutes
Ingredients:

1 lemon	¼ lb. sugar
4 eggs	½ lb. ground almonds
1 tsp cinnamon	

Directions:
Preheat oven to 3500F. Then grease a cake pan and set aside.   On high speed, beat for three minutes the sugar and eggs or until the volume is doubled. Then with a spatula, gently fold in the lemon zest, cinnamon and almond flour until well mixed. Then pour batter on prepared pan and bake for forty minutes or until golden brown.   Let cool before serving.
Nutrition Info: Calorie per Servings: 253; Carbs: 21.1g; Protein: 8.8g; Fats: 16.3g

---

867.   Yogurt Cake

Servings: 1 Piece   Cooking Time: 55 Minutes
Ingredients:

1 cup plain Greek yogurt	1/2 cup vegetable or light olive oil
1 cup sugar	13/4 cups all-purpose flour
2 large eggs	2 tsp. baking powder
1 TB. vanilla extract	1/2 tsp. salt
4 TB. fresh lemon juice	1 cup confectioners' sugar
1 TB. lemon zest	

Directions:
Preheat the oven to 350°F. Lightly coat a 9-inch-round cake pan with cooking spray, and dust the pan using about 2 tablespoons all-purpose flour.   In a large bowl, using an electric mixer on medium speed, blend Greek yogurt, sugar, eggs, vanilla extract, 2 tablespoons lemon juice, lemon zest, and vegetable oil for about 2 minutes.   Add all-purpose flour, baking powder, and salt, and blend for 2 more minutes.   Pour batter into the prepared cake pan, and bake for 55 minutes or until a toothpick inserted in center of cake comes out clean. Cool cake completely.   In a small bowl, whisk together confectioners' sugar and remaining 2 tablespoons lemon juice to make glaze.   When cake is cool, pour glaze over top, cut, and serve.

---

868.   Chunky Apple Sauce

Servings: 16   Cooking Time: 12 Minutes
Ingredients:

4 apples, peeled, cored and diced	2 tbsp cinnamon
1 tsp vanilla	1/4 cup maple syrup
4 pears, diced	3/4 cup water

Directions:

Add all ingredients into the instant pot and stir well. Seal pot with lid and cook on high for 12 minutes. Once done, allow to release pressure naturally for 10 minutes then release remaining using quick release. Remove lid. Serve and enjoy.
Nutrition Info: Calories 75 Fat 0.2 g Carbohydrates 19.7 g Sugar 13.9 g Protein 0.4 g Cholesterol 0 mg

869. Olive Oil Cake

Servings: 1 Piece   Cooking Time: 45 Minutes
Ingredients:

2 large eggs
3/4 cup sugar
1/2 cup light olive oil
1 cup plain Greek yogurt
3 TB. fresh orange juice
2 TB. orange zest

13/4 cups all-purpose flour
1/2 tsp. salt
2 tsp. baking powder
1/2 tsp. baking soda
3/4 cup dried cranberries
2 TB. confectioners' sugar

Directions:
Preheat the oven to 350°F. Lightly coat a 9-inch-round cake pan or Bundt pan with cooking spray, and dust with about 2 tablespoons all-purpose flour. In a large bowl, and using an electric mixer on medium speed, blend eggs and sugar for 2 minutes. Blend in light olive oil, Greek yogurt, orange juice, and orange zest for 2 more minutes. Add all-purpose flour, salt, baking powder, and baking soda and blend for 1 more minute. Using a spatula or wooden spoon, fold cranberries into batter. Pour batter into the prepared pan, and bake for 45 minutes or until a toothpick inserted in center of cake comes out clean. Cool cake completely. Dust top of cake with confectioners' sugar, cut, and serve.

870. Grapes Stew

Servings: 4   Cooking Time: 10 Minutes
Ingredients:

2/3 cup stevia
1 tablespoon olive oil
1 teaspoon vanilla extract

1/3 cup coconut water
1 teaspoon lemon zest, grated
2 cup red grapes, halved

Directions:
Heat up a pan with the water over medium heat, add the oil, stevia and the rest of the ingredients, toss, simmer for 10 minutes, divide into cups and serve.
Nutrition Info:calories 122, fat 3.7, fiber 1.2, carbs 2.3, protein 0.4

871. Lemon Cranberry Sauce

Servings: 8   Cooking Time: 14 Minutes
Ingredients:

10 oz fresh cranberries
3/4 cup Swerve

1/4 cup water
1 tsp lemon zest
1 tsp vanilla extract

Directions:
Add cranberries and water into the instant pot. Seal pot with lid and cook on high for 1 minute. Once done, allow to release pressure naturally for 10 minutes then release remaining using quick release. Remove lid. Set pot on sauté mode.

Add remaining ingredients and cook for 2-3 minutes. Pour in container and store in fridge.
Nutrition Info: Calories 21 Fat 0 g Carbohydrates 25.8 g Sugar 23.9 g Protein 0 g Cholesterol 0 mg

872. Delectable Mango Smoothie

Servings: 2   Cooking Time: 5 Minutes
Ingredients:

2 cups diced mango
1 carrot, peeled and sliced roughly

1 orange, peeled and segmented
Fresh mint leaves

Directions:
Place the mango, carrot, and oranges in a blender. Pulse until smooth. Pour in a glass container and allow to chill before serving. Garnish with mint leaves on top.
Nutrition Info: Calories per serving: 134; Carbs: 33.6g; Protein: 2g; Fat: 0.7g; Sugar

873. Blackberries And Pomegranate Parfait

Servings: 4   Cooking Time: 20 Minutes
Ingredients:

1 cup Plain yogurt
1 tablespoon coconut flakes
1 tablespoon liquid honey

4 teaspoons peanuts, chopped
1 cup blackberries
1 tablespoon pomegranate seeds

Directions:
Mix up together plain yogurt and coconut flakes. Put the mixture in the freezer. Meanwhile, combine together liquid honey and blackberries. Place ½ part of blackberry mixture in the serving glasses. Then add ¼ part of the cooled yogurt mixture. Sprinkle the yogurt mixture with all peanuts and cover with ½ part of remaining yogurt mixture. Then add remaining blackberries and top the dessert with yogurt. Garnish the parfait with pomegranate seeds and cool in the fridge for 20 minutes.
Nutrition Info: Per Serving:calories 115, fat 3.1, fiber 3, carbs 13, protein 5.1

874. Yellow Cake With Jam Topping

Servings: 1 Piece   Cooking Time: 20 Minutes
Ingredients:

5 large eggs
11/4 cups sugar
1 TB. vanilla extract
2 cups all-purpose flour
2 tsp. baking powder
1/2 tsp. salt
1/2 cup whole milk

1/2 cup butter, melted
2 cups apricot or peach jam
1/4 cup sweetened condensed milk
2 TB. hot water

Directions:
Preheat the oven to 350°F. Lightly coat a 9×13-inch cake pan with cooking spray, and dust with about 2 tablespoons all-purpose flour. In a large bowl, and using an electric mixer on medium speed, beat eggs for 3 minutes. Add sugar and vanilla extract, and beat for 2 more minutes. Add all-purpose flour, baking powder, salt, whole milk, and melted butter, and blend for 1 minute. Pour batter into the prepared pan, and bake for 20 minutes or until a toothpick inserted in center of cake comes out clean. Cool cake completely. In a small bowl, whisk together apricot jam, sweetened condensed milk, and hot water. Pour jam icing over cake, letting it run over the edges, cut, and serve.

875. Raspberry Tart

Servings: 6   Cooking Time: 20 Minutes
Ingredients:

3 tablespoons butter, softened
1 cup wheat flour, whole wheat
1 teaspoon baking powder
1 egg, beaten
4 tablespoons pistachio paste
2 tablespoons raspberry jam

Directions:
Knead the dough: combine together softened butter, flour, baking powder, and egg. You should get the non-sticky and very soft dough.   Put the dough in the springform pan and flatten it with the help of the fingertips until you get pie crust.   Bake it for 10 minutes at 365F.   After this, spread the pie crust with raspberry jam and then with pistachio paste.   Bake the tart at 365F for another 10 minutes.   Cool the cooked tart and cut on the servings.
Nutrition Info: Per Serving:calories 311, fat 11, fiber 1.3, carbs 24.7, protein 4.5

876. Mango And Honey Cream

Servings: 6   Cooking Time: 30 Minutes
Ingredients:

2 cups coconut cream, chipped
6 teaspoons honey
2 mango, chopped

Directions:
Blend together honey and mango.   When the mixture is smooth, combine it with whipped cream and stir carefully.   Put the mango-cream mixture in the serving glasses and refrigerate for 30 minutes.
Nutrition Info: Per Serving:calories 272, fat 19.5, fiber 3.6, carbs 27, protein 2.8

877. Raw Truffles

Servings: 6   Cooking Time: 30 Minutes
Ingredients:

½ pound dates, pitted
½ cup water, hot
2 tablespoons raw honey
½ teaspoon vanilla extract
2 tablespoons cocoa powder
1 cup shredded coconut
1 tablespoon chia seeds
1 oz. candied orange, diced
Extra cocoa powder for coating

Directions:
Combine the hot water, dates, honey and vanilla in a food processor and pulse until well mixed.   Add the rest of the ingredients and mix well.   Form small balls and roll them through cocoa powder. Serve right away.
Nutrition Info: Per Serving:Calories:196 Fat:4.8g Protein:1.7g Carbohydrates:41.3g

878. Baked Peaches

Servings: 4   Cooking Time: 30 Minutes
Ingredients:

4 teaspoons stevia
4 peaches, halved and pitted
1 teaspoon vanilla extract
3 tablespoons honey

Directions:
Arrange the peaches on a baking sheet lined with parchment paper, add the stevia, honey and vanilla and bake at 350 degrees F for 30 minutes. Divide them between plates and serve.

Nutrition Info:calories 176, fat 4.5, fiber 7.6, carbs 11.5, protein 5

879. Coconut Risotto Pudding

Servings: 6   Cooking Time: 20 Minutes
Ingredients:

3/4 cup rice
1/2 cup shredded coconut
1 tsp lemon juice
1/2 tsp vanilla
oz can coconut milk
1/4 cup maple syrup
1 1/2 cups water

Directions:
Add all ingredients into the instant pot and stir well. Seal pot with lid and cook on high for 20 minutes. Once done, allow to release pressure naturally for 10 minutes then release remaining using quick release. Remove lid.   Blend pudding mixture using an immersion blender until smooth.   Serve and enjoy.
Nutrition Info: Calories 205 Fat 8.6 g Carbohydrates 29.1 g Sugar 9 g Protein 2.6 g Cholesterol 0 mg

880. Greek Yogurt Muesli Parfaits

Servings: 4   Cooking Time: 10 Minutes
Ingredients:

4 cups Greek yogurt
1 cup whole wheat muesli
2 cups fresh berries of your choice

Directions:
Layer the four glasses with Greek yogurt at the bottom, muesli on top, and berries.   Repeat the layers until the glass is full.   Place in the fridge for at least 2 hours to chill.
Nutrition Info: Calories per serving: 280; Carbs: 36g; Protein:23 g; Fat: 4g

881. Lemon Cream

Servings: 6   Cooking Time: 10 Minutes
Ingredients:

2 eggs, whisked
1 and ¼ cup stevia
10 tablespoons avocado oil
1 cup heavy cream
Juice of 2 lemons
Zest of 2 lemons, grated

Directions:
In a pan, combine the cream with the lemon juice and the other ingredients, whisk well, cook for 10 minutes, divide into cups and keep in the fridge for 1 hour before serving.
Nutrition Info:calories 200, fat 8.5, fiber 4.5, carbs 8.6, protein 4.5

882. Sweet Tropical Medley Smoothie

Servings: 4   Cooking Time: 5 Minutes
Ingredients:

1 banana, peeled
1 sliced mango
1 cup fresh pineapple
½ cup coconut water

Directions:
Place all Ingredients: in a blender.   Blend until smooth.   Pour in a glass container and allow to chill in the fridge for at least 30 minutes.
Nutrition Info: Calories per serving:73 ; Carbs: 18.6g; Protein: 0.8g; Fat: 0.5g.

883. Mediterranean Fruit Tart

Servings: 1/8 Of Tart   Cooking Time: 15 Minutes
Ingredients:

21/4 cups all-purpose flour
1/2 tsp. salt
5 TB. ice water
10 strawberries, sliced

2 TB. sugar
1 cup cold butter
1/2 cup shortening
2 cups Ashta Custard
(recipe earlier in this
chapter)

2 kiwi, peeled and
sliced
1 cup blueberries
1 cup peach or apricot
jam
3 TB. water

Directions:
In a food processor fitted with a chopping blade, pulse 2 cups all-purpose flour, salt, and sugar 5 times. Add butter and shortening, and blend for 1 minute or until mixture is crumbly. Transfer mixture to a medium bowl. Add ice water to batter, and mix just until combined. Place dough on a piece of plastic wrap, form into a flat disc, and refrigerate for 20 minutes. Preheat the oven to 450°F. Dust your workspace with flour, and using a rolling pin, roll out dough to 1/8 inch thickness. Place rolled-out dough into a 9-inch tart pan, press to mold into pan, and cut off excess dough. Bake for 13 minutes. Let tart cool for 10 minutes. Place tart shell on a serving dish, and fill with Ashta Custard. Arrange strawberry slices, kiwi slices, and blueberries on top of tart. In a small saucepan over medium heat, heat peach jam and water, stirring, for 2 minutes. Using a pastry brush, brush top of fruit and tart with warmed jam. Serve chilled and store in the refrigerator.

884. Green Tea And Vanilla Cream

Servings: 4   Cooking Time: 0 Minutes
Ingredients:
14 ounces almond
milk, hot
2 tablespoons green
tea powder
14 ounces heavy
cream

3 tablespoons stevia
1 teaspoon vanilla
extract
1 teaspoon gelatin
powder

Directions:
In a bowl, combine the almond milk with the green tea powder and the rest of the ingredients, whisk well, cool down, divide into cups and keep in the fridge for 2 hours before serving.
Nutrition Info:calories 120, fat 3, fiber 3, carbs 7, protein 4

885. Semolina Pie

Servings: 6   Cooking Time: 1 Hour
Ingredients:
½ cup milk
3 tablespoons
semolina
½ cup butter,
softened
8 Phyllo sheets
2 eggs, beaten
3 tablespoons
Erythritol
1 teaspoon lemon
rind

1 tablespoon lemon
juice
1 teaspoon vanilla
extract
2tablespoons liquid
honey
1 teaspoon ground
cinnamon
¼ cup of water

Directions:
Melt ½ part of all butter. Then brush the casserole glass mold with the butter and place 1 Phyllo sheet inside. Brush the Phyllo sheet with butter and cover it with second Phyllo sheet. Make the dessert filling: heat up milk, and add semolina. Stir it carefully. After this, add remaining softened butter, Erythritol, and vanilla extract. Bring the mixture to boil and simmer it for 2 minutes. Remove it from the heat and cool to the room temperature. Then add beaten eggs and mix up well. Pour the semolina mixture in

the mold over the Phyllo sheets, flatten it if needed. Then cover the semolina mixture with remaining Phyllo sheets and brush with remaining melted butter. Cut the dessert on the bars. Bake galaktoboureko for 1 hour at 365F. Then make the syrup: bring to boil lemon juice, honey, and water and remove the liquid from the heat. Pour the syrup over the hot dessert and let it chill well.
Nutrition Info: Per Serving:calories 304, fat 18, fiber 1.1, carbs 39.4, protein 6.1

886. Vanilla Apple Compote

Servings: 6   Cooking Time: 15 Minutes
Ingredients:
3 cups apples, cored
and cubed
1 tsp vanilla
3/4 cup coconut
sugar

1 cup of water
2 tbsp fresh lime juice

Directions:
Add all ingredients into the inner pot of instant pot and stir well. Seal pot with lid and cook on high for 15 minutes. Once done, allow to release pressure naturally for 10 minutes then release remaining using quick release. Remove lid. Stir and serve.
Nutrition Info: Calories 76 Fat 0.2 g Carbohydrates 19.1 g Sugar 11.9 g Protein 0.5 g Cholesterol 0 mg

887. Cold Lemon Squares

Servings: 4   Cooking Time: 0 Minutes
Ingredients:
1 cup avocado oil+ a
drizzle
2 bananas, peeled
and chopped

1 tablespoon honey
¼ cup lemon juice
A pinch of lemon
zest, grated

Directions:
In your food processor, mix the bananas with the rest of the ingredients, pulse well and spread on the bottom of a pan greased with a drizzle of oil. Introduce in the fridge for 30 minutes, slice into squares and serve.
Nutrition Info:calories 136, fat 11.2, fiber 0.2, carbs 7, protein 1.1

888. Minty Coconut Cream

Servings: 2   Cooking Time: 0 Minutes
Ingredients:
1 banana, peeled
2 cups coconut flesh,
shredded
3 tablespoons mint,
chopped

1 and ½ cups
coconut water
2 tablespoons stevia
½ avocado, pitted
and peeled

Directions:
In a blender, combine the coconut with the banana and the rest of the ingredients, pulse well, divide into cups and serve cold.
Nutrition Info:calories 193, fat 5.4, fiber 3.4, carbs 7.6, protein 3

889. Cherry Cream

Servings: 4   Cooking Time: 0 Minutes
Ingredients:
2 cups cherries,
pitted and chopped
1 cup almond milk
½ cup whipping
cream

1/3 cup stevia
1 teaspoon lemon
juice
½ teaspoon vanilla

3 eggs, whisked   extract

Directions:
In your food processor, combine the cherries with the milk and the rest of the ingredients, pulse well, divide into cups and keep in the fridge for 2 hours before serving.
Nutrition Info:calories 200, fat 4.5, fiber 3.3, carbs 5.6, protein 3.4

---

890. Warm Peach Compote

Servings: 4   Cooking Time: 1 Minute

Ingredients:

4 peaches, peeled and chopped	1/2 tbsp cornstarch
1 tbsp water	1 tsp vanilla

Directions:
Add water, vanilla, and peaches into the instant pot. Seal pot with lid and cook on high for 1 minute. Once done, allow to release pressure naturally. Remove lid. In a small bowl, whisk together 1 tablespoon of water and cornstarch and pour into the pot and stir well. Serve and enjoy.
Nutrition Info: Calories 66 Fat 0.4 g Carbohydrates 15 g Sugar 14.1 g Protein 1.4 g Cholesterol 0 mg

---

891. Honey Walnut Bars

Servings: 8   Cooking Time: 30 Minutes

Ingredients:

5 oz puff pastry	1/3 cup butter, softened
½ cup of water	
3 tablespoons of liquid honey	½ cup walnuts, chopped
1 teaspoon Erythritol	1 teaspoon olive oil

Directions:
Roll up the puff pastry and cut it on 6 sheets. Then brush the tray with olive oil and arrange the first puff pastry sheet inside. Grease it with butter gently and sprinkle with walnuts. Repeat the same steps with 4 puff pastry sheets. Then sprinkle the last layer with walnuts and Erythritol and cove with the sixth puff pastry sheet. Cut the baklava on the servings. Bake the baklava for 30 minutes. Meanwhile, bring to boil liquid honey and water. When the baklava is cooked, remove it from the oven. Pour hot honey liquid over baklava and let it cool till the room temperature.
Nutrition Info: Per Serving:calories 243, fat 19.6, fiber 0.8, carbs 15.9, protein 3.3

---

892. Lime Vanilla Fudge

Servings: 6   Cooking Time: 0 Minutes

Ingredients:

1/3 cup cashew butter	½ teaspoon lime zest, grated
5 tablespoons lime juice	
	1 tablespoons stevia

Directions:
In a bowl, mix the cashew butter with the other ingredients and whisk well. Line a muffin tray with parchment paper, scoop 1 tablespoon of lime fudge mix in each of the muffin tins and keep in the freezer for 3 hours before serving.
Nutrition Info:calories 200, fat 4.5, fiber 3.4, carbs 13.5, protein 5

---

893. Pear Sauce

Servings: 6   Cooking Time: 15 Minutes

Ingredients:

10 pears, sliced	1 1/2 tsp cinnamon

1 cup apple juice   1/4 tsp nutmeg

Directions:
Add all ingredients into the instant pot and stir well. Seal pot with lid and cook on high for 15 minutes. Once done, allow to release pressure naturally for 10 minutes then release remaining using quick release. Remove lid. Blend the pear mixture using an immersion blender until smooth. Serve and enjoy.
Nutrition Info: Calories 222 Fat 0.6 g Carbohydrates 58.2 g Sugar 38 g Protein 1.3 g Cholesterol 0 mg

---

894. Honey Cream

Servings: 2   Cooking Time: 5 Minutes

Ingredients:

½ cup cream	2 teaspoons honey
¼ cup milk	1 tablespoons gelatin
1 teaspoon vanilla extract	2 tablespoons orange juice

Directions:
Mix up together milk and gelatin and leave it for 5 minutes. Meanwhile, pour cream in the saucepan and bring it to boil. Add honey and vanilla extract. Remove the cream from the heat and stir well until honey is dissolved. After this, add gelatin mixture (milk+gelatin) and mix it up until gelatin is dissolved. After this, place 1 tablespoon of orange juice in every serving glass. Add the cream mixture over the orange juice. Refrigerate the pannacotta for 30-50 minutes in the fridge or until it is solid.
Nutrition Info: Per Serving:calories 100, fat 4, fiber 0, carbs 11, protein 4.6

---

895. Dragon Fruit, Pear, And Spinach Salad

Servings: 4   Cooking Time: 3 Minutes

Ingredients:

5 ounces spinach leaves, torn	6 ounces blackberries
	6 ounces raspberries
1 dragon fruit, peeled then cubed	8 tablespoons olive oil
2 pears, peeled then cubed	8 tablespoons red wine vinegar
10 ounces organic goat cheese	1 tablespoon poppy seeds
1 cup pecan, halves	

Directions:
In a mixing bowl, combine all Ingredients: except for the poppy seeds. Place inside the fridge and allow to chill before serving. Sprinkle with poppy seeds on top before serving.
Nutrition Info: Calories per serving:321; Carbs: 27.2g; Protein: 3.3g; Fat: 3.1g

---

896. Kataifi

Servings: 8-10   Cooking Time: 30 Minutes

Ingredients:

1 kilogram almonds, blanched and then chopped	4 tablespoons sugar
	400 g butter
1 teaspoon cinnamon	1 1/2 kilograms sugar
1/4 kilogram kataifi phyllo	1 lemon rind
	1 teaspoon lemon juice
2 eggs	5 cups water

Directions:
Preheat the oven to 170C. Put the sugar, eggs, cinnamon, and the almonds in a bowl. With your fingers, open the kataifi pastry gently. Lay it on a

piece of marble and wood. Put 1 tablespoon of the almond mixture in one end and then roll the pastry into a log or a cylinder. Make sure you fold the pastry a little tight so the filling is enclosed securely. Repeat the process with the remaining pastry and almond mixture.   Melt the butter and put into a baking dish.   Brush the kataifi rolls with the melted butter, covering all the sides.   Place into baking sheets and bake for about 30 minutes. Meanwhile, prepare the syrup.   Except for the lemon juice, cook the rest of the syrup ingredients for about 5-10 minutes. Add the lemon juice and let cook for a few minutes until the syrup is slightly thick.   After baking the kataifi, pour the syrup over the still warm rolls.   Cover the pastry with a clean towel. Let cool as the kataifi absorbs the syrup.

Nutrition Info: Per Serving:1085 cal., 83.3 total fat (24.6 g sat. fat), 119 mg chol., 248 mg sodium, 759 mg pot., 76.6 g total carbs., 12.7 g fiber, 59.1 g sugar, and 22.6 g protein.

897.   Walnuts Kataifi

Servings: 2   Cooking Time: 50 Minutes
Ingredients:

7 oz kataifi dough	4 tablespoons butter, melted
1/3 cup walnuts, chopped	¼ teaspoon ground clove
½ teaspoon ground cinnamon	1/3 cup water
¾ teaspoon vanilla extract	3 tablespoons honey

Directions:
For the filling: mix up together walnuts, ground cinnamon, and vanilla extract. Add ground clove and blend the mixture until smooth.   Make the kataifi dough: grease the casserole mold with butter and place ½ part of kataifi dough.   Then sprinkle the filling over the kataifi dough.   After this, sprinkle the filling with 1 tablespoon of melted butter.   Sprinkle the filling with remaining kataifi dough.   Make the roll from ½ part of kataifi dough and cut it.   Gently arrange the kataifi roll in the tray.   Repeat the same steps with remaining dough. In the end, you should get 2 kataifi rolls.   Preheat the oven to 355F and place the tray with kataifi rolls inside.   Bake the dessert for 50 minutes or until it is crispy.   Meanwhile, make the syrup: bring the water to boil.   Add honey and heat it up until the honey is dissolved. When the kataifi rolls are cooked, pour the hot syrup over the hot kataifi rolls.   Cut every kataifi roll on 2 pieces.   Serve the dessert with remaining syrup.

Nutrition Info: Per Serving:calories 120, fat 1.5, fiber 0, carbs 22, protein 3

898.   Cinnamon Tea

Servings: 1 Cup   Cooking Time: 32 Minutes
Ingredients:

6 cups water	1 (3-in.) cinnamon stick
6 TB. Ahmad Tea, Ceylon tea, or your favorite	3 TB. sugar

Directions:
In a teapot over low heat, bring water and cinnamon stick to a simmer for 30 minutes. Remove cinnamon stick.   Stir in Ahmad tea and sugar, and simmer for 2 minutes.   Remove from heat, and let sit for 10 minutes.   Strain tea into tea cups, and serve warm.

899.   Mediterranean Biscotti

Servings: 3   Cooking Time: 1 Hour
Ingredients:

2 eggs	2 tablespoons sugar
1 cups whole-wheat flour	1/4 cup Kalamata olive, finely chopped
1 cup all-purpose flour	1/3 cup olive oil
3/4 cup parmesan cheese, grated	1/2 teaspoon salt
2 teaspoons baking powder	1/2 teaspoon black pepper, cracked
1/4 cup sun-dried tomato, finely chopped	1 teaspoon dried oregano (preferably Greek)
	1 teaspoon dried basil

Directions:
Into a large-sized bowl, beat the eggs and the sugar together. Pour in the olive; beat until smooth.   In another bowl, combine the flours, baking powder, pepper, salt, oregano, and basil. Stir the flour mix into the egg mixture, stirring until blended.   Stir in the cheese, tomatoes, and olives; stirring until thoroughly combined.   Divide the dough into 2 portions; shape each into 10-inch long logs. Place the logs into a parchment-lined cookie sheet; flatten the log tops slightly.   Bake for about 30 minutes in a preheated 375F oven or until the logs are pale golden and not quite firm to the touch. Remove from the oven; let cool on the baking sheet for 3 minutes. Transfer the logs into a cutting board; slice each log into 1/2-inch diagonal slices using a serrated knife.   Place the biscotti slices on the baking sheet, return into the 325F oven, and bake for about 20 to 25 minutes until dry and firm. Flip the slices halfway through baking. Remove from the oven, transfer on a wire rack and let cool.

Nutrition Info: Per Serving:731.6 Cal, 36.5 g total fat (9 g sat. fat), 146 mg chol., 1238.4 mg sodium, 77.8 g carb., 3.5 g fiber, 10.7 g sugar, and 23.3 g protein.

900.   Tiny Orange Cardamom Cookies

Servings: 80   Cooking Time: 12 Minutes
Ingredients:

1/2 cup whole-wheat flour	1 teaspoon orange zest
1/2 cup all-purpose flour	1 teaspoon vanilla extract
1 large egg	1/2 cup butter, softened
1 tablespoon sesame seeds, toasted, optional (salted roasted pistachios, chopped)	1/2 cup sugar
	1/4 teaspoon ground cardamom

Directions:
Preheat the oven to 375F.   In a medium bowl, blend the orange zest and the sugar thoroughly, and then blend in the cardamom. Add the butter and with a mixer, beat until the mixture is fluffy and light. Beat in the egg and the vanilla into the mixture. With the mixer on low speed, mix in the flours into the mixture. Line 3 baking sheets with parchment paper. Using a level teaspoon measure, drop batter of the cookie mixture onto the sheets. Top each cookie with a pinch of sesame seeds or nuts, if desired; bake for 1bout 10-12 minutes or until the cookies are brown at the edges and crisp. When baked, transfer the cookies on a cooling rack and let them cool completely.

Nutrition Info: Per Serving:113 Cal, 1.4 g protein, 6.5 g total fat (3.8 g sat. fat) 12 g total carbs., 0.3 g fiber, 46 mg sodium, and 29 mg chol.

Other Mediterranean Recipes

901. Sparkling Limoncello

Servings: 1   Cooking Time: 5 Minutes

Ingredients:

4 ounces club soda
1 ounce Limoncello (I used Villa Massa Limoncello)
1 1/2 teaspoon simple syrup

1 ounce vodka
Ice, as needed
Lemon peels, for garnish
Splash lemon juice

Directions:

Combine the lemon juice, simple syrup, club soda, vodka, and limoncello in a cocktail shaker. Fill the shaker 2/3 full with ice. Stir for about 10 to 15 minutes to chill. Strain the ice into a cocktail glass, garnish with the lemon peel, and serve.

Nutrition Info: Per Serving:98 cal., 0 g total fat (0 g sat. fat), 0 mg chol., 33 mg sodium, 10 mg pot., 8.4 g total carbs., 0 g fiber, 0 g sugar, 0 g protein, 0% vitamin A, 0% vitamin C, 1% calcium, and 0% iron.

902. French Baked Brie Recipe With Figs, Walnuts And Pistachios

Servings: 6 To 8   Cooking Time: 10 Minutes

Ingredients:

4 tablespoons fig jam or preserves, divided
1/3 cup walnut hearts, roughly chopped

13 ounces French brie
1/3 cup pistachios, shelled and roughly chopped
1/3 cup dried mission figs, sliced

Directions:

Preheat the oven to 375F.   Place the fig preserves or jam in a microwavable dish; microwave for 30 seconds or until soft.   In a small-sized bowl, combine the nuts and the dried figs. Add in 1/2 of the softened fig preserve; mix well until well combined.   Place the brie into a small-sized ovenproof dish or a cast-iron skillet. With a knife, coat the brie with remaining 1/2 of the softened fig preserve/jam.   Top the brie with the nut and fig mixture.   Place the dish or the skillet in the oven and bake for 10 minutes at 375F or until the brie starts to ooze, but not melt.   Serve warm with your favorite crackers.

Nutrition Info: Per Serving:330 cal.,22.8 g total fat (11.1 g sat. fat), 61 mg chol., 410 mg sodium, 250 mg pot., 18.1 g total carbs., 2 g fiber, 12.3 g sugar, 15.5 g protein, 7% vitamin A, 2% vitamin C, 14% calcium, and 5% iron

903. Creamy Bell Pepper Soup With Cod Fillets

Servings: 6   Cooking Time: 1 Hour

Ingredients:

2 tablespoons olive oil
1 shallot, chopped
2 garlic cloves, chopped
1 jar roasted red bell peppers, sliced
2 cups chicken stock

2 cups water
1 bay leaf
1 thyme sprig
1 rosemary sprig
Salt and pepper to taste
4 cod fillets, cubed

Directions:

Heat the oil in a soup pot and stir in the shallot and garlic. Cook for 2 minutes then add the bell peppers, stock, water and herbs, as well as salt and pepper to taste.   Cook for 15 minutes then remove the herbs and puree the soup with an immersion blender.   Add the cod fillets and place the soup back on heat.   Cook for another 5 minutes. Serve the soup warm and fresh.

Nutrition Info: Per Serving:Calories:48 Fat:5.0g Protein:0.4g Carbohydrates:1.3g

904. Spanish Meatball Soup

Servings: 8   Cooking Time: 1 Hour

Ingredients:

2 tablespoons olive oil
1 onion, chopped
2 garlic cloves, chopped
2 red bell peppers, cored and diced
2 carrots, diced
2 cups vegetable stock

1 celery stalk, diced
6 cups water
1 pound ground veal
1 egg
2 tablespoons chopped parsley
1 can crushed tomatoes
Salt and pepper to taste

Directions:

Heat the oil in a soup pot and stir in the onion, garlic, bell peppers, carrots, celery, stock and water. Season with salt and pepper and bring to a boil. In the meantime, mix the veal, egg and parsley in a bowl. Form small meatballs and place them in the boiling liquid.   Add the tomatoes and adjust the taste with salt and pepper.   Cook on low heat for 20 minutes.   Serve the soup war and fresh.

Nutrition Info: Per Serving:Calories:166 Fat:8.5g Protein:15.6g Carbohydrates:6.5g

905. Eggs Over Kale Hash

Servings: 4   Cooking Time: 20 Minutes

Ingredients:

4 large eggs
1 bunch chopped kale
2 sweet potatoes, cubed

Dash of ground nutmeg
1 14.5-ounce can of chicken broth

Directions:

In a large non-stick skillet, bring the chicken broth to a simmer. Add the sweet potatoes and season slightly with salt and pepper. Add a dash of nutmeg to improve the flavor.   Cook until the sweet potatoes become soft, around 10 minutes. Add kale and season with salt and pepper. Continue cooking for four minutes or until kale has wilted. Set aside. Using the same skillet, heat 1 tablespoon of olive oil over medium high heat.   Cook the eggs sunny side up until the whites become opaque and the yolks have set. Top the kale hash with the eggs. Serve immediately.

Nutrition Info: Calories per serving: 158; Protein: 9.8g; Carbs 18.5g; Fat: 5.6g

906. Leek And Potato Soup

Servings: 8   Cooking Time: 1 Hour

Ingredients:

3 tablespoons olive oil
3 leeks, sliced

2 cups vegetable stock
2 cups water

4 garlic cloves, chopped
6 potatoes, peeled and cubed

1 thyme sprig
1 rosemary sprig
Salt and pepper to taste

Directions:
Heat the oil in a soup pot and stir in the leeks. Cook for 15 minutes until slightly caramelized.   Add the garlic and cook for 2 more minutes.   Add the rest of the ingredients and season with salt and pepper.   Cook on low heat for 20 minutes then remove the herb sprigs and puree the soup with an immersion blender.   Serve the soup fresh.

Nutrition Info: Per Serving: Calories:179 Fat:5.5g Protein:3.4g Carbohydrates:30.6g

907.	**Paleo Chocolate Banana Bread**

Servings: 10   Cooking Time: 50 Minutes

Ingredients:

¼ cup dark chocolate, chopped
½ cup coconut flour, sifted
½ teaspoon cinnamon powder
1 teaspoon baking soda

½ cup almond butter
1 teaspoon vanilla extract
4 bananas, mashed
4 eggs
4 tablespoon coconut oil, melted
A pinch of salt

Directions:
Preheat the oven to 350oF.   Grease an 8" x 8" square pan and set aside.   In a large bowl, mix together the eggs, banana, vanilla extract, almond butter and coconut oil. Mix well until well combined.   Add the cinnamon powder, coconut flour, baking powder, baking soda and salt to the wet ingredients. Fold until well combined. Add in the chopped chocolates then fold the batter again. Pour the batter into the greased pan. Spread evenly. Bake in the oven for about 50 minutes or until a toothpick inserted in the center comes out clean. Remove from the hot oven and cool in a wire rack for an hour.

Nutrition Info: Calories per Serving: 150.3; Carbs: 13.9g; Protein: 3.2g; Fat: 9.1g

908.	**Mast-o Khiar A.k.a Persian Yogurt And Cucumbers)**

Servings: 8   Cooking Time: 10 Minutes

Ingredients:

4 cup yogurt, plain Greek
2 teaspoon mint, dried
2 teaspoon dill, dried

1/4 teaspoon black pepper, ground
1/2 teaspoon salt
1 1/2 cup Persian cucumbers, diced

Directions:
Combine all the ingredients in a medium-sized bowl.

Nutrition Info: Per Serving:62 cal., 4 g total fat (0.8 g sat. fat), 0 mg chol., 1 mg sodium, 81 mg pot., 7.2 g total carbs., 1.3 g fiber, 5.5 g sugar, 0.8 g protein, 0% vitamin A, 0% vitamin C, 1% calcium, and 3% iron.

909.	**Pesto, Avocado And Tomato Panini**

Servings: 4   Cooking Time: 10 Minutes

Ingredients:

2 tbsp extra virgin olive oil

½ lemon

8 oz fresh buffalo mozzarella cheese
2 vine-ripened tomatoes cut into ¼ inch thick slices
2 avocados, peeled, pitted, quartered and cut into thin strips
1 ciabatta loaf
Pepper and salt

1/3 cup extra virgin olive oil
1/3 cup parmesan cheese
1/3 cup pine nuts, toasted
1 ½ bunches fresh basil leaves
2 garlic cloves, peeled

Directions:
To make the pesto, puree garlic in a food processor and transfer to a mortar and pestle and add in basil and smash into a coarse paste like consistency. Mix in the pine nuts and continue crushing. Once paste like, add the parmesan cheese and mix. Pour in olive oil and blend thoroughly while adding lemon juice. Season with pepper and salt. Put aside. Prepare Panini by slicing ciabatta loaf in three horizontal pieces. To prepare Panini, over bottom loaf slice layer the following: avocado, tomato, pepper, salt and mozzarella cheese. Then top with the middle ciabatta slice and repeat layering process again and cover with the topmost ciabatta bread slice.   Grill in a Panini press until cheese is melted and bred is crisped and ridged.

Nutrition Info: Calories per Serving: 577; Carbs: 15.5g; Protein: 24.2g; Fat: 49.3g

910.	**Baba Ganoush**

Servings: 2 Tablespoons   Cooking Time: 50 Minutes

Ingredients:

2 large eggplants
4 TB. extra-virgin olive oil
1 large white onion, chopped
1 TB. minced garlic
3 TB. fresh lemon juice
1 tsp. salt
1/2 tsp. ground black pepper

1/2 medium red bell pepper, ribs and seeds removed, and finely diced
1/2 medium green bell pepper, ribs and seeds removed, and finely diced
3 TB. fresh parsley, finely chopped
1/2 tsp. cayenne

Directions:
3 medium radishes, finely diced   3 whole green onions, finely chopped   Preheat a grill top or a grill to medium-low heat.   Place eggplants on the grill, and roast on all sides for 40 minutes, turning every 5 minutes. Immediately place eggplants on a plate, cover with plastic wrap, let cool for 15 minutes.   Remove eggplant stems, and peel off as much skin as possible. (It's okay if it doesn't all come off.)   In a food processor fitted with a chopping blade, pulse eggplant 7 times. Transfer eggplant to a medium bowl.   In a medium saucepan over low heat, heat 2 tablespoons extra-virgin olive oil. Add white onion, and sauté, stirring occasionally, for 10 minutes. Add onions to eggplant.   Add garlic, lemon juice, salt, black pepper, red bell pepper, green bell pepper, and parsley to eggplant, and stir well.   Spread baba ganoush on a serving plate, and drizzle remaining 2 tablespoons extra-virgin olive oil over top. Sprinkle with cayenne, radishes, and green onions.   Serve cold or at room temperature.

911. Chicken And Mediterranean Tabbouleh

Servings: 2   Cooking Time: 30 Minutes

Ingredients:

6 ounces chicken breast halves, skinless, boneless, broiled or grilled, then sliced

4 large leaves romaine and/or butter head (Bibb or Boston) lettuce

3/4 cup water

3 tablespoons lemon juice

2 tablespoons olive oil

2 tablespoons green onions, thinly sliced

1/8teaspoon ground black pepper

1/4 teaspoon salt

1/4 cup bulgur

1/2 cup tomatoes (1 medium), chopped

1/2 cup seeded cucumber, finely chopped

1/2 cup Italian parsley, finely chopped

1 tablespoon fresh mint, snipped (or 1 teaspoon dried mint, crushed)

Directions:

In a large sized bowl, combine the bulgur and the water; let stand for 30 minutes. After 30 minutes, drain in the sink through a fine sieve; pressing out the excess water from the bulgur using a large spoon. Return the bulgur into the bowl. Stir in the cucumber, tomatoes, green onions, parsley, and the mint.   Prepare the dressing; put the olive oil, lemon juice, salt, and pepper into a screw-top jar. Cover securely and shake well until well mixed. Pour the dressing over the bulgur mixture; lightly toss to coat the bulgur mixture with the dressing. Cover the bowl and refrigerate to chill for at least 4 hours up to 24 hours, occasionally stirring. When ready to serve, bring the bulgur mixture to room temperature. Divide the romaine and/or butterhead lettuce leaves between 2 shallow bowls, top with the broiled or grilled chicken, and then top with the bulgur mixture.

Nutrition Info: Per Serving:294 cal.,13 g total fat (2 g sat. fat,2 g poly. fat, 8 g mono. fat), 72 mg chol., 276 mg sodium, 16 g total carbs., 5 g fiber, 3 g sugar, and 30 g protein.

912. Jew's Mallow Stew (mulukhiya)

Servings: 1 Cup   Cooking Time: 2 Hours

Ingredients:

2 whole chicken thighs, including drumstick

1 (2-in.) cinnamon stick

2 bay leaves

8 cups water

2 tsp. salt

6 cups rehydrated Jew's mallow leaves, drained

1/2 cup extra-virgin olive oil

1 large yellow onion, chopped

6 TB. minced garlic

1 cup fresh cilantro, finely chopped

1/2 tsp. cayenne

1/2 cup fresh lemon juice

Directions:

In a large pot over medium heat, combine chicken thighs, cinnamon stick, bay leaves, water, and 1 teaspoon salt. Cook for 30 minutes. Skim off any foam that comes to the top.   Meanwhile, in another large pot over medium heat, heat 1/4 cup extra-virgin olive oil. Add Jew's mallow leaves, and cook, tossing leaves, for 10 minutes. Remove leaves, and set aside.   Reduce heat to medium-low. Add remaining 1/4 cup extra-virgin olive oil, yellow onion, and 3 tablespoons garlic, and cook for 5 minutes.   Return Jew's mallow leaves to onions. Add 8 cups chicken broth strained to the first pot to onions and Jew's mallow leaves in the second pot. Add remaining 1 teaspoon salt, and cook for 1 hour. Meanwhile, separate chicken meat from bones. Discard bones and remaining contents of first pot. After leaves have been cooking for 1 hour, add chicken, cilantro, cayenne, and remaining 3 tablespoons garlic, and cook for 20 more minutes. Add lemon juice, and cook for 10 more minutes. Serve with brown rice.

913. Homemade Greek Yogurt

Servings: ½ Cup   Cooking Time: 20 Minutes

Ingredients:

2 cups plain Greek yogurt

1 gal. whole milk

Directions:

In a large pot over medium-low heat, bring whole milk to a simmer until a froth starts to form on the surface. If you have a thermometer, bring the milk to 185°F.   Remove from heat, and let milk cool to lukewarm, or 110°F.   Pour all but about 2 cups milk into a large plastic container.   Pour remaining 2 cups milk into a smaller bowl. Add Greek yogurt, and stir until well combined. Slowly pour milk and yogurt mixture into the large bowl of milk, and stir well.   Cover the bowl with a lid, and set aside where it won't be disturbed. Cover it with a towel, and let it sit overnight.   The next morning, gently transfer the bowl to the refrigerator. Chill for at least 1 day.   The next day, gently pour off clear liquid that's formed on top of yogurt, leaving just a little liquid remaining. Serve, or store in the refrigerator for up to 2 weeks.

914. Smoked Ham Split Pea Soup

Servings: 8   Cooking Time: 1 Hour

Ingredients:

2 tablespoons olive oil

4 oz. smoked ham, diced

1 sweet onion, chopped

1 jalapeno pepper, chopped

2 red bell peppers, cored and diced

2 garlic cloves, chopped

2 carrots, diced

1 parsnip, diced

2 tomatoes, peeled and diced

2 cups vegetable stock

6 cups water

½ cup split peas

Salt and pepper to taste

1 lemon, juiced

Crème fraiche for serving

Directions:

Heat the oil in a soup pot and stir in the ham. Cook for 5 minutes then add the rest of the ingredients. Season with salt and pepper and cook on low heat for 30 minutes.   Serve the soup warm, topped with crème fraiche.

Nutrition Info: Per Serving:Calories:139 Fat:5.1g Protein:6.7g Carbohydrates:18.0g

915. Herbed Panini Fillet O'fish

Servings: 4   Cooking Time: 25 Minutes

Ingredients:

4 slices thick sourdough bread

4 slices mozzarella

1 portabella mushroom, sliced

6 tbsp oil

cheese
1 small onion, sliced

4 garlic and herb fish fillets

Directions:
Prepare your fillets by adding salt, pepper and herbs (rosemary, thyme, parsley whatever you like). Then dredged in flour before deep frying in very hot oil. Once nicely browned, remove from oil and set aside.   On medium high fire, sauté for five minutes the onions and mushroom in a skillet with 2 tbsp oil.   Prepare sourdough breads by layering the following over it: cheese, fish fillet, onion mixture and cheese again before covering with another bread slice.   Grill in your Panini press until cheese is melted and bread is crisped and ridged.
Nutrition Info: Calories per Serving: 422; Carbs: 13.2g; Protein: 51.2g; Fat: 17.2g

916.   Aioli Sauce

Servings: 4   Cooking Time: 4 Minutes
Ingredients:

1 cup olive oil	1/2 teaspoon salt
1 lemon, juice	2 large garlic cloves
1 whole egg	(or 3 medium)
1/2 teaspoon mustard, good prepared	White pepper, to taste

Directions:
Except for the oil, put the rest of the ingredients into a food processor with the steel blade attached; process for 2 minutes at HIGH.   With the motor still running, pour the olive oil in the pierced food pusher. Pour in small parts if it is too small to contain all the oil at once.   Let the oil drip in; process 2 minutes more. Open the processor and transfer the aioli into a serving bowl.
Nutrition Info: Per Serving:454 cal., 51.7 g total fat (7.6 g sat. fat), 41 mg chol., 308 mg sodium, 33 mg pot., 0.9 g total carbs., 0 g fiber, 0 g sugar, 1.6 g protein, 1% vitamin A, 6% vitamin C, 1% calcium, and 2% iron.

917.Mediterranean Martini

Servings: 2   Cooking Time: 10 Minutes
Ingredients:

4 pieces fresh strawberries	Chilled sparkling wine, to top
30 ml vodka (Polish rye or French grape)	Few pieces of mint leaves (bruised)
2 pieces fresh gooseberries	Splash of lime juice Splash of sugar syrup

Directions:
Put the gooseberries, strawberries, and the mint leaves into a mixing glass; muddle the ingredients to release the juices.   Put ice into a mixing glass until full. Add in the lime, sugar, and vodka. Shake and then strain into chilled martini glasses. Top with the sparkling wine and then garnish; serve.
Nutrition Info: Per Serving:51 cal., 0.1 g total fat (0 g sat. fat), 0 mg chol., 2 mg sodium, 64 mg pot., 4.6 g total carbs., 1 g fiber, 1.2 g sugar, 0.3 g protein, 1% vitamin A, 29% vitamin C, 1% calcium, and 1% iron.

918.   Sausage & Bacon With Beans

Servings: 12   Cooking Time: 30 Minutes
Ingredients:

12 medium sausages	2 cans baked beans
12 bacon slices	12 bread slices,

8 eggs   toasted
Directions:
Preheat the Airfryer at 325 degrees F and place sausages and bacon in a fryer basket.   Cook for about 10 minutes and place the baked beans in a ramekin.   Place eggs in another ramekin and the Airfryer to 395 degrees F.   Cook for about 10 more minutes and divide the sausage mixture, beans and eggs in serving plates   Serve with bread slices.
Nutrition Info: Calories: 276 Carbs: 14.1g Fats: 17g Proteins: 16.3g Sodium: 817mg Sugar: 0.6g

919.   Creamy Carrot Coriander Soup

Servings: 8   Cooking Time: 50 Minutes
Ingredients:

2 tablespoons olive oil	1 red pepper, sliced
2 shallots, chopped	2 cups vegetable stock
2 garlic cloves, chopped	2 cups water
6 carrots, sliced	Salt and pepper to taste
1 teaspoon coriander seeds	½ cup heavy cream

Directions:
Heat the oil in a soup pot and stir in the shallots, garlic and carrots, as well as coriander seeds. Cook for 5 minutes, then stir in the red pepper, stock, water, salt and pepper.   Cook for another 10-15 minutes on low heat then remove from heat. Add the cream and puree the soup with an immersion blender.   Serve the soup warm and fresh.
Nutrition Info: Per Serving:Calories:84 Fat:6.3g Protein:0.9g Carbohydrates:6.5g

920.   Cucumber, Chicken And Mango Wrap

Servings: 1   Cooking Time: 20 Minutes
Ingredients:

½ of a medium cucumber cut lengthwise	½ of ripe mango
1 tbsp salad dressing of choice	1 whole wheat tortilla wrap
1-inch thick slice of chicken breast around 6-inch in length	2 tbsp oil for frying
	2 tbsp whole wheat flour
	2 to 4 lettuce leaves
	Salt and pepper to taste

Directions:
Slice a chicken breast into 1-inch strips and just cook a total of 6-inch strips. That would be like two strips of chicken. Store remaining chicken for future use.   Season chicken with pepper and salt. Dredge in whole wheat flour.   On medium fire, place a small and nonstick fry pan and heat oil. Once oil is hot, add chicken strips and fry until golden brown around 5 minutes per side.   While chicken is cooking, place tortilla wraps in oven and cook for 3 to 5 minutes. Then remove from oven and place on a plate.   Slice cucumber lengthwise, use only ½ of it and store remaining cucumber. Peel cucumber cut into quarter and remove pith. Place the two slices of cucumber on the tortilla wrap, 1-inch away from the edge.   Slice mango and store the other half with seed. Peel the mango without seed, slice into strips and place on top of

the cucumber on the tortilla wrap.   Once chicken is cooked, place chicken beside the cucumber in a line.   Add cucumber leaf, drizzle with salad dressing of choice.   Roll the tortilla wrap, serve and enjoy.

Nutrition Info: Calories per Serving: 434; Fat: 10g; Protein: 21g; Carbohydrates: 65g

921.   Italian Meatball Soup

Servings: 8   Cooking Time: 1 Hour

Ingredients:

4 cups chicken stock	1 teaspoon dried basil
4 cups water	1 pound ground
1 shallot, chopped	chicken
2 red bell peppers,	2 tablespoons white
cored and diced	rice
1 carrot, diced	1 lemon, juiced
1 celery stalk, diced	Salt and pepper to
2 tomatoes, diced	taste
1 cup tomato juice	2 tablespoons
½ teaspoon dried	chopped parsley
oregano	

Directions:

Combine the stock, water, shallot, bell peppers, carrot, celery, tomatoes, tomato juice, oregano and basil in a soup pot.   Add salt and pepper to taste and cook for 10 minutes.   Make the meatballs by mixing the chicken with rice and parsley.   Form small meatballs and drop them in the hot soup. Continue cooking for another 15 minutes then add the lemon juice.   Serve the soup right away.

Nutrition Info: Per Serving:Calories:150 Fat:4.7g Protein:18.0g Carbohydrates:8.8g

922.   Schug

Servings: 1/2   Cooking Time: 15 Minutes

Ingredients:

3 large hot green	1 teaspoon salt
peppers	5 large hot red
3 tablespoons olive	peppers
oil	5 large garlic cloves,
1 teaspoon ground	peeled
black pepper	3 tablespoons olive
1 tablespoon fresh	oil
lemon juice	1/2 large bunch
1 large bunch	coriander leaves
coriander leaves	1 teaspoon salt
1 head garlic, cloves	1 teaspoon ground
peeled	cumin

Directions:

For both colors of schug: Rinse the coriander leaves and dry them thoroughly. Remove most the stems and then coarsely chop the leaves.   Peel the garlic; chop coarsely.   Rinse and dry the pepper; chop coarsely. Chop with care.   Wash hands thoroughly after handling or use latex gloves. These can be really hot. Avoid touching eyes after handling and chopping the peppers.   Put the peppers, garlic, and coriander into a food processor; process on high for a couple of minutes or until the mixture is a chunky paste.   Add the salt and pepper (and cumin if making red schug); process again to mix.   Stop the processor; by hand, stir in the olive oil. If making the green schug, pour the lemon juice over the surface before storing to preserve the green color.   Serve.   For the green schug:

Nutrition Info: Per Serving: 442 cal., 42.6 g total fat (6.2 g sat. fat), 0 mg chol., 2348 mg sodium,

628 mg pot., 18.3 g total carbs., 3.3 g fiber, 7.5 g sugar, 4 g protein, 54% vitamin A, 570% vitamin C, 6% calcium, and 15% iron.   For the red schug   per serving: 484 cal., 43.6 g total fat (6.1 g sat. fat), 0 mg chol., 2359 mg sodium, 906 mg pot., 26.3 g total carbs., 4.4 g fiber, 12.3 g sugar, 5.9 g protein, 65% vitamin A, 554% vitamin C, 9% calcium, and 24% iron.

923.   Greek Mountain Tea

Servings: 1   Cooking Time: 5 Minutes

Ingredients:

Greek Mountain Tea	Honey or sugar,
1 Cup Water	optional

Directions:

Get about 1 to 2 Greek Mountain Tea leaves and break them into thirds.   Fill a pot or a briki with water. Turn the flame or heat on to medium-high. Put the tealeaves into the pot or briki; bring the water to a boil. When boiling, remove the pot or briki from the heat, and let the tea steep for 7 minutes.   After steeping, pour the tea into a cup over a strainer to catch the tealeaves.   If desired, sweeten with honey and sugar. Enjoy!

Nutrition Info: Per Serving:3 cal., 0 g total fat (0 g sat. fat), 0 mg chol., 8 mg sodium, 19 mg pot., 0.9 g total carbs., 0 g fiber, 0.7 g sugar, 0 g protein, 0% vitamin A, 0% vitamin C, 1% calcium, and 0% iron.

924.   Eggs With Dill, Pepper, And Salmon

Servings: 6   Cooking Time: 15 Minutes

Ingredients:

pepper and salt to	2 tbsp fresh chives,
taste	chopped
1 tsp red pepper	2 tbsp fresh dill,
flakes	chopped
2 garlic cloves,	4 tomatoes, diced
minced	8 eggs, whisked
½ cup crumbled goat	1 tsp coconut oil
cheese	

Directions:

In a big bowl whisk the eggs. Mix in pepper, salt, red pepper flakes, garlic, dill and salmon.   On low fire, place a nonstick fry pan and lightly grease with oil.   Pour egg mixture and whisk around until cooked through to make scrambled eggs.   Serve and enjoy topped with goat cheese.

Nutrition Info: Calories per serving: 141; Protein: 10.3g; Carbs: 6.7g; Fat: 8.5g

925.   Kale And Red Pepper Frittata

Servings: 4   Cooking Time: 23 Minutes

Ingredients:

Salt and pepper to	8 large eggs
taste	1/3 cup onion,
½ cup almond milk	chopped
2 cups kale, rinsed	½ cup red pepper,
and chopped	chopped
3 slices of crispy	1 tablespoon coconut
bacon, chopped	oil

Directions:

Preheat the oven to 350F.   In a medium bowl, combine the eggs and almond milk. Season with salt and pepper. Set aside.   In a skillet, heat the coconut oil over medium flame and sauté the onions and red pepper for three minutes or until

the onion is translucent. Add in the kale and cook for 5 minutes more.   Add the eggs into the mixture along with the bacon and cook for four minutes or until the edges start to set.   Continue cooking the frittata in the oven for 15 minutes.
Nutrition Info: Calories per serving: 242; Protein: 16.5g; Carbs: 7.0g; Fat: 16.45g

926.   Lamb Veggie Soup

Servings: 8   Cooking Time: 1 ½ Hours
Ingredients:

1 ½ pound lamb shoulder, cubed	4 cups vegetable stock
2 tablespoons olive oil	6 cups water
2 shallots, chopped	1 thyme sprig
2 carrots, diced	1 oregano sprig
2 celery stalks, diced	1 basil sprig
¼ teaspoon grated ginger	Salt and pepper to taste
2 cups cauliflower florets	1 can crushed tomatoes
½ cup green peas	2 tablespoons lemon juice

Directions:
Heat the oil in a soup pot and stir in the lamb shoulder.   Cook for 5 minutes on all sides then add the water and stock.   Cook for 40 minutes then add the rest of the ingredients and season with salt and pepper.   Continue cooking for another 20 minutes then serve the soup fresh.
Nutrition Info: Per Serving:Calories:221 Fat:9.9g Protein:25.7g Carbohydrates:6.5g

927.   Avocado And Spinach Breakfast Wrap

Servings: 4   Cooking Time: 10 Minutes
Ingredients:

¼ tsp pepper	4 oz shredded pepper jack cheese
½ tsp salt	4 thin, whole wheat pita bread, 8-inch
1 5-oz box or bag of baby spinach, chopped	Hot sauce, optional
1 avocado, sliced	Nonstick cooking spray
4 egg whites	
4 eggs	

Directions:
On medium high fire, place a nonstick skillet greased with cooking spray.   Once hot, sauté spinach for 2 minutes or until wilted.   Meanwhile, in a small bowl whisk egg whites and eggs. Season with pepper and salt, whisk again. Pour into skillet and scramble. Cook for 3 to 4 minutes or to desired doneness.   Evenly divide egg into 4 equal portions and place in middle of pita bread and add 2 to 4 slices of avocadoes beside the egg and roll tortilla like a burrito.   Serve and enjoy with a side of hot sauce.
Nutrition Info: Calories per Serving: 532; Carbs: 42.7g; Protein: 28.2g; Fat: 27.6g

928.   Tahini Sauce

Servings: 4   Cooking Time: 15 Minutes
Ingredients:

1 cup tahini sesame seed paste, made from light colored seeds	1/4 teaspoon salt, or more to taste
1/4 cup freshly squeezed lemon juice,	3/4 cup lukewarm water, or more for consistency
	2 teaspoon fresh

or more to taste	parsley, minced, optional
3 cloves raw garlic (or	
5 cloves roasted garlic)	

Directions:
Put the tahini paste, lemon juice, lukewarm water, and salt in the food processor; process, scraping the sides periodically until the mixture is ivory-colored and creamy.   If using a blender, break the thick parts of the mixture every 30 seconds using a long-handles spoon; this will prevent the blender blades from clogging.   Process or blend until the sauce turns into a smooth, rich paste.   If the mixture is too thick, slowly add water until the texture is according to your desired consistency. If using tahini as a topping for meat dish or hummus, make the sauce creamy and thick.   If using as a condiment for falafel or fits, make it more liquid.   Taste the sauce often during processing or blending. If desired, add more salt or lemon juice.   Pour the sauce into a bowl once it's blended according to your needed consistency and desired flavor. If desired, stir parley until well mixed or just sprinkle the top with parsley leaves to garnish.
Nutrition Info: Per Serving:364 cal., 32.4 g total fat (4.6 g sat. fat), 0 mg chol., 221 mg sodium, 279 mg pot., 13.8 g total carbs., 5.7 g fiber, 0.6 g sugar, 10.5 g protein, 2% vitamin A, 13% vitamin C, 26% calcium, and 30% iron.

929.   Panini And Eggplant Caponata

Servings: 4   Cooking Time: 10 Minutes
Ingredients:

¼ cup packed fresh basil leaves	4 oz thinly sliced mozzarella
¼ of a 7oz can of eggplant caponata	1 ciabatta roll 6-7-inch length,
1 tbsp olive oil	horizontally split

Directions:
Spread oil evenly on the sliced part of the ciabatta and layer on the following: cheese, caponata, basil leaves and cheese again before covering with another slice of ciabatta.   Then grill sandwich in a Panini press until cheese melts and bread gets crisped and ridged.
Nutrition Info: Calories per Serving: 295; Carbs: 44.4g; Protein: 16.4g; Fat: 7.3g

930.   Lemon Aioli And Swordfish Panini

Servings: 4   Cooking Time: 25 Minutes
Ingredients:

2 oz fresh arugula greens	1 ½ tbsp olive oil
1 loaf focaccia bread	¼ tsp freshly ground black pepper
2 cloves garlic minced	
1 tbsp herbes de Provence	¼ tsp salt
Pepper and salt	1 clove garlic, minced
4 pcs of 6oz swordfish fillet	2 tbsp fresh lemon juice
	1 lemon, zested
	2/3 cup mayonnaise

Directions:
In a small bowl, mix well all lemon Aioli ingredients and put aside.   Over medium high fire, heat olive oil in skillet. Season with pepper,

188

salt, minced garlic and herbs de Provence the swordfish. Then pan fry fish until golden brown on both sides, around 5 minutes per side.   Slice bread into four slices. Smear on the lemon aioli mixture on two bread slices, layer with arugula leaves and fried fish then cover with the remaining bread slices before grilling in a Panini press. Grill until bread is crisped and ridged.
Nutrition Info: Calories per Serving: 433; Carbs: 15.0g; Protein: 36.2g; Fat: 25.1g

931.   Paleo Almond Banana Pancakes

Servings: 3   Cooking Time: 10 Minutes
Ingredients:

¼ cup almond flour	1 banana, mashed
½ teaspoon ground cinnamon	1 teaspoon vanilla extract
3 eggs	1 teaspoon olive oil
1 tablespoon almond butter	Sliced banana to serve

Directions:
Whisk the eggs in a mixing bowl until they become fluffy.   In another bowl mash the banana using a fork and add to the egg mixture.   Add the vanilla, almond butter, cinnamon and almond flour.   Mix into a smooth batter.   Heat the olive oil in a skillet.   Add one spoonful of the batter and fry them from both sides.   Keep doing these steps until you are done with all the batter.   Add some sliced banana on top before serving.
Nutrition Info: Calories per serving: 306; Protein: 14.4g; Carbs: 3.6g; Fat: 26.0g

932.   Mediterranean Wild Mushroom Pie

Servings: 6-8   Cooking Time: 20 Minutes
Ingredients:

250 grams wild mushrooms, sliced or halved	2 tablespoons sundried tomato paste
200 grams squash, sliced into small pieces (or pumpkin)	15 grams fresh parsley, chopped
2 tablespoons vegetable oil	1 large onion, cut in half and slice finely
2 small courgettes or zucchini, cut into thin slices	1 large clove garlic, crushed
100 ml cream, dairy-free (I used Oatly)	1 block (500 grams) vegan short-crust pastry (I used JusRol)
	Salt and pepper

Directions:
Roll out the vegan short-crust pastry and line into a 10-inch baking tray with loose-bottom. Trim off any excess pastry and then blind bake the pastry (see notes) for at 200C for about 15 minutes. Before filling the tart, remove the baking paper carefully. Add vegetable oil into a frying pan. Add the onion and sauté for about 3 to 4 minutes. Put the garlic and the squash; cook for couple of minutes or until squash starts to soften. If necessary, add some water. Add the mushrooms, courgettes, and parsley. Carefully stir and season with salt and generously season with pepper.   Mix the tomato paste with the cream. Stir the mixture into the pan.   Adjust seasoning according to taste and then transfer into the prepared pastry shell; bake for 20 minutes or until the blind baked pastry is golden browned.

Nutrition Info: Per Serving:225 cal.,7 g total fat (1.7 g sat. fat), 2 mg chol., 796 mg sodium, 425 mg pot., 35.7 g total carbs., 2.5 g fiber, 7.4 g sugar, 6.4 g protein, 7% vitamin A, 25% vitamin C, 3% calcium, and 17% iron

933.   Dill And Tomato Frittata

Servings: 6   Cooking Time: 35 Minutes
Ingredients:

pepper and salt to taste	2 tbsp fresh chives, chopped
1 tsp red pepper flakes	2 tbsp fresh dill, chopped
2 garlic cloves, minced	4 tomatoes, diced
½ cup crumbled goat cheese – optional	8 eggs, whisked
	1 tsp coconut oil

Directions:
Grease a 9-inch round baking pan and preheat oven to 3250F.   In a large bowl, mix well all ingredients and pour into prepped pan.   Pop into the oven and bake until middle is cooked through around 30-35 minutes.   Remove from oven and garnish with more chives and dill.
Nutrition Info: Calories per serving: ; Protein: ; g; Fat:

934.   Mixed Bean Minestrone

Servings: 10   Cooking Time: 1 Hour
Ingredients:

2 tablespoons olive oil	2 carrots, diced
2 chicken sausages, sliced	1 can white beans, drained
2 shallots, chopped	4 cups chicken stock
1 green bell pepper, cored and diced	4 cups water
1 garlic clove, chopped	1 cup diced tomatoes
2 celery stalks, sliced	1 tablespoon tomato paste
1 can red beans, drained	Salt and pepper to taste
	½ cup short pasta
	2 tablespoons lemon juice

Directions:
Heat the oil in a soup pot and stir in the sausages. Cook for 5 minutes then add the vegetables. Cook for 10 minutes then add the liquids and season with salt and pepper.   Cook on low heat for 25 minutes.   The soup is best served warm or chilled.
Nutrition Info: Per Serving:Calories:174 Fat:3.5g Protein:9.7g Carbohydrates:27.3g

935.   Italian Flat Bread Gluten Free

Servings: 8   Cooking Time: 30 Minutes
Ingredients:

1 tbsp apple cider	1 tsp baking soda
2 tbsp water	1 ½ tsp baking powder
½ cup yogurt	
2 tbsp butter	½ cup potato starch, not potato flour
2 tbsp sugar	
2 eggs	½ cup tapioca flour
1 tsp xanthan gum	¼ cup brown rice flour
½ tsp salt	
	1/3 cup sorghum flour

Directions:
With parchment paper, line an 8 x 8-inch baking pan and grease parchment paper. Preheat oven to 375oF. Mix xanthan gum, salt, baking soda, baking powder, all flours, and starch in a large bowl. Whisk well sugar and eggs in a medium bowl until creamed. Add vinegar, water, yogurt, and butter. Whisk thoroughly. Pour in egg mixture into bowl of flours and mix well. Transfer sticky dough into prepared pan and bake in the oven for 25 to 30 minutes. If tops of bread start to brown a lot, cover top with foil and continue baking until done. Remove from oven and pan right away and let it cool. Best served when warm.
Nutrition Info: Calories per Serving: 166; Carbs: 27.8g; Protein: 3.4g; Fat: 4.8g

936.	Mediterranean Sunset

Servings: 1   Cooking Time: 2 Minutes
Ingredients:

1 ounce ouzo, or more to taste	Orange juice or lemonade or grapefruit juice
1 tablespoon grenadine	

Directions:
Fill a highball glass with ice cubes. Add all of the ingredients into a shaker; shake to mix. Pour the concoction into the highball glass. Enjoy!
Nutrition Info: Per Serving:47 cal., 0 g total fat (0 g sat. fat), 0 mg chol., 1170 mg sodium, 7 mg pot., 12.4 g total carbs., 0 g fiber, 12.3 g sugar, 0 g protein, 0% vitamin A, 5% vitamin C, 0% calcium, and 0% iron.

937.	Creamy Panini

Servings: 4   Cooking Time: 16 Minutes
Ingredients:

1 jar of 7 oz roasted red peppers, drained and sliced	2 tbsp finely chopped oil-cured black olives
4 slices provolone cheese	¼ cup chopped fresh basil leaves
1 small zucchini, thinly sliced	½ cup Mayonnaise dressing with olive oil, divided
8 slices rustic whole grain bread	

Directions:
In a small bowl, mix together olives, basil and mayonnaise dressing. Spread the dressing evenly on 4 slices of whole grain bread. Then top it with zucchini, bacon, peppers and provolone before covering with another slice of bread. Spread the remaining mayonnaise mixture around the bread and cook over medium heat on a nonstick skillet for two minutes on each side or until bread is golden brown on both sides and cheese is melted.
Nutrition Info: Calories per Serving: 350; Carbs: 24.2g; Protein: 14.4g; Fat: 21.8g

938.	Tuna Melt Panini

Servings: 4   Cooking Time: 10 Minutes
Ingredients:

2 tbsp softened unsalted butter	½ tsp crushed red pepper
16 pcs of 1/8-inch kosher dill pickle	1 tbsp minced basil
8 pcs of ¼ inch thick cheddar or Swiss cheese	1 tbsp balsamic vinegar
	¼ cup extra virgin

Mayonnaise and Dijon mustard	olive oil
4 ciabatta rolls, split	¼ cup finely diced red onion
Pepper and salt	2 cans of 6oz albacore tuna

Directions:
Combine thoroughly the following in a bowl: salt pepper, crushed red pepper, basil, vinegar, olive oil, onion and tuna. Smear with mayonnaise and mustard the cut sides of the bread rolls then layer on: cheese, tuna salad and pickles. Cover with the remaining slice of roll. Grill in a Panini press ensuring that cheese is melted and bread is crisped and ridged.
Nutrition Info: Calories per Serving: 539; Carbs: 27.7g; Protein: 21.6g; Fat: 38.5g

939.	Spiced Breakfast Casserole

Servings: 6   Cooking Time: 35 Minutes
Ingredients:

1 tablespoon nutritional yeast	1 teaspoon coriander
¼ cup water	1 teaspoon cumin
6 large eggs	2 sausages, cooked and chopped
8 kale leaves, stems removed and torn into small pieces	1 large sweet potato, peeled and chopped

Directions:
Preheat the oven to 375oF. Grease an 8" x 8" baking pan with olive oil and set aside. Place sweet potatoes in a microwavable bowl and add ¼ cup water. Cook the chopped sweet potatoes in the microwave for three to five minutes. Drain the excess water then set aside. Fry in a skillet heated over medium flame the sausage and cook until brown. Mix in the kale and cook until wilted. Add the coriander, cumin and cooked sweet potatoes. In another bowl, mix together the eggs, water and nutritional yeast. Add the vegetable and meat mixture into the bowl and mix completely. Place the mixture in the baking dish and make sure that the mixture is evenly distributed within the pan. Bake for 20 minutes or until the eggs are done. Slice into squares.
Nutrition Info: Calories per serving: 137; Protein: 10.1g; Carbs: 10.0g; Fat: 6.6g

940.	Italian Scrambled Eggs

Servings: 1   Cooking Time: 7 Minutes
Ingredients:

1 teaspoon balsamic vinegar	2 large eggs
¼ teaspoon rosemary, minced	½ cup cherry tomatoes
	1 ½ cup kale, chopped
	½ teaspoon olive oil

Directions:
Melt the olive oil in a skillet over medium high heat. Sauté the kale and add rosemary and salt to taste. Add three tablespoons of water to prevent the kale from burning at the bottom of the pan. Cook for three to four minutes. Add the tomatoes and stir. Push the vegetables on one side of the skillet and add the eggs. Season with salt and pepper to taste. Scramble the eggs then fold in the tomatoes and kales.

Nutrition Info: Calories per serving: 230; Protein: 16.4g; Carbs: 15.0g; Fat: 12.4g

941. Simple And Easy Hummus

Servings: 4-5   Cooking Time: 5 Minutes

Ingredients:

1 can (15 ounce) chickpeas, drained and then rinsed
2 garlic cloves
3 tablespoons tahini

3 tablespoons olive oil
2 tablespoons lemon juice
1/2 teaspoon salt

Directions:

Put all the ingredients in a food processor or a blender; process or blend until the texture is pasty.

Nutrition Info: Per Serving:548 cal., 23 g total fat (3.1 g sat. fat), 0 mg chol., 331 mg sodium, 992 mg pot., 67.5 g total carbs., 19.6 g fiber, 11.6 g sugar, 22.6 g protein, 2% vitamin A, 14% vitamin C, 16% calcium, and 43% iron.

942. Grilled Mediterranean Vegetables

Servings: 8   Cooking Time: 25 Minutes

Ingredients:

6 zucchini and/or yellow squash sliced into 1/4-inch thick (about 2 1/2 pounds total),
2 cups couscous
2 bunches scallions, trimmed
1 quart cherry tomatoes (preferably on the vine)

1/2 cup olive oil
1 large eggplant, sliced into 1/4-inch thick (about 1 pound)
Kosher salt and black pepper
Spiced Chili Oil or store-bought harissa (North African chili sauce, found in the international aisle)

Directions:

Cook the couscous according to the directions on the package.   Meanwhile, preheat the grill to medium.   In a large-sized bowl, toss the squash, zucchini, tomatoes, eggplant, and scallions, with 1 teaspoon of salt, 1/2 teaspoon of pepper, and the olive oil.   Working in batches, grill the veggies, covered, occasionally turning, until tender. The squash and the eggplant will be done after about 4-6 minutes. The scallions and the tomatoes will be done after about 1-2 minutes.   Serve with the couscous and drizzle with the spiced chili oil.

Nutrition Info: Per Serving:347 cal.,15 g total fat (2 g sat. fat), 0 mg chol., 269mg sodium, 49 g total carbs., 7 g fiber, 10 g protein, 72 mg calcium, and 2 mg iron.

943. Roasted Mushroom Creamy Soup

Servings: 8   Cooking Time: 55 Minutes

Ingredients:

3 tablespoons olive oil
4 garlic cloves, chopped
1/2 teaspoon chili powder
1/2 teaspoon cumin powder

2 shallots, chopped
1 1/2 pounds mushrooms, halved
2 cups vegetable stock
1/2 cup heavy cream
Salt and pepper to taste

Directions:

Combine the oil, garlic, shallots, chili powder, cumin and mushrooms in a baking tray.   Cook in the preheated oven at 350F for 20 minutes. Transfer the mushrooms in a soup pot and stir in the stock, as well as salt and pepper.   Cook for 10 more minutes then add the cream and puree the soup with an immersion blender.   Serve the soup warm.

Nutrition Info: Per Serving:Calories:96 Fat:8.4g Protein:3.1g Carbohydrates:4.3g

944. Toasted Bagels

Servings: 6   Cooking Time: 10 Minutes

Ingredients:

6 teaspoons butter

3 bagels, halved

Directions:

Preheat the Airfryer to 375 degrees F and arrange the bagels into an Airfryer basket.   Cook for about 3 minutes and remove the bagels from Airfryer.   Spread butter evenly over bagels and cook for about 3 more minutes.

Nutrition Info: Calories: 169 Carbs: 26.5g Fats: 4.7g Proteins: 5.3g Sodium: 262mg Sugar: 2.7g

945. Greek Salad And Mediterranean Vinaigrette

Servings: 2-4   Cooking Time: 15 Minutes

Ingredients:

4 Persian cucumbers, sliced into rounds (or 1 English cucumber)
4 campari tomatoes, cut into wedges
2 tablespoons Vinaigrette

2 ounces feta cheese, crumbled
1/8 cup Kalamata olives
1/4 small red onion, thinly sliced
1 tablespoon capers

Directions:

Except for the vinaigrette, put all of the ingredients into a large-sized salad bowl.   Drizzle with the vinaigrette; toss to evenly coat. Serve.

Nutrition Info: Per Serving:148 cal.,8.1 g total fat (3.1 g sat. fat), 13 mg chol., 271 mg sodium, 751 mg pot., 17.3 g total carbs., 3.3 g fiber, 9.2 g sugar, 5.2 g protein,28% vitamin A, 43% vitamin C, 14% calcium, and 8% iron

946. Cream Of Asparagus Soup

Servings: 6   Cooking Time: 35 Minutes

Ingredients:

2 tablespoons olive oil
1 shallot, chopped
2 garlic cloves, chopped
2 bunches asparagus, trimmed and chopped

2 cups chicken stock
1 cup water
1 teaspoon lemon juice
Salt and pepper to taste
1/2 cup heavy cream

Directions:

Heat the oil in a soup pot and stir in the shallot and garlic. Cook for 2 minutes then add the asparagus, stock, water and lemon juice.   Adjust the taste with salt and pepper and cook for 10 minutes. When done, remove from heat and add the cream. Puree the soup with an immersion blender. Serve the soup warm.

Nutrition Info: Per Serving:Calories:90 Fat:8.6g Protein:1.5g Carbohydrates:2.9g

947. Eggplant Stew

Servings: 1 Cup   Cooking Time: 35 Minutes

Ingredients:

3 TB. extra-virgin

2 large potatoes,

olive oil
1 medium white onion, chopped
2 large carrots, sliced diagonally
4 medium Italian eggplant, trimmed and diced
1 large tomato, diced

peeled and diced
1 (16-oz.) can tomato sauce
1 tsp. garlic powder
1 tsp. paprika
11/2 tsp. salt
1 cup fresh cilantro, chopped

Directions:
In a 3-quart pot over medium heat, heat extra-virgin olive oil. Add white onion and carrots, and cook for 5 minutes. Add Italian eggplant and potatoes, and cook for 7 minutes. Add tomato, and cook for 3 minutes. Add tomato sauce, garlic powder, paprika, and salt, and simmer, stirring occasionally, for 15 minutes. Stir in cilantro, and cook for 5 more minutes. Serve with brown rice.

948. Mediterranean-style Spread

Servings: 14   Cooking Time: 5 Minutes
Ingredients:

1 container (4 ounces) crumbled feta cheese
1 package (8 ounces) cream cheese, softened

1/4 cup sour cream
2 teaspoons dried dill weed
2 teaspoons garlic powder

Directions:
Mix all the ingredients until well blended; cover and chill in the fridge for 30 minutes before serving.
Nutrition Info: Per Serving:88 cal., 8.2 g total fat (5.3 g sat. fat), 27 mg chol., 141 mg sodium, 39 mg pot., 1.3 g total carbs., 0 g fiber, 0 g sugar, 2.6 g protein, 6% vitamin A, 0% vitamin C, 6% calcium, and 2% iron.

949. St. Valentine's Mediterranean Pancakes

Servings: 2   Cooking Time: 20 Minutes
Ingredients:

4 eggs, preferably organic
2 pieces banana, peeled and then cut into small pieces
1 tablespoon milled flax seeds, preferably organic

1/2 teaspoon extra-virgin olive oil (for the pancake pan)
1 tablespoon bee pollen, milled, preferably organic

Directions:
Crack the eggs into a mixing bowl. Add in the banana, flax seeds, and bee pollen. With a hand mixer, blend the ingredients until smooth batter inn texture. Put a few drops of the olive oil in a nonstick pancake pan over medium flame or heat. Pour some batter into the pan; cook for about 2 minutes, undisturbed until the bottom of the pancake is golden and can be lifted easily from the pan. With a silicon spatula, lift and flip the pancake; cook for about 30seconds more and transfer into a plate. Repeat the process with the remaining batter, oiling the pan with every new batter. Serve the pancake as you cook or serve them all together topped with vanilla, strawberry, pine nuts jam.
Nutrition Info: Per Serving:272 cal.,11.6 g total fat (3 g sat. fat), 327 mg chol., 125 mg sodium, 633 mg pot., 32.7 g total carbs., 4.5 g fiber, 17.3 g sugar,

13.3 g protein, 10% vitamin A, 20% vitamin C, 6% calcium, and 12% iron.

950. Garlicky Roasted Sweet Potato Soup

Servings: 8   Cooking Time: 1 Hour
Ingredients:

3 tablespoons olive oil
4 sweet potatoes, peeled and cubed
1 teaspoon dried oregano
1 tablespoon balsamic vinegar

6 garlic cloves
3 cups vegetable stock
1 cup water
Salt and pepper to taste
1 thyme sprig

Directions:
Combine the potatoes, oil, oregano, vinegar and garlic in a baking tray. Season with salt and pepper and cook in the preheated oven at 350F for 25 minutes. Transfer the ingredients in a soup pot and add the remaining ingredients. Adjust the taste with salt and pepper. Cook on low heat for 10 minutes. When done, puree the soup with an immersion blender. Serve the soup warm.
Nutrition Info: Per Serving:Calories:140 Fat:5.4g Protein:1.5g Carbohydrates:22.1g

951. Sandwich With Hummus

Servings: 4   Cooking Time: 0 Minutes
Ingredients:

4 cups alfalfa sprouts
1 cup cucumber sliced 1/8 inch thick
4 red onion sliced 1/4-inch thick
8 tomatoes sliced 1/4-inch thick
2 cups shredded Bibb lettuce
12 slices 1-oz whole wheat bread

1 can 15.5-oz chickpeas, drained
2 garlic cloves, peeled
1/4 tsp salt
1/2 tsp ground cumin
1 tbsp tahini
1 tbsp lemon juice
2 tbsp water
3 tbsp plain fat free yogurt

Directions:
In a food processor, blend chickpeas, garlic, salt, cumin, tahini, lemon juice, water and yogurt until smooth to create hummus. On 1 slice of bread, spread 2 tbsp hummus, top with 1 onion slice, 2 tomato slices, 1/2 cup lettuce, another bread slice, 1 cup sprouts, 1/4 cup cucumber and cover with another bread slice. Repeat procedure for the rest of the ingredients.
Nutrition Info: Calories per Serving: 407; Carbs: 67.7g; Protein: 18.8 g; Fat: 6.8g

952. Spicy Tortilla Soup

Servings: 10   Cooking Time: 1 Hour
Ingredients:

3 tablespoons olive oil
1 sweet onion, chopped
2 garlic cloves, chopped
1/2 teaspoon cumin powder
1/2 teaspoon chili powder
1 celery stalk, sliced
2 carrots, grated
2 tablespoons tomato

1 can diced tomatoes
1 can kidney beans, drained
1 cup canned sweet corn, drained
4 cups vegetable stock
4 cups water
Salt and pepper to taste
1 avocado, peeled and sliced

paste

¼ cup chopped parsley
1 lime, juiced

Directions:
Heat the oil in a soup pot and stir in the onion, garlic, cumin powder, chili powder, celery and carrots. Cook for 5 minutes then add the rest of the ingredients, except the parsley, avocado and lime juice. Continue cooking the soup for 20-25 minutes then add the parsley and avocado slices, as well as lime juice. Serve the soup fresh.
Nutrition Info: Per Serving:Calories:174 Fat:8.6g Protein:5.8g Carbohydrates:21.1g

953. Apple And Ham Flatbread Pizza

Servings: 8   Cooking Time: 15 Minutes
Ingredients:
¾ cup almond flour
½ teaspoon sea salt
2 cups mozzarella cheese, shredded
2 tablespoons cream cheese
1/8 teaspoon dried thyme
4 ounces low carbohydrate ham, cut into chunks

½ small red onion, cut into thin slices
Salt and black pepper, to taste
1 cup Mexican blend cheese, grated
¼ medium apple, sliced
1/8 teaspoon dried thyme

Directions:
Preheat the oven to 425 degrees F and grease a 12-inch pizza pan. Boil water and steam cream cheese, mozzarella cheese, almond flour, thyme, and salt. When the cheese melts enough, knead for a few minutes to thoroughly mix dough. Make a ball out of the dough and arrange in the pizza pan. Poke holes all over the dough with a fork and transfer in the oven. Bake for about 8 minutes until golden brown and reset the oven setting to 350 degrees F. Sprinkle ¼ cup of the Mexican blend cheese over the flatbread and top with onions, apples, and ham. Cover with the remaining ¾ cup of the Mexican blend cheese and sprinkle with the thyme, salt, and black pepper. Bake for about 7 minutes until cheese is melted and crust is golden brown. Remove the flatbread from the oven and allow to cool before cutting. Slice into desired pieces and serve.
Nutrition Info: Calories: 179 Carbs: 5.3g Fats: 13.6g Proteins: 10.4g Sodium: 539mg Sugar: 2.1g

954. Mixed Greens And Ricotta Frittata

Servings: 8   Cooking Time: 35 Minutes
Ingredients:
1 tbsp pine nuts
1 clove garlic, chopped
¼ cup fresh mint leaves
¾ cup fresh parsley leaves
1 cup fresh basil leaves
8-oz part-skim ricotta
1 tbsp red-wine vinegar

½ + 1/8 tsp freshly ground black pepper, divided
½ tsp salt, divided
10 large eggs
1 lb chopped mixed greens
Pinch of red pepper flakes
1 medium red onion, finely diced
1/3 cup + 2 tbsp olive

oil, divided

Directions:
Preheat oven to 350ºF. On medium high fire, place a nonstick skillet and heat 1 tbsp oil. Sauté onions until soft and translucent, around 4 minutes. Add half of greens and pepper flakes and sauté until tender and crisp, around 5 minutes. Remove cooked greens and place in colander. Add remaining uncooked greens in skillet and sauté until tender and crisp, when done add to colander. Allow cooked veggies to cool enough to handle, then squeeze dry and place in a bowl. Whisk well ¼ tsp pepper, ¼ tsp salt, Parmesan and eggs in a large bowl. In bowl of cooked vegetables, add 1/8 tsp pepper, ricotta and vinegar. Mix thoroughly. Then pour into bowl of eggs and mix well. On medium fire, place same skillet used previously and heat 1 tbsp oil. Pour egg mixture and cook for 8 minutes or until sides are set. Turn off fire, place skillet inside oven and bake for 15 minutes or until middle of frittata is set. Meanwhile, make the pesto by processing pine nuts, garlic, mint, parsley and basil in a food processor until coarsely chopped. Add 1/3 cup oil and continue processing. Season with remaining pepper and salt. Process once again until thoroughly mixed. To serve, slice the frittata in 8 equal wedges and serve with a dollop of pesto.
Nutrition Info: Calories per serving: 280; Protein: 14g; Carbs: 8g; Fat: 21.3g

955. Halibut Sandwiches Mediterranean Style

Servings: 4   Cooking Time: 23 Minutes
Ingredients:
2 packed cups arugula or 2 oz.
Grated zest of 1 large lemon
1 tbsp capers, drained and mashed
2 tbsp fresh flat leaf parsley, chopped
¼ cup fresh basil, chopped
¼ cup sun dried tomatoes, chopped
¼ cup reduced fat mayonnaise

1 garlic clove, halved
1 pc of 14 oz ciabatta loaf bread with ends trimmed and split in half, horizontally
2 tbsp plus 1 tsp olive oil, divided
Kosher salt and freshly ground pepper
2 pcs or 6 oz halibut fillets, skinned
Cooking spray

Directions:
Heat oven to 450ºF. With cooking spray, coat a baking dish. Season halibut with a pinch of pepper and salt plus rub with a tsp of oil and place on baking dish. Then put in oven and bake until cooked or for ten to fifteen minutes. Remove from oven and let cool. Get a slice of bread and coat with olive oil the sliced portions. Put in oven and cook until golden, around six to eight minutes. Remove from heat and rub garlic on the bread. Combine the following in a medium bowl: lemon zest, capers, parsley, basil, sun dried tomatoes and mayonnaise. Then add the halibut, mashing with fork until flaked. Spread the mixture on one side of bread, add arugula and cover with the other bread half and serve.
Nutrition Info: Calories per Serving: 125; Carbs: 8.0g; Protein: 3.9g; Fat: 9.2g

956. Ayran A.k.a Tahn A.k.a Refreshing Yogurt Drink

Servings: 4   Cooking Time: 8 Minutes

Ingredients:

2 cups yogurt, good-quality

Salt, to taste

2 cups water

Ice

Directions:

Pour the yogurt into a pitcher. Add the salt; mix thoroughly using a large spoon until the yogurt becomes more liquefied. About 1/2 cup at a time, add in the water, stirring, to remove any lumps. Add water according to your desired texture, thick like a smoothie or silky smooth thin like milk. Add ice, mix well again, and pour into glasses. Serve.

Nutrition Info: Per Serving:87 cal., 1.5 g total fat (1.2 g sat. fat), 7 mg chol., 129 mg sodium, 288 mg pot., 8.6 g total carbs., 0 g fiber, 8.6 g sugar, 7 g protein, 1% vitamin A, 2% vitamin C, 23% calcium, and 1% iron.

957. Baked Mediterranean Halibut

Servings: 2   Cooking Time: 12 Minutes

Ingredients:

100 grams (3 1/2 ounces) watercress

142 ml double cream

2 pieces (175 grams or 6 ounce each) halibut steaks

2 tablespoons extra-virgin olive oil

25 g (1 ounce) parmesan cheese, grated

2 tablespoons lemon juice

25 grams (1 ounce) olives, pitted, chopped

25 grams (1 ounce) sundried tomatoes, chopped

Basil leaves, to garnish

Salt and black pepper, to season

Directions:

Preheat the oven to 190C or fan to 170C or gas to 6. Lightly grease a small-sized oven-safe dish. Season both sides of the halibut steaks with salt and pepper. Place the seasoned halibut steaks into the prepared dish.   Pour the cream over the fish and dot each halibut steak with the sundried tomatoes and the olive. Sprinkle with the parmesan cheese. Cook in the oven for about12 to 15 mnutes or until the fish flakes when you gently press them and the cheese is golden.   Mix the olive oil and the lemon juice; season with salt and pepper. Add the watercress; toss to coat.   Place the halibut steaks into serving plates, divide the watercress mixture between each serving, and if desired, garnish with the basil leaves.

Nutrition Info: Per Serving:7231 cal.,187.9 g total fat (39.9 g sat. fat), 2085 mg chol., 3930 mg sodium, 801 mg pot., 23.8 g total carbs., 13 g fiber, 8.9 g sugar, 7.7 g protein, 3% vitamin A, 30% vitamin C, 17% calcium, and 21% iron

958. Fig Relish Panini

Servings: 4   Cooking Time: 40 Minutes

Ingredients:

Grated parmesan cheese, for garnish

Olive oil

Fig relish (recipe follows)

Arugula

4 ciabatta slices

1 tsp dry mustard

Pinch of salt

1 tsp mustard seed

½ cup apple cider vinegar

Basil leaves

Toma cheese, grated or sliced

Sweet butter

½ cup sugar

½ lb. Mission figs, stemmed and peeled

Directions:

Create fig relish by mincing the figs. Then put in all ingredients, except for the dry mustard, in a small pot and simmer for 30 minutes until it becomes jam like. Season with dry mustard according to taste and let cool before refrigerating.   Spread sweet butter on two slices of ciabatta rolls and layer on the following: cheese, basil leaves, arugula and fig relish then cover with the remaining bread slice. Grill in a Panini press until cheese is melted and bread is crisped and ridged.

Nutrition Info: Calories per Serving: 264; Carbs: 55.1g; Protein: 6.0g; Fat: 4.2g

959. Santorini Sunrise

Servings: 1   Cooking Time: 5 Minutes

Ingredients:

2 1/4 cups vodka, unflavored, plus more

1 pink grapefruit, sliced

2 ounce Pink Grapefruit-infused Vodka

2 slices pink grapefruit, quartered (8 total pieces)

1 ounces Campari

2 teaspoons honey (or Greek honey, if available)

3 ounces freshly squeezed pink grapefruit juice

4 mint leaves, plus more for garnish

Directions:

For the grapefruit-infused vodka: Put the grapefruit in a sterilized 1-quart glass jar, stuffing them tight. Pour the vodka over the grapefruit. Add more vodka, if needed, to submerge the grapefruit completely. Seal the jar with a tight lit; let sit at room temperature for 3 days. After 3 days, strain the infused-vodka through a coffee filter into another sterilized glass jar; store with other spirits for up to 2 months.   For the cocktail: In a highball glass, muddle 7 pieces of the quartered grapefruit slices with the honey and mint leaves. Add ice until the glass is filled. Add the vodka, Campari, and grapefruit juice. Stir. Garnish with the remaining 1 grapefruit slice and mint leaves; serve.

Nutrition Info: Per Serving:284 cal., 0.6 g total fat (0 g sat. fat), 0 mg chol., 14 mg sodium, 606 mg pot., 38.3 g total carbs., 6.2 g fiber, 31.4 g sugar, 3.3 g protein, 89% vitamin A, 173% vitamin C, 12% calcium, and 31% iron.

960. Pink Lady Mediterranean Drink

Servings: 1   Cooking Time: 5 Minutes

Ingredients:

1 1/2 ounces London dry gin,

1 large egg white

1/2 ounce Cointreau

1/2 ounce freshly squeezed lemon juice

1/4 ounce Campari

1/4 ounce limoncello

3-4 lemon zest, thin strips, for garnish

Ice

Directions:

Except for the ice and garnish, combine all the ingredients in a cocktail shaker; shake well. Add the ice; shake again. Strain the drink into a chilled coupe. Garnish with the strips of lemon zest.

Nutrition Info:Per Serving:163 cal., 0.2 g total fat (0 g sat. fat), 0 mg chol., 39 mg sodium, 72 mg pot., 0.5 g total carbs., 0 g fiber, 0.5 g sugar, 3.7g protein, 0% vitamin A, 11% vitamin C, 1% calcium, and 0% iron.

961. Mediterranean Baba Ghanoush

Servings: 4   Cooking Time: 25 Minutes

Ingredients:

1 bulb garlic	1 tsp black pepper
1 red bell pepper, halved and seeded	2 eggplants, sliced lengthwise
1 tbsp chopped fresh basil	2 rounds of flatbread or pita
1 tbsp olive oil	Juice of 1 lemon

Directions:
Grease grill grate with cooking spray and preheat grill to medium high.   Slice tops of garlic bulb and wrap in foil. Place in the cooler portion of the grill and roast for at least 20 minutes.   Place bell pepper and eggplant slices on the hottest part of grill.   Grill for at least two to three minutes each side.   Once bulbs are done, peel off skins of roasted garlic and place peeled garlic into food processor.   Add olive oil, pepper, basil, lemon juice, grilled red bell pepper and grilled eggplant. Puree until smooth and transfer into a bowl. Grill bread at least 30 seconds per side to warm. Serve bread with the pureed dip and enjoy.
Nutrition Info: Calories per Serving: 213.6; Carbs: 36.3g; Protein: 6.3g; Fat: 4.8g

962. Red Beet Soup

Servings: 8   Cooking Time: 1 Hour

Ingredients:

2 tablespoons olive oil	1 parsnip, diced
2 leeks, sliced	1 cup diced tomatoes
1 celery stalk, sliced	2 cups shredded cabbage
2 carrots, diced	2 cups water
3 red beets, peeled and diced	1 bay leaf
4 cups vegetable stock	1 thyme sprig
	1 rosemary sprig
	Salt and pepper to taste

Directions:
Heat the oil in a soup pot and stir in the leeks, celery, carrots, parsnip and beets, as well as cabbage.   Cook for 5 minutes then add the rest of the ingredients and season with salt and pepper. Cook for 20-25 minutes.   Serve the soup warm or chilled.
Nutrition Info: Per Serving:Calories:91 Fat:3.8g Protein:1.9g Carbohydrates:13.9g

963. Egg Muffin Sandwich

Servings: 2   Cooking Time: 10 Minutes

Ingredients:

1 large egg, free-range or organic	2 tbsp water
1/4 cup almond flour (25 g / 0.9 oz)	pinch salt
	1 tbsp ghee
1/4 cup flax meal (38 g / 1.3 oz)	1 tsp Dijon mustard
1/4 cup grated cheddar cheese (28 g / 1 oz)	2 large eggs, free-range or organic
	2 slices cheddar cheese or other hard type cheese (56 g / 2 oz)
1/4 tsp baking soda	

2 tbsp heavy whipping cream or coconut milk	Optional: 1 cup greens (lettuce, kale, chard, spinach, watercress, etc.)
1 tbsp butter or 2 tbsp cream cheese for spreading	salt and pepper to taste

Directions:
Make the Muffin: In a small mixing bowl, mix well almond flour, flax meal, baking soda, and salt. Stir in water, cream, and eggs. Mix thoroughly.   Fold in cheese and evenly divide in two single-serve ramekins.   Pop in the microwave and cook for 75 seconds.   Make the filing: on medium the fire, place a small nonstick pan, heat ghee and cook the eggs to the desired doneness. Season with pepper and salt.   To make the muffin sandwiches, slice the muffins in half. Spread cream cheese on one side and mustard on the other side.   Add egg and greens. Top with the other half of sliced muffin. Serve and enjoy.
Nutrition Info: Calories per serving: 639; Protein: 26.5g; Carbs: 10.4g; Fat: 54.6g

964. Buffalo Chicken Crust Pizza

Servings: 6   Cooking Time: 25 Minutes

Ingredients:

1 cup whole milk mozzarella, shredded	1 large egg
	1/4 teaspoon salt
1 teaspoon dried oregano	1 stalk celery
2 tablespoons butter	3 tablespoons Franks Red Hot Original
1 pound chicken thighs, boneless and skinless	1 stalk green onion
	1 tablespoon sour cream
1/4 teaspoon black pepper	1 ounce bleu cheese, crumbled

Directions:
Preheat the oven to 400 degrees F and grease a baking dish.   Process chicken thighs in a food processor until smooth.   Transfer to a large bowl and add egg, 1/2 cup of shredded mozzarella, oregano, black pepper, and salt to form a dough. Spread the chicken dough in the baking dish and transfer in the oven   Bake for about 25 minutes and keep aside.   Meanwhile, heat butter and add celery, and cook for about 4 minutes.   Mix Franks Red Hot Original with the sour cream in a small bowl.   Spread the sauce mixture over the crust, layer with the cooked celery and remaining 1/2 cup of mozzarella and the bleu cheese.   Bake for another 10 minutes, until the cheese is melted
Nutrition Info: Calories: 172 Carbs: 1g Fats: 12.9g Proteins: 13.8g Sodium: 172mg Sugar: 0.2g

965. Muhammara Spread

Servings: 2 Tablespoons   Cooking Time: 30 Minutes

Ingredients:

2 large red bell peppers	3 TB. pomegranate molasses
11/2 cups walnuts	1 TB. paprika
1/4 cup plain breadcrumbs	1 tsp. cumin
1 TB. crushed red pepper flakes	1 tsp. salt
3 cloves garlic	1/2 tsp. ground black pepper
3 TB. lemon juice	2 TB. extra-virgin olive oil

Directions:

Preheat a grill top or a grill to medium heat. Place red bell peppers on the grill, and cook on all sides for about 20 minutes or until charred. Immediately place peppers on a plate, cover with plastic wrap, let cool for 10 minutes.   Preheat the oven to 450°F.   When peppers are cool enough to handle, peel off skin. (It's okay if it doesn't all come off.) Remove stalks and seeds.   Spread walnuts evenly on a baking sheet, and bake for 7 minutes or until they're lightly toasted. Be sure not to burn them.   In a food processor fitted with a chopping blade, blend roasted red bell peppers, toasted walnuts, breadcrumbs, crushed red pepper flakes, garlic, lemon juice, pomegranate molasses, paprika, cumin, salt, black pepper, and extra-virgin olive oil for 2 minutes or until well combined, intermittently scraping down the sides of the food processor bowl with a rubber spatula.   Serve cold or at room temperature.

966.   Mediterranean Bloody Mary

Servings: 2   Cooking Time: 5 Minutes
Ingredients:

4 teaspoons hot sauce	3 ounces vodka
2 teaspoons Worcestershire sauce	Cubed feta, for garnish
2 tablespoons red wine vinegar	Ice
12 ounces tomato juice	Pepperoncini, for garnish
1 teaspoon fresh oregano, chopped	Pitted Kalamata olives, for garnish

Directions:
Put the tomato juice, vodka, red wine vinegar, hot sauce, Worcestershire sauce, and oregano into a cocktail shaker; shake. Fill 2 pint glasses with ice. Pour the bloody Mary mixture into the glasses. Garnish with the olives, feta, and pepperoncini.
Nutrition Info: Per Serving:139 cal., 0.2 g total fat (0 g sat. fat), 0 mg chol., 770 mg sodium, 428 mg pot., 9 g total carbs., 1 g fiber, 7.3 g sugar, 1.4 g protein, 17% vitamin A, 64% vitamin C, 3% calcium, and 6% iron.

967.   Greek Bean Soup

Servings: 8   Cooking Time: 1 Hour
Ingredients:

3 tablespoons olive oil	1 cup diced tomatoes
2 sweet onions, chopped	½ teaspoon dried mint
2 garlic cloves, chopped	½ teaspoon dried oregano
2 celery stalks, sliced	½ teaspoon dried basil
2 carrots, diced	2 cups vegetable stock
1 can red beans, drained	4 cups water
	Salt and pepper to taste

Directions:
Heat the oil in a soup pot and stir in the onions. Cook for 5 minutes then add the garlic and cook for 1 more minute.   Add the rest of the ingredients and season with salt and pepper.   Cook for 20 minutes.   The soup is best served warm.
Nutrition Info: Per Serving:Calories:147 Fat:5.6g Protein:6.0g Carbohydrates:19.7g

968.   Quinoa Pizza Muffins

Servings: 4   Cooking Time: 30 Minutes
Ingredients:

1 cup uncooked quinoa	2 tsp garlic powder
2 large eggs	1/8 tsp salt
½ medium onion, diced	1 tsp crushed red peppers
1 cup diced bell pepper	½ cup roasted red pepper, chopped*
1 cup shredded mozzarella cheese	Pizza Sauce, about 1-2 cups
1 tbsp dried basil	
1 tbsp dried oregano	

Directions:
Preheat oven to 350°F.   Cook quinoa according to directions.   Combine all ingredients (except sauce) into bowl. Mix all ingredients well.   Scoop quinoa pizza mixture into muffin tin evenly. Makes 12 muffins.   Bake for 30 minutes until muffins turn golden in color and the edges are getting crispy.   Top with 1 or 2 tbsp pizza sauce and enjoy!
Nutrition Info: Calories per Serving: 303; Carbs: 41.3g; Protein: 21.0g; Fat: 6.1g

969.   Cod Potato Soup

Servings: 8   Cooking Time: 1 Hour
Ingredients:

2 tablespoons olive oil	1 cup diced tomatoes
2 shallots, chopped	1 bay leaf
1 celery stalk, sliced	1 thyme sprig
1 carrot, sliced	½ teaspoon dried marjoram
1 red bell pepper, cored and diced	2 cups chicken stock
2 garlic cloves, chopped	6 cups water
1 ½ pounds potatoes, peeled and cubed	Salt and pepper to taste
	4 cod fillets, cubed
	2 tablespoons lemon juice

Directions:
Heat the oil in a soup pot and stir in the shallots, celery, carrot, bell pepper and garlic.   Cook for 5 minutes then stir in the potatoes, tomatoes, bay leaf, thyme, marjoram, stock and water.   Season with salt and pepper and cook on low heat for 20 minutes.   Add the cod fillets and lemon juice and continue cooking for 5 additional minutes.   Serve the soup warm and fresh.
Nutrition Info: Per Serving:Calories:108 Fat:3.9g Protein:2.2g Carbohydrates:17.1g

970.   Eggless Spinach & Bacon Quiche

Servings: 8   Cooking Time: 20 Minutes
Ingredients:

1 cup fresh spinach, chopped	4 dashes Tabasco sauce
4 slices of bacon, cooked and chopped	1 cup Parmesan cheese, shredded
½ cup mozzarella cheese, shredded	Salt and freshly ground black pepper, to taste
4 tablespoons milk	

Directions:
Preheat the Airfryer to 325 degrees F and grease a baking dish.   Put all the ingredients in a bowl and mix well.   Transfer the mixture into prepared

196

baking dish and cook for about 8 minutes. Dish out and serve.

Nutrition Info: Calories: 72 Carbs: 0.9g Fats: 5.2g Proteins: 5.5g Sodium: 271mg Sugar: 0.4g

971.Pumpkin Pancakes

Servings: 8   Cooking Time: 20 Minutes

Ingredients:

2 squares puff pastry
6 tablespoons pumpkin filling
2 small eggs, beaten
¼ teaspoon cinnamon

Directions:

Preheat the Airfryer to 360 degrees F and roll out a square of puff pastry.   Layer it with pumpkin pie filling, leaving about ¼-inch space around the edges.   Cut it up into equal sized square pieces and cover the gaps with beaten egg.   Arrange the squares into a baking dish and cook for about 12 minutes.   Sprinkle some cinnamon and serve.

Nutrition Info: Calories: 51 Carbs: 5g Fats: 2.5g Proteins: 2.4g Sodium: 48mg Sugar: 0.5g

972.   Chicken Green Bean Soup

Servings: 8   Cooking Time: 45 Minutes

Ingredients:

3 tablespoons olive oil
2 chicken breasts, cubed
1 shallot, chopped
1 garlic clove, chopped
1 red bell pepper, cored and diced
1 celery stalk, diced
2 carrots, diced
1 pound green beans, sliced
3 cups vegetable stock
4 cups water
1 bay leaf
1 thyme sprig
1 can diced tomatoes
Salt and pepper to taste

Directions:

Heat the oil in a soup pot and stir in the chicken. Cook for 5 minutes then add the shallot, garlic, bell pepper, celery and carrots.   Cook for 5 more minutes then stir in the green beans, stock, water, bay leaf, thyme sprig and tomatoes.   Add salt and pepper and cook for 25 minutes.   Serve the soup warm and fresh.

Nutrition Info: Per Serving:Calories:149 Fat:8.1g Protein:11.9g Carbohydrates:8.2g

973.   Cauliflower Stew

Servings: 2 Cups   Cooking Time: 25 Minutes

Ingredients:

1/2 lb. ground beef
2 tsp. salt
1 tsp. black pepper
1 (16-oz.) can plain tomato sauce
1 (16-oz.) can crushed tomatoes
2 cups water
1 TB. fresh thyme
1 tsp. garlic powder
1/2 tsp. onion powder
4 cups cauliflower florets
2 large potatoes
2 large carrots, finely diced
1 (16-oz.) can chickpeas, rinsed and drained

Directions:

In a small bowl, combine beef, 1/2 teaspoon salt, and 1/2 teaspoon black pepper. Form mixture into 20 to 30 mini meatballs about 1 teaspoon each. In a large, 3-quart pot over medium heat, add meatballs. Cover and cook for 5 minutes.   Add tomato sauce, crushed tomatoes, water, thyme, garlic powder, onion powder, remaining 11/2

teaspoons salt, and remaining 1/2 teaspoon black pepper, and simmer for 5 minutes.   Stir in cauliflower, potatoes, carrots, and chickpeas, and simmer for 20 minutes.   Serve with brown rice.

974.   Mediterranean Lamb Kebabs

Servings: 4   Cooking Time: 40 Minutes

Ingredients:

2 tablespoons scallions, chopped
2 tablespoons extra-virgin olive oil
2 tablespoons of crème fraîche
12 large-sized shallots; peel, halved lengthwise, and then trim root ends but keep intact
1/2 teaspoon black pepper, freshly ground
1 pound ground lamb
1/3 cup of water
1 teaspoon freshly squeezed lemon juice
1 tablespoon parsley, flat-leaf, chopped
1 garlic clove, minced
1 1/4 teaspoons salt
1 1/2 teaspoons pomegranate molasses, divided
Warm pita bread, for serving

Directions:

Light an outdoor grill.   In medium-sized bowl, gently mix the ground lamb, garlic, crème fraîche, salt, and the pepper until combined.   With moistened hands, roll lamb mixture to form 16 balls.   Into 8 pieces 10-inch or less metal skewers, alternate skewer 3 halves shallots and 2 pieces lamb balls. Brush kebabs with olive oil. Place on the grill and cook over medium high heat for about 3 minutes, turning once, until the outside of the lamb balls and the shallots are browned but are not cooked all the way through.   Transfer the semi-cooked kebabs into very large-sized deep skillet, about 12-14 inches. Add water, the lemon juice, and 1 teaspoon pomegranate molasses to the water; bring the water mixture to a boil. When boiling, cover and gently simmer for about 30 minutes over low flame or heat or until the meatballs are cooked through and the shallots are very tender.   Uncover the skillet; increase heat to high. Add remaining 1/2 teaspoon pomegranate molasses. Continue cooking for 5 minutes more, basting the shallots and the meatballs occasionally until they are glazed.   Transfer kebabs into a serving platter. Drizzle with the remaining sauce from the skillet. Garnish with parsley and scallions. Serve with warmed pita bread.

Nutrition Info: Per Serving:379   cal.,16.9 g total fat (4.8 g sat. fat), 909 mg sodium, 105 mg chol., 665 mg pot., 21.3   g total carbs., 0.5 g fiber, 1.7 g sugar, 35.1   g protein, 17% vitamin A, 13% vitamin C, 7% calcium, and 23% iron

975.   Bbq Chicken Pizza

Servings: 4   Cooking Time: 30 Minutes

Ingredients:

Dairy Free Pizza Crust
6 tablespoons Parmesan cheese
6 large eggs
3 tablespoons psyllium husk powder
Salt and black pepper, to taste
1½ teaspoons Italian
Toppings
6 oz. rotisserie chicken, shredded
4 oz. cheddar cheese
1 tablespoon mayonnaise
4 tablespoons tomato sauce
4 tablespoons BBQ sauce

seasoning

Directions:
Preheat the oven to 400 degrees F and grease a baking dish. Place all Pizza Crust ingredients in an immersion blender and blend until smooth. Spread dough mixture onto the baking dish and transfer in the oven. Bake for about 10 minutes and top with favorite toppings. Bake for about 3 minutes and dish out.

Nutrition Info: Calories: 356 Carbs: 2.9g Fats: 24.5g Proteins: 24.5g Sodium: 396mg Sugar: 0.6g

976.   Mushroom, Spinach And Turmeric Frittata

Servings: 6   Cooking Time: 35 Minutes

Ingredients:

½ tsp pepper	1 lb fresh spinach
½ tsp salt	6 cloves freshly
1 tsp turmeric	chopped garlic
5-oz firm tofu	1 large onion,
4 large eggs	chopped
6 large egg whites	1 lb button
¼ cup water	mushrooms, sliced

Directions:
Grease a 10-inch nonstick and oven proof skillet and preheat oven to 3500F. Place skillet on medium high fire and add mushrooms. Cook until golden brown. Add onions, cook for 3 minutes or until onions are tender. Add garlic, sauté for 30 seconds. Add water and spinach, cook while covered until spinach is wilted, around 2 minutes. Remove lid and continue cooking until water is fully evaporated. In a blender, puree pepper, salt, turmeric, tofu, eggs and egg whites until smooth. Pour into skillet once liquid is fully evaporated. Pop skillet into oven and bake until the center is set around 25-30 minutes. Remove skillet from oven and let it stand for ten minutes before inverting and transferring to a serving plate. Cut into 6 equal wedges, serve and enjoy.

Nutrition Info: Calories per serving: 166; Protein: 15.9g; Carbs: 12.2g; Fat: 6.0g

977.   Breakfast Egg On Avocado

Servings: 6   Cooking Time: 15 Minutes

Ingredients:

1 tsp garlic powder	1/4 tsp black pepper
1/2 tsp sea salt	3 medium avocados
1/4 cup Parmesan cheese (grated or shredded)	(cut in half, pitted, skin on)
	6 medium eggs

Directions:
Prepare muffin tins and preheat the oven to 3500F. To ensure that the egg would fit inside the cavity of the avocado, lightly scrape off 1/3 of the meat. Place avocado on muffin tin to ensure that it faces with the top up. Evenly season each avocado with pepper, salt, and garlic powder. Add one egg on each avocado cavity and garnish tops with cheese. Pop in the oven and bake until the egg white is set, about 15 minutes. Serve and enjoy.

Nutrition Info: Calories per serving: 252; Protein: 14.0g; Carbs: 4.0g; Fat: 20.0g

978.   Fresh Bell Pepper Basil Pizza

Servings: 3   Cooking Time: 25 Minutes

Ingredients:

Pizza Base	
2 tablespoons cream	½ cup almond flour
cheese	1 large egg
1 teaspoon Italian seasoning	½ teaspoon salt
½ teaspoon black pepper	Toppings
6 ounces mozzarella cheese	4 ounces cheddar cheese, shredded
2 tablespoons psyllium husk	¼ cup Marinara sauce
2 tablespoons fresh Parmesan cheese	2/3 medium bell pepper
	1 medium vine tomato
	3 tablespoons basil, fresh chopped

Directions:
Preheat the oven to 400 degrees F and grease a baking dish. Microwave mozzarella cheese for about 30 seconds and top with the remaining pizza crust. Add the remaining pizza ingredients to the cheese and mix together. Flatten the dough and transfer in the oven. Bake for about 10 minutes and remove pizza from the oven. Top the pizza with the toppings and bake for another 10 minutes. Remove pizza from the oven and allow to cool.

Nutrition Info: Calories: 411 Carbs: 6.4g Fats: 31.3g Proteins: 22.2g Sodium: 152mg Sugar: 2.8g

979.   Spicy Silan A.k.a Date Syrup

Servings: 10   Cooking Time: 5 Minutes

Ingredients:

1 cup silan (date honey)	1 teaspoon salt
1 teaspoon hot Spanish paprika	1/2 teaspoon black pepper
1 teaspoon parsley flakes	1 tablespoon garlic powder

Directions:
Simply mix the date honey with 1-2 teaspoons of the grilling sauce.

Nutrition Info: Per Serving:107 cal., 0 g total fat (0 g sat. fat), 0 mg chol., 234 mg sodium, 34 mg pot., 28.7 g total carbs., 0 g fiber, 28.1 g sugar, 0.3 g protein, 2% vitamin A, 1% vitamin C, 0% calcium, and1% iron.

980.   White Bean Kale Soup

Servings: 8   Cooking Time: 1 Hour

Ingredients:

2 tablespoons olive oil	2 tablespoons lemon juice
1 shallot, chopped	1 can diced tomatoes
2 garlic cloves, chopped	2 cups vegetable stock
1 red pepper, chopped	6 cups water
1 celery stalk, diced	Salt and pepper to taste
2 carrots, diced	1 bunch kale, shredded
1 can white beans, drained	

Directions:
Heat the oil in a soup pot and stir in the shallot, garlic, red pepper, celery and carrots. Cook for 2 minutes until softened. Add the rest of the ingredients and season with salt and pepper. Cook on low heat for 30 minutes. Serve the soup warm or chilled.

Nutrition Info: Per Serving:Calories:136 Fat:3.8g Protein:6.8g Carbohydrates:19.8g

981. White Wine Fish Soup

Servings: 8   Cooking Time: 50 Minutes

Ingredients:

3 tablespoons olive oil
2 shallots, chopped
2 garlic cloves, chopped
1 celery stalk, sliced
2 red bell peppers, cored and sliced
2 carrots, sliced
2 tomatoes, sliced
1 cup diced tomatoes
½ cup tomato juice

2 cups chicken stock
2 cups water
1 cup dry white wine
2 cod fillets, cubed
2 flounder fillets, cubed
1 pound fresh mussels, cleaned and rinsed
1 bay leaf
1 thyme sprig
Salt and pepper to taste

Directions:

Heat the oil in a soup pot and stir in the shallots, garlic, celery, bell peppers and carrots.   Cook for 10 minutes then add the tomatoes and tomato juice, as well as stock, water and wine.   Cook for 15 minutes then add the cod, flounder and fresh mussels, as well as the bay leaf and thyme. Adjust the taste with salt and pepper and cook for another 5 minutes.   Serve the soup warm and fresh.

Nutrition Info: Per Serving: Calories:190 Fat:7.4g Protein:15.8g Carbohydrates:10.0g

982. Chicken Soup

Servings: 2 Cups   Cooking Time: 1 Hour 10 Minutes

Ingredients:

1 (3-lb.) whole chicken
3 bay leaves
5 whole allspice
1 (2-in.) cinnamon stick
1/2 medium yellow onion, sliced
11/2 tsp. salt
10 cups water
5 medium carrots, chopped

3 medium stalks celery, chopped
5 TB. extra-virgin olive oil
1/2 medium yellow onion, chopped
1 cup vermicelli noodles
1 large potato, peeled and diced
1/2 cup fresh parsley, chopped

Directions:

In a large pot over high heat, combine chicken, bay leaves, allspice, cinnamon stick, sliced yellow onion, 1 teaspoon salt, and water. Bring to a boil, reduce heat to medium-low, and simmer for 40 minutes, skimming any foam that rises to the top. Remove chicken from the pot, and set aside to cool enough to handle. Pick chicken apart, removing skin and bones, and cut into bite-size pieces. Strain broth, discard solids, and return broth and boneless chicken pieces to the pot over medium-low heat.   Add carrots and celery, and cook for 10 minutes.   In a small saucepan over medium heat, heat 3 tablespoons extra-virgin olive oil. Add chopped yellow onion, and sauté for 5 minutes. Add to the pot.   In the same small saucepan over medium heat, heat remaining 2 tablespoons extra-virgin olive oil. Add vermicelli noodles, and cook, stirring to brown evenly, for 3 minutes.   Add toasted vermicelli noodles and diced potato to the pot, and cook for 10 minutes. Add parsley, remove from heat, and serve.

983. Avocado And Turkey Mix Panini

Servings: 2   Cooking Time: 8 Minutes

Ingredients:

2 red peppers, roasted and sliced into strips
¼ lb. thinly sliced mesquite smoked turkey breast
2 slices provolone cheese

1 cup whole fresh spinach leaves, divided
1 tbsp olive oil, divided
2 ciabatta rolls
¼ cup mayonnaise
½ ripe avocado

Directions:

In a bowl, mash thoroughly together mayonnaise and avocado. Then preheat Panini press.   Slice the bread rolls in half and spread olive oil on the insides of the bread. Then fill it with filling, layering them as you go: provolone, turkey breast, roasted red pepper, spinach leaves and spread avocado mixture and cover with the other bread slice.   Place sandwich in the Panini press and grill for 5 to 8 minutes until cheese has melted and bread is crisped and ridged.

Nutrition Info: Calories per Serving: 546; Carbs: 31.9g; Protein: 27.8g; Fat: 34.8g

984. Breakfast Egg-artichoke Casserole

Servings: 8   Cooking Time: 35 Minutes

Ingredients:

16 large eggs
14 ounce can artichoke hearts, drained
10-ounce box frozen chopped spinach, thawed and drained well
1 cup shredded white cheddar
1 garlic clove, minced

1 teaspoon salt
1/2 cup parmesan cheese
1/2 cup ricotta cheese
1/2 teaspoon dried thyme
1/2 teaspoon crushed red pepper
1/4 cup milk
1/4 cup shaved onion

Directions:

Lightly grease a 9x13-inch baking dish with cooking spray and preheat the oven to 3500F.   In a large mixing bowl, add eggs and milk. Mix thoroughly. With a paper towel, squeeze out the excess moisture from the spinach leaves and add to the bowl of eggs.   Into small pieces, break the artichoke hearts and separate the leaves. Add to the bowl of eggs.   Except for the ricotta cheese, add remaining ingredients in the bowl of eggs and mix thoroughly.   Pour egg mixture into the prepared dish.   Evenly add dollops of ricotta cheese on top of the eggs and then pop in the oven.   Bake until eggs are set and doesn't jiggle when shook, about 35 minutes.   Remove from the oven and evenly divide into suggested servings. Enjoy.

Nutrition Info: Calories per serving: 302; Protein: 22.6g; Carbs: 10.8g; Fat: 18.7g

985. Hearty Brown Lentil Soup

Servings: 2 Cups   Cooking Time: 1 Hour 20 Minutes

Ingredients:

2 cups brown lentils, picked over and rinsed

3 TB. extra-virgin olive oil
1 medium yellow

14 cups water
2 tsp. salt
1/4 cup long-grain rice
1/2 lb. lean ground beef
1 tsp. ground black pepper

onion, chopped
1 TB. cumin
1/2 cup fresh parsley, chopped
2 medium potatoes, peeled and medium diced

Directions:
In a large pot over medium-low heat, combine brown lentils, water, and 1 teaspoon salt. Bring to a simmer, and cook, stirring occasionally, for 1 hour. Remove the pot from heat. Using a handheld immersion blender or in a food processor fitted with a chopping blade, blend lentils for 1 or 2 minutes or until smooth. If desired, strain soup to remove any pulp from lentil skins. Set the pot over low heat, add long-grain rice, and cook, stirring occasionally to stop rice from clumping, for 10 minutes. In a small bowl, combine ground beef, 1/2 teaspoon salt, and 1/2 teaspoon black pepper. Form mixture into about 20 to 30 (1/2-inch) meatballs. In a small skillet over medium heat, cook meatballs for 6 minutes, turning over every 2 minutes until browned on all sides. Add cooked meatballs to soup. In the small skillet, heat extra-virgin olive oil. Add yellow onion, and sauté for 5 minutes. Add onion to soup. Add remaining 1/2 teaspoon salt, remaining 1/2 teaspoon black pepper, cumin, parsley, and potatoes to soup, and stir to combine. Cook for 5 minutes. Remove from heat, and serve.

986.   Thin Crust Low Carb Pizza

Servings: 6   Cooking Time: 25 Minutes
Ingredients:
2 tablespoons tomato sauce
1/8 teaspoon black pepper
1/8 teaspoon chili flakes
1 piece low-carb pita bread
2 ounces low-moisture mozzarella cheese

1/8 teaspoon garlic powder
Bacon, roasted red peppers, spinach, olives, pesto, artichokes, salami, pepperoni, roast beef, prosciutto, avocado, ham, chili paste, Sriracha

Directions:
Preheat the oven to 450 degrees F and grease a baking dish. Mix together tomato sauce, black pepper, chili flakes, and garlic powder in a bowl and keep aside. Place the low-carb pita bread in the oven and bake for about 2 minutes. Remove from oven and spread the tomato sauce on it. Add mozzarella cheese and top with your favorite toppings. Bake again for 3 minutes and dish out.
Nutrition Info: Calories: 254 Carbs: 12.9g Fats: 16g Proteins: 19.3g Sodium: 255mg Sugar: 2.8g

987.   Cheesy Vegetable Soup

Servings: 8   Cooking Time: 1 Hour
Ingredients:
2 tablespoons olive oil
2 garlic cloves, chopped
2 shallots, chopped
2 carrots, diced
1 celery stalk,

1 cup diced tomatoes
2 cups vegetable stock
6 cups water
1/2 teaspoon dried basil

chopped
2 red bell peppers, cored and diced
1 zucchini, cubed
1 red pepper, sliced

1/2 teaspoon dried oregano
Salt and pepper to taste
4 oz. grated Cheddar cheese

Directions:
Heat the oil in a soup pot and stir in the garlic, shallots, carrots and celery. Cook for 5 minutes then add the bell pepper, zucchini, red pepper, tomatoes, stock and water. Season with salt and pepper, as well as basil and oregano and cook for 20 minutes on low heat. When done, pour into serving bowls and top with cheese. Serve the soup warm and fresh.
Nutrition Info: Per Serving:Calories:120 Fat:8.5g Protein:4.8g Carbohydrates:7.1g

988.   Garlic-rosemary Dinner Rolls

Servings: 8   Cooking Time: 20 Minutes
Ingredients:
2 garlic cloves, minced
1 tsp dried crushed rosemary
1/2 tsp apple cider vinegar
2 tbsp olive oil
2 eggs
1 1/4 tsp salt

1 3/4 tsp xanthan gum
1/2 cup tapioca starch
3/4 cup brown rice flour
1 cup sorghum flour
2 tsp dry active yeast
1 tbsp honey
3/4 cup hot water

Directions:
Mix well water and honey in a small bowl and add yeast. Leave it for exactly 7 minutes. In a large bowl, mix the following with a paddle mixer: garlic, rosemary, salt, xanthan gum, sorghum flour, tapioca starch, and brown rice flour. In a medium bowl, whisk well vinegar, olive oil, and eggs. Into bowl of dry ingredients pour in vinegar and yeast mixture and mix well. Grease a 12-muffin tin with cooking spray. Transfer dough evenly into 12 muffin tins and leave it 20 minutes to rise. Then preheat oven to 375oF and bake dinner rolls until tops are golden brown, around 17 to 19 minutes. Remove dinner rolls from oven and muffin tins immediately and let it cool. Best served when warm.
Nutrition Info: Calories per Serving: 200; Carbs: 34.3g; Protein: 4.2g; Fat: 5.4g

989.   Tomato-bacon Quiche

Servings: 6   Cooking Time: 47 Minutes
Ingredients:
2 small medium sized tomatoes, sliced
1/4 tsp black pepper
1/4 tsp salt
1/2 cup fresh spinach, chopped
2/4 cups cauliflower, ground into rice
5 slices nitrate free bacon, cooked and chopped
3 tbsp unsweetened plain almond milk

1/4 tsp ground mustard
1/2 cup organic white eggs
5 eggs, beaten
1/8 tsp sea salt
1 tbsp butter
1 tsp flax meal
1 1/2 tbsp coconut flour
1 egg, beaten
2 small to medium sized organic

zucchini, grated

Directions:
Grease a pie dish and preheat oven to 400oF. Grate zucchini, drain and squeeze dry. In a bowl, add dry zucchini and remaining crust ingredients and mix well. Place in bottom of pie plate and press down as if making a pie crust. Pop in the oven and bake for 9 minutes. Meanwhile in a large mixing bowl, whisk well black pepper, salt, mustard, almond milk, egg whites, and egg. Add bacon, spinach, and cauliflower rice. Mix well. Pour into baked zucchini crust, top with tomato slices. Pop back in the oven and bake for 28 minutes. If at 20 minutes baking time top is browning too much, cover with parchment paper for remainder of cooking time. Once done cooking, remove from oven, let it stand for at least ten minutes. Slice into equal triangles, serve and enjoy.
Nutrition Info: Calories per serving: 154; Protein: 11.6g; Carbs: 3.4g; Fat: 10.3g

990. Dill, Havarti & Asparagus Frittata

Servings: 4   Cooking Time: 20 Minutes
Ingredients:

1 tsp dried dill weed or 2 tsp minced fresh dill	6 eggs, beaten well
	3 tsp. olive oil
4-oz Havarti cheese cut into small cubes	2/3 cup diced cherry tomatoes
Pepper and salt to taste	6-8 oz fresh asparagus, ends trimmed and cut into
1 stalk green onions sliced for garnish	1 ½-inch lengths

Directions:
On medium-high the fire, place a large cast-iron pan and add oil. Once oil is hot, stir-fry asparagus for 4 minutes. Add dill weed and tomatoes. Cook for two minutes. Meanwhile, season eggs with pepper and salt. Beat well. Pour eggs over the tomatoes. Evenly spread cheese on top. Preheat broiler. Lower the fire to low, cover pan, and let it cook for 10 minutes until the cheese on top has melted. Turn off the fire and transfer pan in the oven and broil for 2 minutes or until tops are browned. Remove from the oven, sprinkle sliced green onions, serve, and enjoy.
Nutrition Info: Calories per serving: 244; Protein: 16.0g; Carbs: 3.7g; Fat: 18.3g

991. Fattoush Salad –middle East Bread Salad

Servings: 6   Cooking Time: 15 Minutes
Ingredients:

2 loaves pita bread	5 Roma tomatoes, chopped
1 tbsp Extra Virgin Olive Oil	
1/2 tsp sumac, more for later	2 cups chopped fresh parsley leaves, stems removed
Salt and pepper	1 cup chopped fresh mint leaves
1 heart of Romaine lettuce, chopped	
1 English cucumber, chopped	1 1/2 lime, juice of
	1/3 cup Extra Virgin Olive Oil
5 green onions (both white and green parts), chopped	Salt and pepper
	1 tsp ground sumac
5 radishes, stems removed, thinly	1/4 tsp ground cinnamon
	scant 1/4 tsp ground

sliced   allspice

Directions:
For 5 minutes toast the pita bread in the toaster oven. And then break the pita bread into pieces. In a large pan on medium fire, heat 3 tbsp of olive oil in for 3 minutes. Add pita bread and fry until browned, around 4 minutes while tossing around. Add salt, pepper and 1/2 tsp of sumac. Remove the pita chips from the heat and place on paper towels to drain. Toss well the chopped lettuce, cucumber, tomatoes, green onions, sliced radish, mint leaves and parsley in a large salad bowl. To make the lime vinaigrette, whisk together all ingredients in a small bowl. Drizzle over salad and toss well to coat. Mix in the pita bread. Serve and enjoy.
Nutrition Info: Calories per Serving: 192; Carbs: 16.1g; Protein: 3.9g; Fats: 13.8g

992. Fried Caprese Pistachio Bites

Servings: 10   Cooking Time: 1 Minutes
Ingredients:

20 pieces bocconcini cheese	1/3 cup pistachios, crushed
2 tablespoons of protein packed nut free hemp basil pesto (or store bought)	1/2 cup of all-purpose flour (for gluten free use rice flour)
	1 pint of grape tomatoes
2 Tablespoons of Balsamic Vinegar	Baby mini mushrooms, optional
1/3 cup panko breadcrumbs (or gluten free breadcrumbs, rice cereal)	Fresh minced basil for sprinkling
	2 pinches salt, divided
1/2 of an egg	

Directions:
Line a tray with wax paper or parchment paper. Put the bocconcini in the tray and cover with a plastic wrap; freeze for at least 6 hours or overnight or until the cheeses are completely hard. Put the flour in a bowl. In another bowl, add the pesto, egg, vinegar, and a pinch of salt. In another bowl, mix the pistachio with the breadcrumbs. Preheat an electric fryer or fill a small pot with oil half full until the heat is 375F. Dredge each bocconcini cheese in the flour, shaking off any excess. Drop into the basil pesto mix, rolling it well to coat. Finally, roll in the bowl with pistachio, making sure the entire surface is covered with the coating well. Put the coated balls on a plate mined with wax paper. Repeat the process with the rest of the cheese balls and the coatings. If you want some fried mushrooms, follow the process to coat them. Fry the coated bocconcini and, if adding, the mushrooms for about1 minute and, if needed, 30 seconds more, depending the temperature of your oil or how crowded the pot is. Drain each on paper towels and sprinkle with a pinch of salt.
Nutrition Info: Per Serving:105 cal., 7.3 g total fat (3.1 g sat. fat), 22 mg chol., 182.7 mg sodium, 3.9 g total carbs., 0.5 g fiber, 0.9 g sugar, 6.1 g protein, 6% vitamin A, 4% vitamin C, 13% calcium, and 3% iron.

993. Cream Of Artichoke Soup

Servings: 6   Cooking Time: 45 Minutes
Ingredients:

2 tablespoons olive	2 shallots, chopped

oil
2 garlic cloves, chopped
1 jar artichoke hearts, chopped
2 pears, peeled and cubed

2 cups vegetable stock
1 cup water
Salt and pepper to taste
¼ cup heavy cream

Directions:
Heat the oil in a soup pot and stir in the shallots and garlic. Cook for 2 minutes until softened. Add the artichoke hearts, pears, stock and water, as well as salt and pepper. Cook for 15 minutes then remove from heat and stir in the cream. Puree the soup with an immersion blender and serve the soup fresh.
Nutrition Info: Per Serving:Calories:116 Fat:6.7g Protein:1.5g Carbohydrates:14.8g

---

994. Tuscan Cabbage Soup

Servings: 8   Cooking Time: 1 Hour
Ingredients:
2 tablespoons olive oil
2 sweet onions, chopped
2 carrots, grated
1 celery stalk, chopped
1 can diced tomatoes
1 cabbage, shredded

2 cups vegetable stock
2 cups water
1 lemon, juiced
1 thyme sprig
1 oregano sprig
1 basil sprig
Salt and pepper to taste

Directions:
Heat the oil in a soup pot and stir in the onions, carrots and celery. Cook for 5 minutes then stir in the rest of the ingredients. Season with salt and pepper to taste and cook on low heat for 25 minutes. Serve the soup warm.
Nutrition Info: Per Serving:Calories:58 Fat:3.6g Protein:1.0g Carbohydrates:6.6g

---

995. Smoky Sausage Soup

Servings: 8   Cooking Time: 45 Minutes
Ingredients:
2 tablespoons olive oil
2 smoked chicken sausages, sliced
2 fresh chicken sausages, sliced
2 carrots, sliced
1 sweet onion, chopped
1 celery stalk, sliced

1 can diced tomatoes
½ cup short pasta
2 cups vegetable stock
4 cups water
Salt and pepper to taste
2 tablespoons chopped parsley
2 tablespoons chopped cilantro

Directions:
Heat the oil in a soup pot and stir in the sausages. Cook for 5 minutes then add the carrots, sweet onion, celery and tomatoes and continue cooking for another 5 minutes. Add the stock, pasta, water, salt and pepper and cook for 20 minutes. When done, stir in the parsley and cilantro and serve the soup warm and fresh.
Nutrition Info: Per Serving:Calories:48 Fat:3.6g Protein:0.6g Carbohydrates:4.0g

---

996. Cucumber Yogurt Gazpacho

Servings: 6   Cooking Time: 20 Minutes
Ingredients:
4 cucumbers,

2 tablespoons cream

partially peeled
1 cup seedless white grapes
2 tablespoon sliced almonds
1 cup ice cubes
2 garlic cloves
1 tablespoon chopped dill

cheese
½ cup plain yogurt
2 tablespoons extra virgin olive oil
Salt and pepper to taste
1 tablespoon lemon juice

Directions:
Combine the cucumbers with the rest of the ingredients in a blender. Add salt and pepper and pulse until smooth and creamy. Serve the gazpacho as fresh as possible.
Nutrition Info: Per Serving:Calories:111 Fat:7.3g Protein:3.3g Carbohydrates:9.9g

---

997. Turkish Chicken Skewers

Servings: 4   Cooking Time: 12 Minutes
Ingredients:
2 pounds chicken breasts, boneless skinless, cut into 1 inch cubes
2 tablespoons sumac spice, for sprinkling
2 lemons, thinly sliced, for skewering
For the marinade:
5 cloves garlic
2 roma tomatoes
2 tablespoons olive oil

1 lemon, juiced
1/4 cup yogurt (low fat, full, or fat free)
1/4 cup total fresh cilantro and parsley leaves
1/2 teaspoon salt
1/2 teaspoon pepper
1/2 teaspoon allspice
1 teaspoon oregano
1 teaspoon cinnamon

Directions:
Preheat the oven to 375F or a grill to medium high heat. Put the marinade ingredients into a food processor; pulse until smooth. Toss the chicken with the marinade. Thread the chicken cubes in skewers, alternating with a thin slice of lemon between chicken cubes. Grill the skewers for about 3-5 minutes per side, covered. When cooked, sprinkle the skewers with generously with the sumac. Serve with plenty of Aryan.
Nutrition Info: Per Serving:303 cal., 11.1 g total fat (2.1 g sat. fat), 134 mg chol., 247.5 mg sodium, 8 g total carbs., 2.5 g fiber, 2.4 g sugar, 42.5 g protein, 9% vitamin A, 48% vitamin C, 6% calcium, and 9% iron.

---

998. Creamy Roasted Vegetable Soup

Servings: 8   Cooking Time: 45 Minutes
Ingredients:
2 red onions, sliced
1 zucchini, sliced
2 tomatoes, sliced
2 potatoes, sliced
2 garlic cloves
2 tablespoons olive oil
1 teaspoon dried basil

1 teaspoon dried oregano
4 cups vegetable stock
8 cups water
Salt and pepper to taste
1 bay leaf
1 thyme sprig

Directions:
Combine the onions, zucchini, tomatoes, potatoes, garlic, oil, basil and oregano in a deep dish baking pan. Season with salt and pepper and cook in the preheated oven at 400F for 30 minutes or until golden brown. Transfer the vegetables in a soup pot and add the stock and water. Stir in the bay

leaf and thyme sprig and cook for 15 minutes. When done, remove the thyme and bay leaf and puree the soup with an immersion blender. Serve the soup warm and fresh.

Nutrition Info: Per Serving:Calories:92 Fat:3.8g Protein:2.0g Carbohydrates:13.9g

999. Green Pea Stew (bazella)

Servings: 1 Cup   Cooking Time: 43 Minutes
Ingredients:

1/2 lb. ground beef
3 TB. extra-virgin olive oil
1 large yellow onion, finely chopped
2 TB. garlic, minced
2 cups fresh or frozen green peas
2 large carrots, diced (1 cup)
1 (16-oz.) can plain tomato sauce
2 cups water
11/2 tsp. salt
1 tsp. ground black pepper
1/2 cup fresh Italian parsley, finely chopped

Directions:

In a 3-quart pot over medium heat, brown beef for 5 minutes, breaking up chunks with a wooden spoon.   Add extra-virgin olive oil, yellow onion, and garlic, and cook for 5 minutes.   Add peas and carrots, and cook for 3 minutes.   Add tomato sauce, water, salt, and black pepper, and simmer for 25 minutes.   Stir in Italian parsley, and simmer for 5 more minutes.   Serve warm with brown rice.

1000. Pistachio Oil Drizzled Robiola, And Pickled Fig Crostini

Servings: 12   Cooking Time: 15 Minutes
Ingredients:

6 dried figs
2 tablespoons sugar
2 tablespoons pistachios, toasted and shelled
12 slices ciabatta bread
1/4 cup extra-virgin olive oil
1/2 cup red wine vinegar
1/4 cup water
Robiola cheese, at room temperature

Directions:

In a saucepan, combine the sugar, red wine vinegar, dried figs, and water; bring the mixture to a simmer. When simmering, remove from the heat; let sit for about 30 minutes or until the figs are soft. When the figs are soft, cut the figs into halves in a lengthwise manner. Alternatively, you can use 6 pieces fresh figs halve d lengthwise.   Crush the pistachios into fine pieces and then combine with the olive oil.   Grill the slices of ciabatta bread. Spread the cheese over the warm toasted bread slices. Top with each with a fig half and then drizzle with the pistachio oil.

Nutrition Info: Per Serving:132.8 cal., 5.8 g total fat (1 g sat. fat), 120.7 mg sodium, , 1.2 mg chol., 18.44 g total carbs., 1 g fiber, 4.7 g sugar, and 2.8 g protein.

30-Day Meal Plan

Day 1
Breakfast: 1. Zucchini And Quinoa Pan
Lunch: 101. Chili Oregano Baked Cheese
Dinner: 143. Chicken And Rice Soup

Day 2
Breakfast: 2. Peas Omelet
Lunch: 102. Mediterranean-style Vegetable Casserole
Dinner: 144. Spicy Salsa Braised Beef Ribs

Day 3
Breakfast: 3. Low Carb Green Smoothie
Lunch: 103. Creamy Smoked Salmon Pasta
Dinner: 145. Pork And Prunes Stew

Day 4
Breakfast: 4. Fig With Ricotta Oatmeal
Lunch: 104. Spiced Eggplant Stew
Dinner: 146. Low-carb And Paleo Mediterranean Zucchini Noodles

Day 5
Breakfast: 5. Raspberry Pudding
Lunch: 105. Shrimp Soup
Dinner: 147. Pork And Rice Soup

Day 6
Breakfast: 6. Walnuts Yogurt Mix
Lunch: 106. Halloumi, Grape Tomato And Zucchini Skewers With Spinach-basil Oil
Dinner: 148. Tomato Roasted Feta

Day 7
Breakfast: 7. Mediterranean Egg-feta Scramble
Lunch: 107. Beef Bourguignon
Dinner: 149. Fettuccine With Spinach And Shrimp

Day 8
Breakfast: 8. Spiced Chickpeas Bowls
Lunch: 108. Mediterranean Flank Steak
Dinner: 150. Sage Pork And Beans Stew

Day 9
Breakfast: 9. Orzo And Veggie Bowls
Lunch: 109. Spiced Grilled Flank Steak
Dinner: 151. Broccoli Pesto Spaghetti

Day 10
Breakfast: 10. Vanilla Oats
Lunch: 110. Pan Roasted Chicken With Olives And Lemon
Dinner: 152. Chorizo Stuffed Chicken Breasts

Day 11
Breakfast: 11. Mushroom-egg Casserole
Lunch: 111. Creamy Salmon Soup
Dinner: 153. Grilled Mediterranean-style Chicken Kebabs

Day 12
Breakfast: 12. Bacon Veggies Combo
Lunch: 112. Grilled Salmon With Cucumber Dill Sauce
Dinner: 154. Sumac Salmon And Grapefruit

Day 13
Breakfast: 13. Brown Rice Salad
Lunch: 113. Grilled Basil-lemon Tofu Burgers
Dinner: 155. Bean Patties With And Salsa Avocado

Day 14
Breakfast: 14. Olive And Milk Bread
Lunch: 114. Creamy Green Pea Pasta
Dinner: 156. Raisin Stuffed Lamb

Day 15
Breakfast: 15. Breakfast Tostadas
Lunch: 115. Meat Cakes
Dinner: 157. Spinach Orzo Stew

Day 16
Breakfast: 16. Chicken Souvlaki
Lunch: 116. Herbed Roasted Cod
Dinner: 158. Grapes, Cucumbers And Almonds Soup

Day 17
Breakfast: 17. Tahini Pine Nuts Toast
Lunch: 117. Mushroom Soup
Dinner: 132. Mediterranean Scones

Day 18
Breakfast: 18. Eggs And Veggies
Lunch: 118. Salmon Parmesan Gratin
Dinner: 133. Mixed Olives Braised Chicken

Day 19
Breakfast: 20. Pear Oatmeal
Lunch: 120. Rosemary Roasted New Potatoes
Dinner: 134. Coconut Chicken Meatballs

Day 20
Breakfast: 22. Mediterranean Egg Casserole
Lunch: 121. Artichoke Feta Penne
Dinner: 135. Grilled Turkey With White Bean Mash

Day 21
Breakfast: 23. Milk Scones
Lunch: 122. Grilled Chicken And Rustic Mustard Cream
Dinner: 136. Vegetable Turkey Casserole

Day 22
Breakfast: 24. Herbed Eggs And Mushroom Mix
Lunch: 123. Balsamic Steak With Feta, Tomato, And Basil
Dinner: 137. Mediterranean Grilled Pork With Tomato Salsa

Day 23
Breakfast: 25. Leeks And Eggs Muffins
Lunch: 124. Fried Chicken With Tzatziki Sauce

Dinner: 138. Beef And Macaroni Soup

Day 24
Breakfast: 26. Mango And Spinach Bowls
Lunch: 125. Spiced Lamb Patties
Dinner: 139. Provencal Beef Stew

Day 25
Breakfast: 27. Veggie Quiche
Lunch: 126. Chicken And Orzo Soup
Dinner: 140. Greek Beef Meatballs

Day 26
Breakfast: 28. Tuna And Cheese Bake
Lunch: 127. Sweet And Sour Chicken Fillets
Dinner: 141. Sausage And Beans Soup

Day 27
Breakfast: 29. Tomato And Cucumber Salad
Lunch: 128. Salt Crusted Salmon
Dinner: 142. Jalapeno Grilled Salmon With Tomato Confit

Day 28
Breakfast: 30. Cream Olive Muffins
Lunch: 129. Sun-dried Tomato Pesto Penne
Dinner: 163. Chicken And Spaghetti Soup

Day 29
Breakfast: 31. Roasted Asparagus With Prosciu6tto And Poached Egg
Lunch: 130. Herbed Marinated Sardines
Dinner: 164. Mediterranean Flounder

Day 30
Breakfast: 32. Figs Oatmeal
Lunch: 131. Spicy Tomato Poached Eggs
Dinner: 165. Crunchy Baked Mussels

CPSIA information can be obtained
at www.ICGtesting.com
Printed in the USA
LVHW100143190121
676861LV00009B/86

9 781922 572332